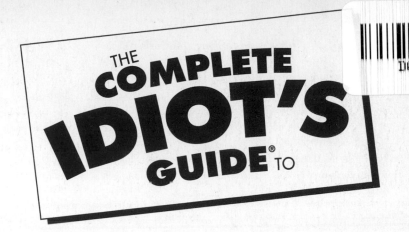

THE

COMPLETE IDIOT'S GUIDE® TO

Vegan Living

WITHDRAWN

by Beverly Lynn Bennett and Ray Sammartano

A member of Penguin Group (USA) Inc.

To all the creatures we share this world with.

ALPHA BOOKS

Published by the Penguin Group

Penguin Group (USA) Inc., 375 Hudson Street, New York, New York 10014, U.S.A.

Penguin Group (Canada), 10 Alcorn Avenue, Toronto, Ontario, Canada M4V 3B2 (a division of Pearson Penguin Canada Inc.)

Penguin Books Ltd, 80 Strand, London WC2R 0RL, England

Penguin Ireland, 25 St Stephen's Green, Dublin 2, Ireland (a division of Penguin Books Ltd)

Penguin Group (Australia), 250 Camberwell Road, Camberwell, Victoria 3124, Australia (a division of Pearson Australia Group Pty Ltd)

Penguin Books India Pvt Ltd, 11 Community Centre, Panchsheel Park, New Delhi—10 017, India

Penguin Group (NZ), cnr Airborne and Rosedale Roads, Albany, Auckland 1310, New Zealand (a division of Pearson New Zealand Ltd)

Penguin Books (South Africa) (Pty) Ltd, 24 Sturdee Avenue, Rosebank, Johannesburg 2196, South Africa

Penguin Books Ltd, Registered Offices: 80 Strand, London WC2R 0RL, England

International Standard Book Number: 1-59257-417-3
Library of Congress Catalog Card Number: 2005930932

07 06 05   8 7 6 5 4 3 2 1

Interpretation of the printing code: The rightmost number of the first series of numbers is the year of the book's printing; the rightmost number of the second series of numbers is the number of the book's printing. For example, a printing code of 05-1 shows that the first printing occurred in 2005.

Printed in the United States of America

Note: This publication contains the opinions and ideas of its authors. It is intended to provide helpful and informative material on the subject matter covered. It is sold with the understanding that the authors and publisher are not engaged in rendering professional services in the book. If the reader requires personal assistance or advice, a competent professional should be consulted.

The authors and publisher specifically disclaim any responsibility for any liability, loss, or risk, personal or otherwise, which is incurred as a consequence, directly or indirectly, of the use and application of any of the contents of this book.

Most Alpha books are available at special quantity discounts for bulk purchases for sales promotions, premiums, fund-raising, or educational use. Special books, or book excerpts, can also be created to fit specific needs.

For details, write: Special Markets, Alpha Books, 375 Hudson Street, New York, NY 10014.

Publisher: *Marie Butler-Knight*
Editorial Director: *Mike Sanders*
Senior Managing Editor: *Jennifer Bowles*
Senior Acquisitions Editor: *Randy Ladenheim-Gil*
Development Editor: *Christy Wagner*
Production Editor: *Megan Douglass*
Copy Editor: *Nancy Wagner*
Cartoonist: *Jody Schaeffer*
Cover/Book Designer: *Trina Wurst*
Indexer: *Heather McNeil*
Layout: *Ayanna Lacey*
Proofreading: *John Etchison*

Contents at a Glance

Contents

Foreword

When I was first asked to write the foreword to a book titled *The Complete Idiot's Guide to Vegan Living*, I experienced two distinct feelings. On the one hand, I know how many people today are interested in vegan living, and having an easy-to-understand, simple-to-follow guide available seemed like a fine idea. And I knew Beverly Lynn Bennett and Ray Sammartano would do an excellent job.

At the same, though, I am aware that most of the vegans I know are actually quite intelligent people who are sensitive to suffering and want to live healthy and compassionate lives. Something about "an idiot's guide" to the subject seemed a contradiction—not that being a vegan is like being a brain surgeon. Being a vegan is easy to do when you know how, and Beverly and Ray are wonderful guides to learning.

Why do people become vegans? For many reasons, but a common denominator seems to be an enhanced sensitivity to the cruelty inflicted upon animals in modern meat production. Compassion plays a large role in the experiences of most people who have an interest in vegan living. Vegans are people who want to see an end to cruelty to animals.

It can be hard to look at sometimes, and disturbing. I've been so blind myself. I remember watching the release of hundreds of beautiful white doves at the opening and closing ceremonies of the Olympic games, enthralled by the spectacle. I didn't think about the birds as animals and what they might be going through. I didn't know they had been trucked in, crowded underground, and then propelled upward. Nor did I know they were terrified and confused in completely strange surroundings. At the Korean games, many of the frightened and disoriented doves actually flew into the Olympic flame, and millions watching were treated to the far-from-inspiring spectacle of seeing the birds burned alive.

I remember, when I was a child, thinking that fur coats were fabulous. I never imagined that wild, fur-bearing animals who are caught in traps suffer slow, agonizing deaths. Or that when we purchase the products of fur farms, we support massive animal pain and death. But slowly it dawned on me that, as beautiful as furs are, they look a lot better on their original owners—the foxes, minks, and other animals from whom they were taken. Now I don't buy furs.

I also remember when I was a child going to a friend's house where there were deer heads on the walls. I thought they were cool. But comedian Ellen DeGeneres has a point when she says, "You ask people why they have deer heads on the wall. They always say, 'Because it's such a beautiful animal.' There you go. I think my mother's attractive, but I have photographs of her."

There's something about our society that makes it hard to see animal suffering, even when, or maybe particularly when, it's your own actions that are causing pain. It's not always easy to break through the wall of denial.

But many of the people who are drawn to a vegan way of life are doing so. And with this awareness comes the motivation to bring your life into greater alignment with your heart. If you are the kind of person who knows there is wisdom in your heart and wants to live by it, this book's for you.

John Robbins

John Robbins is the author of numerous best-sellers, including *Diet for a New America*, *The Food Revolution*, and the forthcoming *Healthy at 100*. He has been a featured and keynote speaker at major conferences sponsored by Physicians for Social Responsibility, Beyond War, Oxfam, the Sierra Club, the Humane Society of the United States, the United Nations Environmental Program, UNICEF, and many other organizations dedicated to creating a healthy, just, and sustainable way of life. He is the recipient of the Rachel Carson Award, the Albert Schweitzer Humanitarian Award, and the Peace Abbey's Courage of Conscience Award.

Introduction

People are drawn to living a vegan lifestyle for various reasons, and this book explores many of them. Going vegan often stems from a love and compassion toward animals and a deeper understanding that all creatures experience the same pain and suffering we humans do, along with a desire not to contribute to it anymore. This is actually what brought the authors of this book to veganism in the first place. In addition, in the 15 years we've been vegan, we have also discovered many of the positive effects veganism can have on our health and the environment.

Eliminating animal foods from one's diet has gone from being thought of as a strange, "health nut" fad to receiving wide acknowledgment as a nutritionally sound, healthful, and even optimal way of eating. In comparison to the Standard American Diet (SAD), eating vegan is much richer in nutrients, lower in fat, and higher in fiber. It's definitely not just another crazy fad diet that's here today and forgotten tomorrow.

Many people seem to think vegans are unhealthy, too thin, and have some pretty strange thoughts about things, but these are stereotypes that couldn't be further from the truth. Vegans come from all walks of life and are mothers, fathers, doctors, lawyers, teachers, preachers, politicians, actors, athletes, factory workers, students, and yes, some tree-hugging environmentalists and animal rights activists as well. We come in all shapes, sizes, and cultural backgrounds from all corners of the globe.

The one thing vegans really do all have in common is a desire to lessen humanity's negative impact on our fellow creatures and a willingness to try to do something about it. More and more people are becoming aware of how the things they buy, eat, wear, and do affect animals, other people, and the environment. They're making conscious decisions to eliminate animal cruelty from their lives, and positive changes are happening all over the place. The numbers of vegans are increasing every year—already in the millions—and there seems to be no stopping us!

In this book, we provide you with some tips to help you begin your transition into being, living, and surviving as a vegan. We also give you some practical advice on how to handle answering the many questions, from the ridiculous to the insightful, which will most certainly come your way. Remember, the word *vegan* and our approach to living and eating can be a new and confusing concept to some people. After we have filled you in on what it means to live as a vegan, maybe you can do your best to help spread the word to others.

As a new or aspiring vegan, be confident in knowing you're one of millions of vegans out there in the world. They think and feel as you do. Find comfort in knowing that you're not alone in your feelings or your decision to eliminate animal use and abuse from your life. Stand strong and proud as a vegan, and know you're helping make a difference, and a better world for all the creatures that inhabit it!

How This Book Is Organized

This book is divided into seven parts. Each part focuses on a different aspect of what it means to live as a vegan, from the philosophical and nutritional to the practical and functional. We provide you with the knowledge and tools necessary to transition into a vegan lifestyle and apply compassion and caring to all parts of your day-to-day life, including what you buy, eat, and wear. By taking small steps, being true to yourself, and taking the time to analyze the various issues surrounding living a compassionate lifestyle, you are sure to be successful as a vegan and as a great human being!

Part 1, "Compassion for All," explains some of the spiritual, moral, and environmental issues behind being vegan. You learn the history of the vegetarian and vegan movements and take a quick quiz to determine if going vegan might be right for you. We discuss some of the many added health benefits of a vegan diet, as well as some of the medical and dietary reasons that lead some people to eliminating animal products from their diet. We also offer a few tips to get you started on your transition into becoming a vegan.

Part 2, "Clearing Up the Misconceptions," alleviates any concerns you and your loved ones may have regarding the nutritional adequacy and healthfulness of a vegan diet. Discover the many delicious vegan foods you can enjoy that supply your body with all the protein, calcium, and carbohydrates it requires to stay healthy and fit. Learn about the benefits of getting your calcium and protein from plant-based sources, as well as the importance of good carbs. Malnutrition and overconsumption are two opposite sides of the spectrum of the problem of world hunger; bet you didn't know eating vegan can greatly impact both of them in a positive way.

Part 3, "A Vegan Survival Guide," gives you some essential information you need to be a healthy vegan. We give you a history and brief explanation of various food guidelines, as well as the development of the current USDA Food Pyramid. We take a look at the Standard American Diet (SAD) and all its drawbacks. To set you on course for eating right, we cover the basics of a proper, well-balanced vegan diet, including how to eat wisely if you want to drop a few pounds. We help you cover your nutritional bases with supplementation, and for you mothers- and fathers-to-be, we offer you some advice and information you can use before, during, and after pregnancy. We also explore the topic of raw foods and their many benefits and give you some tips on incorporating more of them into your diet.

Part 4, "Veggin' It: Tips for Maintaining a Vegan Lifestyle," helps you with the various issues that arise after you have begun your journey into veganism. We give you some advice on handling the veg-curious you will encounter. We provide some tips on handling family get-togethers and holidays, eating out at restaurants, hosting your own gatherings, and even sharing kitchen space with meat-eaters. Being a wise shopper is important for saving time and money, getting your money's worth, and maybe even avoiding future problems with your health. To help you further embrace the vegan lifestyle, we offer tips on how and where to shop. We cover the advantages of buying in bulk, the joys of shopping at natural foods stores, the concept of fair trade, and the importance of reading food labels; plus, we look at a few vegan goodies that can make your life easier and tastier.

Part 5, "Substitution Is the Mother of Invention," helps get you primed for vegan cooking and hopefully gets your creative culinary juices flowing. Starting with protein sources, you get the lowdown on how to cook and use beans, grains, and greens in your vegan dishes. You'll become soy savvy when it comes to using tofu, tempeh, and TVP. We also take a look at the versatile seitan, which you can use to create many a marvelous mock meat. Get the facts about fats, including which ones to use and avoid and why. Find out how to use prepackaged alternatives, like nondairy milks, yogurts, sour cream, cream cheeses, and assorted varieties of vegan cheese. We even offer some help in making your own "cheesy" creations! If vegan baking is your thing, then you'll probably appreciate some vegan baking advice, including the various ways to replace butter, dairy, eggs, and gelatin or how to use tofu and fruit to make some spectacular baked goods.

Part 6, "Vegan Food for the Soul," provides you with wonderful vegan recipe ideas for every meal of the day, from breakfast to lunch, dinner, and desserts. The recipes are easy to follow, and most of them contain ingredients you may already have on hand or can easily obtain. There are recipes to suit all tastes, food allergies and sensitivities, and even some treats for the raw foodist in you. Several recipes take less than 5 minutes of preparation time and contain only a few ingredients, which is perfect for when you need to dine and dash or eat on the go. If you're in need of a big meal with all the fixings, roll up your sleeves and take a whirl at making the Baked Seitan Roast or Baked Breaded Tofu Cutlets with Mouthwatering Mashed Potatoes and Groovy Onion Gravy in Chapter 22. Satisfy your sweet tooth and impress your friends with a Raw Mixed Berry and Mango Pie, Vegan New York–Style Tofu Cheesecake, or a batch of Orange Chocolate Chunk and Cashew Cookies in Chapter 23!

Part 7, "Vegan Lifestyle Choices," provides you with some information to further assist and empower you to live as a new vegan. We focus on the things you put on your body, including what you use to wash your face or brush your hair or to cover your skin or feet. You learn about compassionate alternatives that can help you veganize your wardrobe and your personal care items. We examine some issues relating to animal companions, from whether or not it's safe to feed a cat a vegan diet, to where to adopt your next furry friend. We take a look around the house at some household items that may be derived from animal sources, and offer some plant-based alternatives. Last but not least, you'll pick up a few traveling tips that will help you make the most out of your traveling experiences while not going hungry in the process.

After Part 7, we include some appendixes we think you'll find helpful in your future vegan endeavors. Appendix A contains a list of defined terms used in the book, and Appendix B features lists of vegan books, websites, and contact information for various pro-veg organizations.

Extras

In every chapter you'll find boxes that give you extra information, helpful tips, or just fun facts:

Vegan 101

Vegan 101 boxes feature definitions that teach you the meaning of some terms you might not be familiar with.

Golden Apple

Golden Apple boxes contain quotes and words of wisdom on a wide assortment of topics.

In a Nutshell

In a Nutshell boxes offer useful information or tips relating to the issues discussed in the text.

Hot Potato

Hot Potato boxes alert you to potential problems or pitfalls.

Acknowledgments

We wish to express our heartfelt appreciation to the people who helped make this book possible: to our agent Jacky Sach and BookEnds Literary Agency; to Senior Acquisitions Editor Randy Ladenheim-Gil and Development Editor Christy Wagner for their invaluable advice, input, and support; and to John Robbins for graciously agreeing to write the foreword to this book. Mr. Robbins has greatly influenced millions of people to go vegan and vegetarian through his work with Earthsave and his many books, including *Diet for a New America* and *The Food Revolution*. We would also like to thank our family and friends for their enthusiasm, guidance, and support while we were immersed in the writing of this book. Beverly would like to give a special thanks to three vegan writers and thinkers whose works have had a profound effect on her development as a vegan, a chef, and a woman: Carol J. Adams, Joanne Stepaniak, and Nava Atlas. Thank you for the endless inspiration.

Special Thanks to the Technical Reviewer

The technical reviewer for the recipes in Part 6 was Ellen Brown, a Providence, Rhode Island–based cookbook author, caterer, and food authority. The founding food editor of *USA Today*, she has written 10 cookbooks, including *The Complete Idiot's Guide to Slow Cooker Cooking*, *The Complete Idiot's Guide to Smoothies*, and *The Complete Idiot's Guide to Cover and Bake Meals*. Her articles have appeared in more than two dozen publications, including *Bon Appétit*, *The Washington Post*, and *The Los Angeles Times*. *The Gourmet Gazelle Cookbook* won the IACP award in 1989, and she is a member of the prestigious "Who's Who of Cooking in America."

Trademarks

All terms mentioned in this book that are known to be or are suspected of being trademarks or service marks have been appropriately capitalized. Alpha Books and Penguin Group (USA) Inc. cannot attest to the accuracy of this information. Use of a term in this book should not be regarded as affecting the validity of any trademark or service mark.

Part 1

Compassion for All

Compassion for all: this sounds like some sort of pledge taken by the Three Musketeers or something you might find in the Hippocratic Oath. In a way, it *is* a little like a pledge or an oath. Vegans base many of their life choices on compassion and consider the well-being of others whenever possible.

So you think you want to be a vegan? Well then, read on about the roots, history, and benefits of veganism, and prepare to begin your journey into a cruelty-free lifestyle!

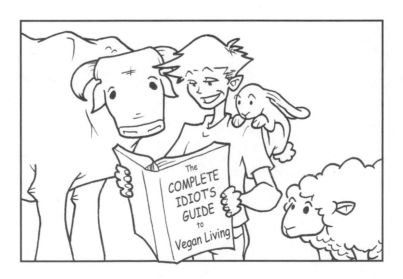

Why Be Vegan?

In This Chapter

- Understanding the role of compassion in veganism
- What is a vegan? Is it the right choice for you?
- Questions to ask yourself regarding animal issues
- Growing as a vegan—at your own speed
- Making choices and staying the vegan course

What are vegans? A tofu-eating race of extra-terrestrial beings from the planet Vega who have come to Earth to surprise, confuse, befuddle, and conquer unsuspecting Earthlings? Well, they might as well be, considering the lack of understanding the average person seems to have about vegans and their way of approaching life. In actuality, vegans are just plain ol' humans who have made a conscious decision to live their lives with a compassion directed toward all living creatures.

Compassion: Emotion in Motion

The definition of *compassion*, in simple terms, involves being sympathetic to the suffering or distress of others—but it doesn't stop there. It also includes a desire to help alleviate or eliminate that suffering. According to the definition of compassion, without the desire to make things better, compassion can't really exist. This concept actually forms the basis of what being *vegan* is all about: being aware that there is suffering, feeling a responsibility to do something about it, and acting upon that feeling. Veganism is compassion in action.

> **Vegan 101**
>
> A **vegan** is one who avoids causing harm or exploiting other living beings as much as humanly possible. This involves excluding all animal foods and animal-based items from their lives.

Compassion is purely an emotional response. Most people feel compassion toward something or someone on some basic level. Living and showing compassion to all creatures big and small as much as possible is at the heart of being and living as a vegan.

It's common that many of us feel disconnected from the fellow creatures we share this planet with. We, as a species, seem to forget that other creatures are actually our distant relatives, forever linked to us by millions of years of evolution.

For many, it's hard to take the time to ponder this and other great truths of the universe while trying to meet all the daily commitments of a job, school, friends, family, and so on. But for those who do make it a point to try to understand who we are as a species, where we came from, and where we're going, it can be the start of a lifetime of increasing awareness and a positive struggle for internal and external change. As Gandhi said, "We must become the change we want to see."

Putting Forth Positive Energy

When you become aware that there is much needless animal suffering going on in the world and you become determined that you will no longer contribute to it, you have already taken the first step in bringing your compassion to the next level.

> **Golden Apple**
>
> Man did not weave the web of life, he is merely a strand in it. Whatever he does to the web, he does to himself.
>
> —Chief Seattle, leader of the Suquamish people, in a letter to the American government, 1854

You and every other living creature on the planet only get one shot at this life you're living right now, and it only seems logical to make the most positive impact possible at this place in time. The possibility of reincarnation aside, it could be your only chance. *Carpe diem!*

Putting positive energy out into the universe brings more back to you. Doing your best to help effect positive change can cause a chain reaction of good things, the ripples of which can reach out into places previously unimagined.

Searching Your Soul

As the saying goes, a mind is a terrible thing to waste, and as humans, we have very developed minds that are often not used to their full potential. We really owe it to ourselves to be the best we can be on all levels: physical, mental, emotional, and spiritual. Doing a little soul searching can be a catalyst for good things, particularly when you think about how you view yourself and your role in society, as well as how you fit within the bigger scheme of things.

It's okay to take some time to invest in yourself and your own growth. It's good to question things. The world around you is in a constant state of change, and it makes sense that you should be as well, particularly in developing who you are and the kind of person you want to be.

Looking around and really analyzing your life and the world around you can reveal pleasant and happy images, along with those that are more harsh and brutal. Some of what you see and experience will most likely upset and concern you. If, how, and to what extent you react will be up to you. Some people prefer to follow a safe and steady course, not questioning or getting involved but rather just existing. Others are impassioned to action to try to make a change when they are faced with injustice.

That's how it is with compassion—some people have a little bit; others have a lot. Some choose to talk about it; some do nothing; and others make tremendous strides to right the wrongs of the world. It's all up to you.

Is Vegan Living for You?

If you're wondering if living a vegan lifestyle might be for you, ask yourself the following questions:

- ◆ Do you love animals?

- ◆ Do you oppose the use of animals in entertainment?

- ◆ Do you feel sad seeing animals in pet store windows?

- ◆ Do you sometimes find eating meat or dairy unappetizing?

- ◆ Do you find yourself gravitating toward the veggie side dishes on your plate first?

- Does your leather coat ever suddenly seem unappealing?

- Do you have any health concerns that may be diet-related?

- Do you suffer from any food allergies or sensitivities?

- Does the knowledge that your lotion or mascara was tested on an animal make you think twice about using it?

If you answered yes to any of these questions, you could be a potential vegan in the making, and this book is certainly for you. We hope to educate, inform, and guide you through all the phases necessary to becoming, being, and living as a vegan.

These questions reflect some of the issues you may encounter as you begin to ponder the issues surrounding veganism and living compassionately. They should also spark more questions, whet your curiosity, and drive you to expand your knowledge base and thought processes. As you arrive at the answers to your questions, you may or may not be faced with making some major life choices to reconcile your feelings.

If you are compassionate and empowered to begin making decisions based on compassionate living, the vegan way of life could be for you. But only you know what is best for you.

> **In a Nutshell**
>
> Move at your own speed and level. Sometimes an accumulation of small steps makes for a profound journey. As the Chinese proverb goes, a journey of 1,000 miles begins with the first step!

Decisions, Decisions

By now you probably realize that transitioning to a vegan lifestyle is all about making decisions and choices. It's like getting a chance at remaking yourself from scratch; you get to decide how you will live your life and by which moral or ethical codes. You and you alone decide how you will sustain yourself on a physical, emotional, and spiritual level. It's all up to you, so take your time and really ponder. If or when you feel you are ready, move forward and transition into your new vegan lifestyle. Do it in your own way and at your own pace.

Lifestyle Choices and Quandaries

Begin by taking small steps and making decisions on basic issues first. Being a vegan is about trying to live as compassionately as possible and applying this to all the choices you make concerning your life, whether it's what to wear, what to buy, what to put in and on your body, and most important, how you choose to treat your fellow creatures on Earth. Transition at your own speed and level.

Never forget that with all your small yet positive changes, you are making a difference in the lives of other creatures. You may never know the results of the ripples of compassion you are causing to spread or how far they will eventually reach.

Spiritual Connection

For many people, the compassion of a vegan lifestyle lays the foundation for the moral and ethical codes they choose to follow and to base their life choices on. To many vegans, this way of life is a little like a religion, similar to Christianity or Hinduism. It is deserving of the same respect, as the roots of compassion are just as old and ancient and provide the practitioner with guidance and wisdom. Personal morals and ethics are what define our spirituality for us. Compassion, respect, and reverence for life are at the root of many of the great religious beliefs of our time.

The great Albert Schweitzer spoke freely of his views on the reverence for life, which became a guiding force in his life as well as the inspiration for a group of writings on the subject. His writings were inspired by those of veg-heads before him, and the cycle continues, as these writings have inspired and will continue to inspire future generations of veg-heads.

Throughout history, many different cultures and religions have been supportive of veganism and vegetarianism (see Chapter 2 for more information on vegetarianism). Most vegans try to live by the Golden Rule and treat others the way they themselves wish to be treated.

> **Golden Apple**
>
> By having a reverence for life, we enter into a spiritual relation with the world. By practicing reverence for life, we become good, deep, and alive.
> —Albert Schweitzer

Do's and Don'ts of Veganism

As you move toward a vegan lifestyle, you will have to make your own individual choices about what you will and will not feel comfortable doing in your life. For instance, will you continue to go to the zoo or circuses or support other forms of entertainment that use animals or keep them in confined areas? It might not bother you much in your first stages of becoming vegan, but you will probably feel much different later on. Perceptions often change over time and when the time is right.

You also might have a problem sticking to your new dietary choices or vegan standards 100 percent of the time as you transition into the vegan way of approaching the various aspects of your life. If you slip, don't beat up on yourself. Just try your best and do as much as you can!

One of the most important things to remember during your transition process is not to take a superior attitude or "holier-than-thou" approach to those around you who aren't vegan. If there's some aspect of your life that you have not fully "veganized" yet, someone who doesn't understand your choice to become a vegan or who is angered by your superior attitude is sure to call you out on it.

Just try to do your best, and take slow and steady steps. Remind yourself that you are making a difference, however small it may seem. Every time you live up to a vegan ideal, you are helping to limit suffering and hopefully saving an innocent life. It's hard for anyone to be 100 percent vegan when you start to scrutinize every aspect of your life. Remember, you can only do the best you can with the things you have control over.

Cruelty-Free Living

As vegans, we choose to do no harm and live what we call a cruelty-free lifestyle. That is, we make a conscious effort to ensure that no animal had to suffer, in any way, in the creation of the products we use and the foods we consume. We believe we can better sustain ourselves and the planet by using plant-based renewable resources and by doing no harm to animals.

Vegans take consumerism very personally and are very careful about the products and services we support with our money. From a vegan perspective, it isn't right to put another creature through something we ourselves would not be willing to go through. There are almost always alternatives to anything that has its roots in cruelty, and if not, there may be ways to avoid the product or practice altogether.

> **In a Nutshell**
>
> When purchasing personal or household items, look for the phrase "No animal testing" often accompanied by a drawing of a bunny on the product packaging. These signify that the product was produced using cruelty-free means.

Vegans practice *ahimsa*, which is an ancient Sanskrit word meaning "nonviolence," or more specifically, "to cause no harm or injury to another living creature." It is at the heart of cruelty-free living and forms much of the foundation veganism is built upon. (See Chapter 2 for more on ahimsa.)

Vegans: Square Pegs in Round Holes?

When you first decide to go vegan, you might feel at odds with the world and people around you. But just like anything in life, you can figure out things for yourself if you remain patient and persevere. It helps to know that you as a vegan are not alone. Millions of other people in the world think very much like you do. You may not know any of them at first, but you eventually will. You will run into veg-heads in unexpected places—often when you least expect it!

We Come in All Shapes and Sizes

Vegans and vegetarians come in all shapes and sizes, just like all the other creatures in the animal kingdom. Big, tall, short, fat, petite, long-lived, or gone in a blink of an eye—like any subculture or religion, it's impossible to stereotype vegans into one boilerplate form. Vegans are hippies, yuppies, Republicans, hip-hoppers, grandmothers, and regular Janes and Joes.

People arrive at their chosen compassionate lifestyle for their own personal reasons, often in their own roundabout way. Some start out by being concerned with animal issues, while others come to a vegan lifestyle after first exploring seemingly unconnected issues. Sometimes dietary or medical concerns, including food allergies and weight-loss issues, start a person down a road that eventually leads him to veganism.

Then there are the raw foodists, the religious-minded, and those who view their bodies as temples and discover that eating vegan is the healthiest way to worship at that temple. Some just stumble into it out of pure curiosity while pursuing any one of the various issues surrounding it or maybe due to peer or celebrity influence. We're all unique, and the paths we take to get here are equally unique!

It's important to remember that some vegans may have arrived at their life choices in a different manner than you. It's best not to be judgmental about how anyone got to where he or she is. We are each on our own journey, with many paths to choose from along the way. Allow others to meander, as you did, and they may soon be beside you on your journey.

Same Thoughts, Different Places

The concept of compassion, respect, and reverence for life on all levels is present in many cultures and religions both past and current. Humans have pondered these concepts many times over, and many of these ideas are timeless and almost universally held. Across many different locations and throughout the span of history, humans seem to have come to the same conclusions or have had the same thoughts about how to treat our fellow creatures.

In a Nutshell

Ellen White, vegetarian and one of the founders of the Seventh-day Adventist Church, was responsible for making vegetarianism a part of the teaching of the Adventists. Today, about half of more than 10 million Adventists living in the world are vegetarians.

Many different religious sects and cultures from all corners of the globe hold in their roots concepts of compassion and kindness that are designed to lead to inner peace or salvation and bring true balance. Moral codes of conduct relating to animals were addressed in the writings of the Buddhist, Hindu, Judaic, Islamic, and Christian faiths, all by people who were separated by time and distance but who were all linked by a common thought: that it is wrong to needlessly take a life or to cause suffering because life is sacred and should be respected.

Finding the Perfect Fit

Many vegans have found, after they make the transition to a vegan lifestyle, that they have a newfound sense of belonging and inner peace. Making contact with others who share your thoughts and beliefs or learning that you aren't alone in the way you feel toward other living creatures can be so empowering. It's like finding the perfect fit or your just-right place in the world.

It might take time for you to find your place in the world as a vegan, but be patient. The search for your own perfect place, which may be a physical or mental state, can take some time. If you don't find it in your present location, you can relocate to a better place. For the time being, you can still keep it in your state of mind.

You can live in your own little vegan utopia mentally even though you may still be swimming upstream in a nonvegan society, searching out the kind of life you want. Your local library and bookstore likely have quite a few books and other materials on veganism and animal issues you will find helpful. Use the Internet and local resources to seek out like-minded people. Having support and someone in your life who shares your ideals can help you stay the course and also empower you as a vegan.

The Least You Need to Know

- Compassion is a combination of being aware of the distress or suffering of others and wanting to help alleviate it.
- Many religions have compassion at the root of their beliefs, and veganism is really no different.
- When transitioning to a vegan lifestyle, you'll face many decisions. Just do the best you can, at your own pace.
- People often take different paths toward becoming vegan. Try not to be judgmental of the way others approach their own journey.
- Finding support for your beliefs can be important in helping you stay the course.

Chapter 2

Vegan 101

In This Chapter

◆ The difference between vegans and vegetarians

◆ Illustrious veg-heads through history

◆ The birth of the Vegan and Vegetarian Societies

◆ The spread of the vegan movement

The transition to a vegan lifestyle usually involves a gradual progression, although for some it happens almost overnight. As they learn more and more about the positive impact of a cruelty-free lifestyle and the wonderful health benefits gained from a plant-based diet, many people feel compelled to move further toward a complete vegan lifestyle. Enter, the veg-heads.

Veg-Heads

When a person decides to become a "veg-head"—a vegetarian, vegan, or someone who avoids animal-based products or foods to varying degrees—it's usually at his own speed and comfort level. Let's begin by taking a look at the similarities and differences between vegans and vegetarians, two of the main types of veg-heads.

The Vegetarians

Vegetarians choose not to eat animals, but they do often consume and use other animal products. For instance, some vegetarians wear leather shoes, eat dairy products, and use animal-based beauty products.

Foods such as milk, cheese, butter, eggs, honey, and other animal-sourced substances are often considered a normal part of a vegetarian diet. In fact, these products often form the basis of many a vegetarian's diet. When a new or inexperienced vegetarian is unaware of other nonanimal sources for protein, creaminess, and flavor, he often gravitates toward an increase in eggs and dairy. For this and other reasons, most vegetarians fall into the *lacto-ovo* category.

Vegan 101

The term *lacto-ovo* is derived from the Latin words for milk and eggs. This moniker is given to those vegetarians who also include dairy products and eggs in their diets.

Some people who call themselves vegetarians even eat fish and poultry. These are the pesco-vegetarians (vegetarian fish-eaters) and pollo-vegetarians (vegetarian poultry-eaters).

Labeling oneself a vegetarian while still eating meat is often a source of controversy and discussion among vegans and vegetarians alike. Many see it as a contradiction in terms, similar to that of being a war-supporting pacifist or a polluting environmentalist. Others feel that an increase in people trying to be "mostly vegetarian" is ultimately better for the animals, as well as for individual and planetary health, than if they had remained unrestrained meat-eaters.

The Vegans

Veganism takes the dietary compassion of vegetarianism to the next level as it concerns itself with all aspects of a living creature's existence. Vegans do not use or consume anything that comes from an animal. That includes flesh, milk in all its forms, and even things like honey, silk, or feathers. If something came from an animal source—insects included—or involved something from an animal source used in the production of a product, vegans don't use or consume it.

Vegans are faced with many daily choices that are based on whether or not animal suffering or exploitation is present or involved. As much as possible, a vegan abstains from any activity, food, business, or product that involves causing harm in any way to any living, feeling, and sentient creatures. This applies to human as well as nonhuman beings.

So Close, and Yet So Far

Both vegans and vegetarians agree that we should consume more of a plant-based, rather than animal-based, diet. But they disagree fundamentally when it comes to consuming animal-based foods at all. Much of being vegetarian centers on the dietary realm and does not spill over into other areas of life as much as being vegan does.

Using and wearing products that come from animal sources, such as leather, wool, fur, and feathers, is often not considered inconsistent with the vegetarian lifestyle. From a vegan perspective, much of this use is based on a lack of information and understanding of the underlying factors involved in the production of those items. It's wrongly assumed that just because the animal isn't killed (or at least directly killed) in the production of any given thing, that the story ends there.

> **Hot Potato**
>
> By continuing to consume dairy products and eggs, vegetarians are, unwittingly, still supporting the factory farm system and the corporations that profit from them. Vegans tend to "vote with their dollars" by not giving their money to industries that conflict with their cruelty-free outlook.

Some vegetarians think that moving toward a vegan lifestyle is difficult or inconvenient, and often they aren't quite sure how they would go about replacing the animal products in their lives. How can you find good nonleather shoes or get enough calcium and protein in your diet if you don't consume dairy products? Have no fear. It's actually quite simple if you're armed with the right information. These are the types of issues and life factors we address in this book.

Veg-Heads Through the Ages

Many influential people throughout history were either vegetarian or vegan. Veg-heads abound and run rampant throughout all phases of history.

Recent studies have shown that some of the earliest humans were mostly vegetarians who ate meat only during extreme circumstances or while in hostile climates. Instead of the "hunter-gatherer" image we learned of in elementary school and beyond, our early ancestors were far more likely to be primarily gatherers.

In addition to the many gifts the ancient Greeks gave the world, they also did quite a bit to develop and spread the concept of vegetarianism. Among the influential Greek vegetarians was philosopher and "father of mathematics" Pythagoras of Samos (580 B.C.E.), who is remembered most for his Pythagorean Theorem, which has helped and/or frustrated first-year geometry students for centuries. Other notable ancient Greek vegetarians included Plato, Porphyry, Epicurus, Plutarch, and Diogenes.

> **Golden Apple**
>
> He who harms animals has not understood or renounced deeds of sin … Those whose minds are at peace and who are free from passions do not desire to live at the expense of others.
> —Mahavira (599–527 B.C.E.), Hindu teacher and founder of Jainism

Major Eastern religions such as Buddhism and Jainism have, at their core, a strong advocacy of vegetarian and vegan values. Siddhartha Gautama, who later became *the* Buddha and founder of Buddhism, was a vegetarian. Through many spiritual writings, he mandated a vegetarian diet rooted in compassion. Mahavira, founder of the Jain religion in the sixth century B.C.E., advocated nonviolence toward human and nonhumans alike and mandated a strict veganism for all followers.

The quintessential Renaissance Man himself, Leonardo da Vinci, was also a vegetarian. He wrote in his journal that "I have from an early age adjured the use of meat, and the time will come when men such as I will look upon the murder of animals as they now look upon the murder of men." While the man who gave the world so many inventions and great works of art was busy painting, discovering, and writing, he was fueling his body and mind with a vegetarian diet.

Many famous writers have also led meatless lives. Through their writings, vegetarian poets Percy Bysshe Shelley, Ralph Waldo Emerson, and Lord Byron influenced others, including playwright George Bernard Shaw, to "go veggie." Percy's wife, Mary Shelley, herself a vegetarian, weaved vegetarian and anti–animal experimentation themes throughout her novel *Frankenstein*. Renowned Russian writer Leo Tolstoy was also a strong vegetarian advocate, as were Franz Kafka and H. G. Wells.

The complete list of other illustrious vegetarians and vegans throughout history is much too long to include here, but consider this small sampling:

- Albert Einstein, scientist
- Albert Schweitzer, humanitarian
- Charlotte Brontë, novelist
- Harriet Beecher Stowe, writer
- Henry David Thoreau, writer
- Isaac Bashevis Singer, writer
- Mohandas Gandhi, humanitarian
- Sir Isaac Newton, scientist and mathematician
- Susan B. Anthony, women's suffrage pioneer
- Thomas Edison, inventor
- Vincent van Gogh, painter

The British Invasion: The Vegetarian Society

During the 1800s, more and more people who shared some of the same ideals started organizing meetings and publishing writings about their views and feelings toward animals. A monumental meeting took place on September 30, 1847, in London, when 140 people gathered to voice their feelings regarding the consumption of animals. This was the beginning of the Vegetarian Society of the United Kingdom. Members chose to call themselves "vegetarians" based on the Latin word *vegetus*, meaning "whole," "sound," "fresh," and "lively." (It wasn't based on *vegetable*, as many people think!)

The Vegetarian Society started the *Vegetarian Messenger* as a way to publish its writings that supported its positions and challenged the status quo. This publication helped further expand vegetarians' influence throughout the world as well as bring people together.

Members of the Vegetarian Society came from all walks of life. Some held political, religious, and esteemed positions within society. As members traversed the globe, their influences helped shape public opinions throughout the world. Many Christian religious leaders embraced the *natural hygiene* and vegetarian movements, helping further spread the good message of compassionate living.

Reverend William Metcalfe was one of the first religious leaders to help the British vegetarian message spread to the Americas when he emigrated to the United States in 1817. He influenced many people, including Bronson Alcott, father of the famous American writer and herself vegetarian Louisa May Alcott, who established one of the first vegan communities in America.

> ### In a Nutshell
>
> The natural hygiene movement's principles date back centuries, but the 1800's saw the most advances in this new area of emerging medicine. This new approach suggested many "revolutionary" concepts for the time, such as consuming whole natural foods, receiving sufficient rest and sleep, getting enough fresh air and sunshine, and bathing regularly.

Metcalfe also influenced Sylvester Graham, who preached the "good book" as well as natural hygiene, raw and whole foods, and vegetarianism. He was also the creator of the famous "graham cracker" made from graham flour, both of which are named after him. As the vegetarian movement grew in the United States, the America Vegetarian Society and others also grew.

The Vegan Society Emerges

A diverse group of people made up the Vegetarian Society. As members' conscious-ness raised and eyes opened to the suffering of animals, further questions and quandaries arose. Many began to question the practices they had once supported, including eating animal-based foods such as dairy products and eggs, and to examine the many moral issues tied to the raising and using of animals for various facets of life.

Donald Watson: Vegan Revolutionary

Articles that addressed these new issues and concerns began appearing in the *Vegetarian Messenger*. Many members opposed these "radical new views," which caused dissension in the ranks of the Vegetarian Society. In December 1943, Donald Watson spoke freely about his views in a lecture titled "Should Vegetarians Eat Dairy Products?" This lecture sparked questioning and contemplation for some of the members of the society, but for the most part, it was met with opposition.

> **Vegan 101**
>
> Donald Watson first coined the word **vegan**. He took the first three letters of *vegetarian* (*veg*) and the last two letters (*an*) because, as he plainly put it, "veganism starts with vegetarian-ism and carries it through to its logical conclusion."

In November 1944, Watson and several others gathered to discuss the formation of a society that supported their ideals of compassion for all crea-tures. From that gathering came the Vegan Society. Members first referred to themselves as "total vege-tarians" and then later shortened it to "vegans."

The Aims of the Vegan Society

Members of the Vegan Society believed in living as humanely and compassionately as possible, thus eliminating practices and products from their lives that lead to the exploitation or cruelty of animals. The aims of the Vegan Society were and continue to be as follows:

◆ To advocate that man's food should be derived from fruits, nuts, vegetables, grains, and other wholesome nonanimal products, and that it should exclude flesh; fowl; eggs; honey; and animal's milk, butter, and cheese.

◆ To encourage the manufacture and use of alternatives to animal commodities.

Donald Watson's and the Vegan Society's first newsletter was titled the *Vegan News*. Starting with only 30 subscribers, it soon became known as simply *The Vegan*. Today, thousands worldwide read the quarterly magazine.

In 2005, the Vegan Society is still doing its part to spread the vegan message by providing educational material on veganism to schools, organizations, and individuals. It also publishes the *Animal Free Shopper* and various books and videos on animal issues, lifestyle choices, cooking, and nutrition. It recently helped establish World Vegan Day as November 1 and developed a trademarked vegan logo that appears on products that adhere to vegan standards.

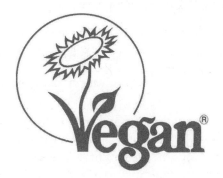

This symbol is the trade mark of The Vegan Society, which it permits to be used on products which fulfill their no animal ingredients, no animal testing criteria. It must not be used without permission.

The Grassroots Spreading of Veganism

The Vegan Society's work eventually helped spread the concept of veganism to other shores as well, influencing people in Asia, India, Australia, New Zealand, and the Americas. Little did the founding Vegan Society members know how far-reaching their message would eventually be!

Coming to America

Just a few years after the creation of the Vegan Society, Dr. Catherine Nimmo and Rubin Abramowitz started a branch in California. Their work caused a snowballing effect for veganism on North American shores.

In 1960, Jay Dinshah began the American Vegan Society, better known as AVS, and accepted as its first member Catherine Nimmo, who remained a member until her passing. The writings of Jay and others were featured in *Ahimsa* (defined by AVS as "dynamic harmlessness"), the organization's magazine from 1960 to 2000. In 2001, it became the quarterly magazine *American Vegan*. Jay also founded the North American Vegetarian Society, better known as NAVS.

In a Nutshell
In 2004, the vegan population in the United Kingdom was well over a quarter million. In a 2000 Zogby Poll, the vegan population in the United States was estimated to be around 2.9 million or 1 percent of the total population.

The AVS spells out *ahimsa* as an acronym, creating a moral code that can help guide a vegan through life. It is made up of "six pillars of the compassionate way." They are as follows:

- **A**bstinence from animal products

- **H**armlessness with reverence for life

- **I**ntegrity of thought, word, and deed

- **M**astery over oneself

- **S**ervice to humanity, nature, and creation

- **A**dvancement of understanding and truth

When Jay died in 2000, he was still working to spread the message of veganism and compassion. He was posthumously awarded the Mankar Memorial Award at the 34th World Vegetarian Congress in Toronto. At each congress, this award is given to those who have made a significant contribution to the cause of vegetarianism. Jay was honored for his work with the AVS, NAVS, American Natural Hygiene Society (known as the National Health Association since 1998), International Vegetarian Union (IVU), and Vegetarian Union of North America (VUNA). Jay's wife and children continue his work, as well as their own, of spreading the message of dynamic harmlessness.

Oh, Canada!

The first records of organized vegetarianism in Canada are the formation of the Toronto Vegetarian Association (TVA). In 1945, a small group of 20 or so vegetarians gathered at the home of Esther Greenburg to discuss their views. They came away with the basis of their organization, as well as a president, J. Don Scott. Within a year, their numbers had grown to 150, and they helped send surplus soy grits and vegetable-based oils to those in need in the throes of war in Europe. A few years later, members organized the Vegetarian Fund for India to help fight famine in the region.

The TVA is, to date, Canada's largest vegetarian organization. Its work has inspired other grassroots organizations, including the newly founded Vegan Canada. This organization is dedicated to working with individuals and other vegan and vegetarian groups to educate, inform, and encourage a vegan lifestyle.

> **In a Nutshell**
>
> For more information, or to find addresses and websites for the organizations discussed in this chapter, see Appendix B.

The Least You Need to Know

◆ Vegetarianism is mainly concerned with diet, while veganism focuses on all aspects relating to animal cruelty and usage.

◆ Many influential thinkers, writers, and doers throughout history were either vegetarian or vegan.

◆ Donald Watson founded the Vegan Society in 1944 as an offshoot of the Vegetarian Society due to differences of opinion surrounding the use of animals in the diet and beyond.

◆ Watson also coined the term *vegan* from the first three and last two letters of *vegetarian*.

◆ Through the work of Catherine Nimmo, Jay Dinshah, and others, the Vegan Society's message spread to the Americas and beyond.

◆ The Toronto Vegetarian Association (TVA) is Canada's largest and oldest established vegetarian organization.

Key to Good Health

In This Chapter

- ◆ Health concerns surrounding animal-based diets
- ◆ Healthful benefits of plant-based diets
- ◆ Preventive medicine and its proponents
- ◆ The China Project

Many new vegans, as well as their friends and family, are sometimes concerned that their new way of eating, sans animal products, will not be as healthy as their previous diet. Although you should always be conscious of whether or not your nutritional intake is adequately meeting your needs, eating a well-balanced vegan diet is actually *more* healthful than eating one that includes animal products. All you need is a little information to help arm and guide you along the way, and soon you'll be thriving on a vegan diet!

Meat Mayhem

Consuming food from animal sources has many pitfalls, and serious health concerns are certainly among them. We've discussed the spiritual and emotional reasons behind being vegan and the history of the veggie movement. Now we come to perhaps the strongest argument for a vegan lifestyle: the health disadvantages of eating meat and the health benefits that one can obtain by eating and living as a vegan.

Food-Borne Illness Concerns

Food-borne illnesses are of serious concern to all of us, whether we eat meat or not. People often think they have the "24-hour flu" or the stomach flu, when in actuality they are having an intestinal reaction to food-borne or water-borne bacteria that has invaded the body and taken up residence. The most commonly known food- or water-borne bacteria are E-coli, salmonella, campylobacter, and listeria. Each takes varying lengths of time to rear its ugly and painful head, but the most common symptoms are abdominal pain and cramps, vomiting, and diarrhea often accompanied by blood.

> **CAUTION**
> **Hot Potato**
>
> If you're leaning toward a vegan diet but have any hesitations or health concerns, talk to a nutritionist or physician before making any changes. These professionals can help you with your transition and to be sure you're covering all your nutritional bases.

According to U.S. government statistics, E-coli is present in about half of all cattle, which is 10 times higher than previously thought. Campylobacter infects more than 70 percent of chickens and 90 percent of turkeys, and between 20 to 80 percent of all chickens are also infected with salmonella.

Improper food handling can be blamed for the spreading of bacteria, but the most numerous and serious of incidents can all be traced back to animal-based contamination. Much of the meat, eggs, and dairy products consumed by Americans is infected with some sort of food-borne bacteria, which is then passed on to the humans when the food is consumed. Even when plant foods appear to be the source of an outbreak, the true source is often traced back to water that was contaminated by infected livestock or to improper handling of tainted meat.

What Is Mad Cow Disease?

In the past few years, you may have heard of mad cow disease, but many people aren't really sure what it is. Are cows going crazy and running wild in the streets, causing chaos and wreaking havoc all around us? Are they like some sort of horror flick zombies, out to eat humans or take some sort of revenge on us? Actually, mad cow disease is a transmissible spongiform encephalopathy (TSE), which is found in several species. In humans, it's called Creutzfeld-Jacob Disease (CJD); in sheep it's called scrapies; in elk and deer herds, it's referred to as chronic wasting; and in cattle, it's called bovine spongiform encephalopathy (BSE), or more commonly, mad cow disease.

Whatever you label it, TSE affects the central nervous system, causing disintegration of the brain or little holes to appear in its composition, and it is fatal. Consuming infected meat and other parts, specifically brains and other organ meats, and spinal cord material most commonly transmits TSE. Problems occur when contaminated animals go undetected and get into the "food chain" of modern farming. The infected meat contains prions, small infected proteins that transmit the disease, that can pass from animal to animal and even species to species.

Mad cow crosses over to our species when humans eat the infected beef. Symptoms of the human version, CJD, can lie dormant for 20 years before making themselves apparent. Because the symptoms of CJD mimic those of other brain-wasting conditions such as Alzheimer's, CJD usually goes undiagnosed. At the time of this writing, the only way to positively test for the presence of the CJD prion is to take a tissue sample from the brain.

> **In a Nutshell**
>
> In 1996, Texas cattle ranchers sued Oprah Winfrey and Howard Lyman, author of *Mad Cowboy*, for remarks they made involving mad cow disease and not eating hamburgers anymore. Oprah and Howard won against the ranchers, who said they slandered beef's good name. The pair were the first defendants sued under the then-new Texas Food Disparagement Act.

The Connection Between Diet and Disease

Heredity determines if you have a genetic predisposition for a particular illness or disease, but many other factors help determine the quality of your health. Getting adequate rest and plenty of fresh air and sunshine; drinking pure, filtered water; exercising regularly; and most important, consuming a well-balanced vegan diet rich in plant-based foods is necessary to your physical and emotional well-being.

Many health organizations, such as the American Cancer Society, the American Dietetic Association, the American Heart Association, the American Diabetic Association, and even the Senate Select Committee on Nutrition, have stated that diet and lifestyle play a major role in developing certain illnesses and diseases. Studies have shown that many chronic diseases are indeed diet-related, including cancer, diabetes, hypertension, heart disease, kidney and liver disease, strokes, obesity, arthritis, gastrointestinal disorders, and osteoporosis.

The medical community is doing more research than ever before into the links between health and diet. They are most concerned about diets that are high in cholesterol and saturated fat, low in dietary fiber and complex carbohydrates, and lacking in adequate vitamins and minerals. Animal-based diets are high in saturated fat and very low in dietary fiber. In contrast, plant-based diets contain large amounts of dietary fiber and vital nutrients, have low levels of saturated fats, and are cholesterol-free. Eating like a veg-head can actually decrease your risk of disease.

Golden Apple

Over consumption of certain dietary components is now a major concern for Americans. While many foods are involved, chief among them is the disproportionate consumption of foods high in fats, often at the expense of foods high in complex carbohydrates and fiber that may be more conducive to health.

—Surgeon General C. Everett Koop, in his 1994 report *Nutrition and Health in the United States*

Links to Cancer

Meat-eaters have higher incidences of cancer than plant-eaters have. Why? According to the American Cancer Society, one third of all cancer deaths in the United States are attributable to nutritional factors. Diets high in animal fat raise estrogen levels, which promote the growth of cancer cells and could lead to breast or ovarian cancer. Diets based heavily on meat and dairy products also tend to be lacking in estrogen-reducing fiber, which just exacerbates the problem.

It has also been suggested that meat-eaters get too much testosterone from their meat-based diet. A high-fat, meat-based diet increases the body's testosterone levels, and a link has been proven between prostate and other cancers and increased testosterone levels. In addition, nearly 80 percent of all livestock in the United States are fed some sort of hormones, including synthetic growth hormones, to increase and extend production. When humans eat the hormone-fed meat, the hormones are also passed on and wreak havoc on our systems.

According to the Physicians Committee for Responsible Medicine, "vegetarians are about 40 percent less likely to get cancer than non-vegetarians, regardless of other risks such as smoking, body size, and socioeconomic status." A study published by the American Cancer Society in early 2005 showed that eating large amounts of red or processed meat over a long period of time can also raise the risk of colorectal cancer. The study defined "large amounts" as 3 or more ounces of meat per day for men and 2 ounces per day for women—equivalent to the amount of meat found in a fast-food hamburger.

Obesity on the Rise

The United States has the highest obesity rate in the world. Obesity has reached epidemic proportions, with 64.5 percent of Americans being classified as overweight or obese. While more and more people go on diets to lose weight, 25 percent of the world's population is malnourished. High-fat fast-food diets, sedentary lifestyles, and plain old lack of energy all contribute to ever-expanding waistlines and rising numbers on the scale.

On average, one in three Americans is obese. To be considered obese you only have to be 20 percent above the average weight of someone your height and age. So you can see how easy it is to find yourself in the obese category. As your weight increases, you also increase your chances of developing diabetes, cancer, heart disease, kidney disease, high blood pressure, high cholesterol, and breathing and sleep disorders.

If you are overweight, it is because you are taking in more fuel (food) than you expend as energy, and your body stores the excess as fat. Making serious dietary and lifestyle changes are the only nonsurgical ways to win the battle of the bulge. Let's face facts: fats make you fat. It isn't just sugars and other carbohydrates, as some diet books would have you believe. Overindulge on fatty foods on a regular basis, and surprise, surprise, you'll probably gain weight.

Hot Potato

The State of the World 2000 Report declared that the number of underfed people worldwide is 1.2 billion, which is also equal to the number of overweight people worldwide. Also, if trends continue, it is believed that by 2025, 75 percent of the population of North America will be overweight.

Most animal-based foods contain several kinds of fats, but most troubling are the high concentrations of *saturated fats*. Saturated fats clog your arteries and add a layer of fat to your outsides as well. What you put in your body really does affect how it looks on the outside, so be sure to eat the best nature has to offer: luscious healthful veggies, whole grains, and succulent fruits!

Veg-Head Vitality

After many years of speculation, it has finally become widely accepted that a well-balanced vegan diet provides adequate nutrition and helps in the prevention and treatment of illness. The idea of diet and health being tied together isn't new. Hippocrates, the Greek vegetarian man of wonder, saw the connection centuries ago. The "father of modern medicine" even reportedly cured many illnesses with fasting and raw foods.

Plant Life Benefits

Across the board, vegans have lower incidences of cancer, stroke, heart disease, kidney disease, diabetes, and arthritis and lower blood pressure and cholesterol levels, just to name a few.

In the last few decades, much research has been conducted on the ties between various diseases and our diets, both in the United States and abroad. In study after study, the benefits of plant-based foods outweighed those of animal-based selections. This knowledge empowered people to take the prevention or treatment of disease into their own hands by nourishing their bodies with a diet high in the kinds of vitamins, minerals, and other important nutrients that only come from fresh fruits, veggies, grains, and other plant foods.

In addition to the many vital nutrients fruits and veggies are loaded with, including vitamins and much-needed fiber, *phytochemicals* are included in the plant-based foods we eat. These chemical compounds are produced naturally by plants and are extremely beneficial in keeping the body happy and healthy. They provide our bodies with an arsenal of natural weapons we need to fight off cancer and other diseases.

Consider these examples of phytochemicals, along with the foods they are found in and the benefits they give us:

◆ **Sulforphane.** Found in broccoli, sulforphane helps fight cancer.

◆ **Limonoids.** Found in citrus fruits, limonoids increase the activity of enzymes that eliminate carcinogens.

◆ **Indoles.** Found in cruciferous vegetables like cauliflower, cabbages, and greens, indoles lower the risk of cancer, especially breast cancer.

◆ **Carotenoids, including lycopene, beta-carotene, and lutein.** Found in carrots, tomatoes, fruits, and greens, carotenoids lower the risk of cancer, heart disease, premature aging, and degenerative eye disease.

◆ **Flavonoids.** Found in cranberries and other berries, grapes, nuts, seeds, and olives, flavonoids lower the risk of cancer and heart disease and also lower cholesterol levels.

◆ **Isoflavones.** Found in beans, especially in soybeans, isoflavones lower the risk of cancers, attack free radicals, and balance estrogen and hormone levels.

Longer and Healthier Lives

On average, vegans and vegetarians live 6 to 10 years longer than meat-eaters. That's primarily due to the many health benefits of eating a plant-based diet. We tend to have lower cholesterol and blood pressure levels, consume less saturated fat and more fiber, and get lots of good disease-fighting plant compounds. As a result, on average, vegans also tend to be more fit.

We tend to be more conscious of and concerned with what we put into our bodies, whether it be clean air, clean water, or good foods from organic sources whenever possible. We also tend to be more active, which helps keep our bones stronger for longer throughout our lives and joints and muscles moving as they should.

We are all familiar with how fat and cholesterol affect our health, but so do excess amounts of protein and calcium, especially where our internal organs are concerned. By not consuming excess amounts of meat and dairy, vegans have a better shot at avoiding those pitfalls. (We touch more on this in Chapters 5 and 6, where we discuss our body's protein and calcium requirements and take a look at some good sources from food.)

An Ounce of Prevention: Preventive Medicine

The medical community is finally starting to alert the public to the preventative aspects of a plant-based diet. Some physicians have taken it a step further and have become leaders in a field of medicine known as *preventive medicine*, with various clinics, organizations, and literature to support it.

Preventive medicine is not really a new concept, but it has recently been winning over many within the medical community. Most doctors entered the medical profession out of a desire to help others, and giving patients the information and guidance needed for them to stay healthy in the first place is certainly one of the best ways to help them.

A number of doctors are on the forefront of this exciting field and advocate plant-based diets in their disease prevention techniques. Let's meet a few.

Vegan 101

Preventive medicine is primarily concerned with helping healthy people *stay* healthy and providing the tools and information needed to keep disease at bay. It explores the environmental and dietary effects on disease and health and works to determine the root causes instead of reaching for quick fixes.

Reversing Heart Disease with Dr. Ornish

Dr. Dean Ornish is the president and director of the Preventive Medical Research Institute in Sausalito, California. Throughout his many years of dedication, he has proven with research and through work with his many patients that coronary artery disease is reversible with a cholesterol-free diet, stress management, meditation, and yoga, as outlined in his best-selling book, *Dr. Dean Ornish's Program for Reversing Heart Disease*.

His Reversal and Prevention Diets encourage people to adopt a more vegetarian and vegan way of eating to help dramatically reduce fat and cholesterol levels. Dr. Ornish and his program have had tremendous success in changing people's lives and health for the better.

Lifestyle Changes with Dr. McDougall

Dr. John McDougall, along with his wife, Mary, developed *The McDougall Plan*, which guides people through making changes in their diet and lifestyle to achieve healthful living. Among the many positive lifestyle changes they recommend to their patients and their readers, the McDougalls' programs advocate a diet free of animal foods. They have devoted their lives to helping people improve their health, diet, and overall well-being, also without the use of medications or surgeries.

> **In a Nutshell**
>
> John and Mary McDougall are the authors of several best-selling books, including *The McDougall Plan: 12 Days to Dynamic Health*, *The McDougall Program for Maximum Weight Loss*, *The McDougall Program for Women*, and *The McDougall Program for a Healthy Heart*.

At the McDougall Health Center in Santa Rosa, California, patients can be part of a 10-day live-in program as they make transitional changes to their lifestyle and dietary habits. The center's program is vegan, and it even has a line of prepackaged vegan foods to make it convenient to eat healthful, vegan foods on the go, as part of school lunches, or at the office.

The Healthy-Hearted Dr. Pinckney

When Dr. Neal Pinckney's cardiologist told him the main arteries to his heart were almost completely blocked, Pinckney (a self-professed "devout coward") refused surgery and instead began to research his condition on his own. Fortunately, he happened upon the works of Dr. Ornish and Dr. McDougall and made some serious changes to his lifestyle, including adopting a vegan diet.

More than a decade later—and without any surgery—Dr. Pinckney is free of blockage and going stronger than ever. Because he also believes that community helps in the healing process, he organized support groups in association with both Castle Medical Center and Kaiser Permanente in Hawaii, known as the Healing Heart Foundation, to assist those with heart disease concerns. He is also the author of the *Healthy Heart Handbook*, in which he instructs on how to prevent and reverse heart disease, lower the risk of heart attack and cancer, reduce stress, and lose weight without hunger, all by adopting a vegan diet and making lifestyle changes.

The Physicians Committee for Responsible Medicine and Dr. Barnard

The Physicians Committee for Responsible Medicine (PCRM) is a nonprofit organization comprised of well-known physicians, laypersons, and grassroots individuals. Founded in 1985, it promotes preventive medicine, conducts clinical research, and encourages higher standards for ethics and effectiveness in research.

The big deal about PCRM is that it focuses on preventive medicine and advocates taking conscious steps and making lifestyle changes, if necessary, to prevent a health crisis from settling on your shoulders. It employs these preventive techniques first, instead of gravitating toward medications or surgeries for quick fixes.

The members are also developing a proposal for "The New Four Food Groups," which will feature truly healthy choices as recommendations for our daily dietary needs, all of which form the basis of a well-balanced vegan diet. The group also provides free informational brochures such as its *Vegetarian Starter Kit*, *Vegetarian Starter Kit for Restaurants*, and *Replacing Animals in Research* for use as educational tools.

Dr. Neal Barnard is the president of PCRM and author of *Turn Off the Fat Genes; Foods That Fight Pain; Eat Right, Live Longer; Food for Life;* and other books on preventive medicine. In all his books he tries to show how following a plant-based diet, exercising, and taking direct control of your own health will ensure that your life and health are all they should be.

PCRM's advisory board includes 11 well-known health-care professionals from a broad range of specialties:

- T. Colin Campbell, Ph.D., Cornell University

- Caldwell B. Esselstyn Jr., M.D., Cleveland Clinic

- Suzanne Havala, Ph.D., M.S., R.D., L.D.N., F.A.D.A., Vegetarian Resource Group

- Henry J. Heimlich, M.D., Sc.D., Heimlich Institute
- Lawrence Kushi, Sc.D., Division of Research, Kaiser Permanente
- Virginia Messina, M.P.H., R.D., Nutrition Matters, Inc.
- John McDougall, M.D., McDougall Program, St. Helena Hospital

---

In a Nutshell

For more information on PCRM and its informative website, see Appendix B.

- Milton Mills, M.D., Gilead Medical Group
- Myriam Parham, R.D., L.D., C.D.E., East Pasco Medical Center
- William Roberts, M.D., Baylor Cardiovascular Institute
- Andrew Weil, M.D., University of Arizona

The China Project and Dr. T. Colin Campbell

Dr. T. Colin Campbell of Cornell University and Dr. Richard Peto of Oxford University have conducted a research project studying thousands of patients in China. The Cornell-Oxford-China Project, or the China Project, as it's more commonly referred to, is one of the most comprehensive studies done to date on the correlation between diet and disease.

Dr. Campbell and Dr. Peto chose to study the Chinese because in comparison to other cultural or ethnic groups throughout the world, a majority of Chinese people tend to remain in one area for many decades, even generations. They also tend to consume certain types of foods, regionally and routinely, that have sustained them and formed the basis of their diets for centuries.

Chinese diets generally contain only about 0 to 20 percent animal-based foods, compared to 60 to 80 percent for the standard American diet. The study has shown that the more westernized their diet becomes and the farther they stray from their former mostly plant-based diet, the more they experience an increase of heart disease, cancer, obesity, diabetes, and so on.

The study also found that the Chinese have fewer incidences of breast and ovarian cancer than people in Western countries. This may have a tie to soy, which is quite prevalent in the average Chinese diet and also contains beneficial cancer-fighting *phytoestrogens*.

In addition, the study showed that a diet high in animal protein affects the rate at which young people grow and mature sexually, and that hormones contained in animal foods, including bovine growth hormone, make humans grow taller and larger in disproportional and increased rates.

The many findings of the study discovered that chronic degenerative diseases, such as diabetes, cancers, and heart disease, occur most in areas where diets are higher in animal products and fat, such as in industrialized and urbanized Chinese locales. It also found that even adding small amounts of animal foods to an otherwise all-plant-based diet significantly raises cholesterol levels as well as the risk for related diseases.

Vegan 101

Phytoestrogens are naturally occurring plant compounds similar to estradiol, the most potent form of human estrogen. The effects of phytoestrogens are not as strong as most estrogens and are very easily broken down and eliminated. They help regulate the estrogen levels in the body.

Lactose and Lactose Intolerance

Some people find their way to a plant-based diet because of allergies or intolerances to foods. Milk, dairy, eggs, shellfish, and even certain fruits, vegetables, and nuts are common allergens and negatively impact millions of people each year in the United States alone.

One of the most predominant food intolerances is to dairy products. If a person is lactose intolerant, his or her body is unable to break down lactose into glucose, which the body uses to provide energy and fuel.

All mammals breast-feed until a certain age, and then when they are weaned, their bodies no longer need to produce lactase, the protein enzyme needed to break down the lactose into glucose. For humans, this begins happening around age 2. So when we consume dairy products beyond that age, our bodies may no longer be able to digest the lactose they contain, thus causing some people symptoms of lactose intolerance.

Lactose intolerance is a common concern throughout the modern world that sustains itself on a diet of dairy-rich foods. In fact, only a small part of the world population can even digest cow's lactose throughout their entire lives, and it's mostly those of Eastern European descent. For the rest, nearly 75 percent of the population worldwide, consuming dairy products may start out as a harmless act but soon ends in pain and discomfort.

Symptoms of lactose intolerance include gas, bloating, cramping, nausea, and diarrhea and are experienced by many who consume dairy products in the form of milk, cheese, yogurt, ice cream, and so on. Left unchecked, it could lead to extreme weight loss and malnutrition.

Protecting Your Heart from Disease

Heart disease is becoming the number-one killer of men and women throughout the world. It was once thought that one's only options when diagnosed with this disease were either to wait and see, take costly medications, or face a series of risky surgeries. Now doctors and laypersons are beginning to understand that you can do something to reduce your risks. By making changes in your diet and lifestyle, you can greatly reduce your risks of having a heart attack and facing a lifelong battle with heart disease. In many cases, a person can actually reverse heart disease through diet and exercise alone.

Begin by getting enough rest, reducing your stress levels, and enjoying some form of regular exercise, hopefully outdoors so you can breathe in fresh air. Then analyze your diet and be sure it's low in excess saturated fats, sugars, and sodium and includes good sources of protein, complex carbohydrates, and fiber. Check your weight, blood pressure, and cholesterol levels; heart disease is affected by all those factors. If you want to reduce your chances of having a heart attack and reverse the symptoms of heart disease, you can take a proactive approach and adopt a plant-based diet. Consult with your doctor for other advice on helping keep heart disease at bay.

Foods that are part of a vegan diet tend to be high in fiber and low in fat, especially saturated fats, which will help you maintain a proper weight. Plant foods are cholesterol-free, as something has to have a liver to produce cholesterol, and carrots didn't have livers the last time we checked. So if you don't increase your cholesterol levels with your food intake and you combine that with eating cholesterol-fighting plant foods like oats, you'll be on your way to lowering your cholesterol naturally.

The average cholesterol level for someone who follows the Standard American Diet (SAD) is around 210. Your chances of having a heart attack decrease as your cholesterol levels dip below 150. As a vegan, unless you have a strong genetic predisposition for having high cholesterol, your levels will be 125 and below. Your chances of having a heart attack at that level are virtually nil.

In a Nutshell

The director of the nonprofit Institute of Nutrition Education and Research, Dr. Michael Klaper, believes that animal fats clog us up (our arteries, that is) and make us fat, and that we have no nutritional requirements for animal protein or products. Because plant foods help lower our cholesterol levels, which helps us fight heart disease, he and other doctors are instructing heart patients to cut their cholesterol and adopt a heart-healthy, low-fat, vegan diet.

The Least You Need to Know

◆ A diet high in animal fats, proteins, and cholesterol can lead to a plethora of health problems.

◆ A completely plant-based diet gives the body all the nutritional ammunition it needs to fight disease.

◆ Preventive medicine works at helping healthy people stay healthy and solving potential health problems before they arise.

◆ The China Project was a comprehensive study that showed a correlation between consumption of animal products and disease.

◆ Many people find their way to a plant-based diet due to food allergies or intolerances.

Chapter 4

Starting Your Vegan Transition

In This Chapter

- ◆ Beginning your journey to a vegan lifestyle
- ◆ Transitioning tips
- ◆ Out with the old and in with the new
- ◆ Detoxing and cleansing
- ◆ Being kind to yourself

Transitioning is a necessary part of your personal evolution to veganism. It involves your sense of awareness of the world around you and your place within it. The rate and level at which you evolve is personal to you and you alone and should come naturally to you. Some people might be able to transition to a vegan lifestyle in one fell swoop, but for others it may take many months, and many even have a few stumbles along the way.

It's best to be like the turtle (another illustrious plant-eater), slow and steady to win the race. And for you, winning the race is reaping all the benefits of a vegan lifestyle. Go at your own pace and with what makes you feel comfortable. This chapter helps you transition from a meat-eating or vegetarian diet to a vegan lifestyle.

Taking Small Steps

For many, making life changes can seem intimidating; others embrace it and become energized by the process. However you approach your transition into veganism, think of it as taking small steps in making a positive change for yourself, the animals, and the planet. We discuss many of the health, physical, environmental, and social benefits of adopting a vegan lifestyle throughout the pages of this book. Take and absorb the information; then make changes in your diet and lifestyle as you see fit, at your own speed.

You decide which part of your life to change first, what goes into your body, onto it, or surrounding it. Having patience with yourself can really help empower you during the times you may stumble or falter in your transitioning process. But be confident and stay the course. No one is perfect; we all make mistakes and go astray along the way on our journey into veganism.

Getting Your Diet in Order

One of the first transitional changes the vegan-curious make is to their diet. They often give up added cheese or butter toppings or avoid eating a burger and opt instead for a salad at lunch. These are positive steps in the right direction to changing your diet to a vegan one. If you find you don't miss the eliminated food, keep going and try other eliminations or substitutions (see Part 5 for more on substitutions). Begin with small changes, like giving up animal-based foods for one meal, then another, until you find you no longer have the need or taste buds for these foods. Soon you will feel the positive affects of clean, vegan living.

Detoxing Your System

After eliminating animal-based foods from your diet, you will definitely feel some physical changes as your body eliminates much of the excess fats, mucus, cholesterol, and various toxins from your system. Detoxification is the body's way of cleansing itself and rejuvenating organs, cells, and body tissues.

When you're first transitioning yourself away from animal-based foods, it's a good idea to go on a cleanse or detox to help thoroughly clean your body on the inside and speed along its adjustment to eating a better diet. Many do this by not consuming any foods for one day, several days, or a week. Some people experiencing extreme health crises detox for several weeks under medical supervision. They do drink plenty of water, and some even consume fruit juices, soups, or broths as part of the detox cleansing process.

In a Nutshell

The most well-known detox is the Lemonade Master Cleanse:

2 TB. fresh organic lemon juice	Cayenne to taste
2 TB. Grade B maple syrup	10 oz. filtered water

Mix lemon juice, syrup, cayenne, and water, and drink as often as you want throughout the day, along with additional filtered water. You can stay on this cleanser for as long as you like; the average is 1 to 10 days.

You can expect to feel a bit odd during a detox—after all, you are purging yourself of unneeded toxins and other substances. You might experience such symptoms as nausea, increased bowel movements, abdominal discomfort, headaches, nervousness, even dizziness. But these often subside as the process goes along, and the benefits far outweigh any unpleasantness you may experience. Excess mucus in the body is quickly eliminated, which can help alleviate many bronchial and sinus-related problems.

Detoxing can also improve your kidney functions; aid digestion; ease pain in your joints; remove excess calcium, protein, and fat deposits; and clean your blood of excess cholesterol. Stay on a detox as long as you feel comfortable and deem necessary. It's best to gradually return to eating by drinking fruit and vegetable juices and eating small, easily digestible servings of food.

Eating Lots of Raw Goodness

After coming off a detox, you should try to increase your consumption of raw fruits and vegetables. The vitamins and nutrients in these raw foods are left more intact, even after cutting and washing, than their cooked food counterparts. Especially, more of the beneficial digestive enzymes are left intact. These aid in your digestion processes.

A great and relatively easy way to get more servings of fruits and veggies into your daily diet is through the consumption of juices and smoothies. You can also blend a variety of raw fruits and vegetables to increase your consumption of beneficial phyto-chemicals and encourage their symbiotic relationships.

Transitioning Out Certain Foods

While increasing your consumption of fruits and veggies, you could start transition-ing animal-based foods out of your diet. Start by eliminating the foods you don't particularly care for or enjoy eating. Then begin making other small changes, like leaving the sour cream and butter off your baked potato and using a little nonhydrogenated margarine or olive oil instead. Or buy a cartoon of soy milk for use on your morning cereal instead of using cow's milk.

Hot Potato

Don't let your food cravings derail your new vegan diet. Keep your freezer stocked with convenience vegan food items like frozen veggie burgers, veggie dogs, and dairy-free piz-zas. When a craving hits you for one of your former favorite non-vegan foods, you'll be prepared with a vegan alternative.

Approach it one item and one meal at a time. Don't beat yourself up if you stumble and give in to a craving for a cheeseburger or pizza at first. Keep at it, and soon you will find yourself choosing vegan selections naturally and eating all your meals as a vegan.

Getting Your House in Order

When making the decision to become a vegan, you have to analyze many of your past and present choices about how you eat, what you wear, and what products you use. Often this means getting rid of the old and buying all new. We offer some sugges-tions in the following sections, but ultimately, what you do with those no-longer-accepted vegan items is a personal decision.

Sorting Your Pantry

What should you do with your nonvegan food items? Your choices are basically consuming them one last time, giving them away, or discarding them altogether. We have often been faced with this choice when we have been given or inadvertently purchased nonvegan foods. Depending on how "unhealthy" or "wrong" the item is, we either pass them along to nonvegan friends, food banks, or as a last resort, the landfill.

We choose to throw things away as a last resort because it is wasteful. We acknowledge that the item has already been prepared, thus the wrong has already been done to the animal and we can't change it. We may be showing the animal further disrespect for the suffering it had to endure by just discarding the item when someone could receive a benefit from it. This is one of the tough personal calls you will have to make for yourself.

> **In a Nutshell**
>
> There's a Native American line of reasoning that you should pay homage to the life that has given its own to sustain yours. You should not show it disrespect in the giving of its gift, which would be an injustice and not in balance with nature.

Cleaning Out Your Closet

When it comes to clothing and accessories, you can apply the same type of reasoning as with foods. If the items are worn out, discard or recycle them. If they still have some use, pass them along to others who can put them to use. If you don't know someone who could use the items, donate them to charity. We feel best passing on these nonvegan items to those who can use them.

As you rid your closet and drawers of any leather, fur, wool, or other animal ingredients, you can seek out vegan-friendly substitutes. That means shopping! You can find many natural and plant-based fabrics used in clothing, coats, and accessories in most retailers and department stores.

Man-made materials are also used in these same types of clothing and in footwear, from sandals to dress shoes to boots. Begin by reading labels and feeling fabrics when you're in doubt of their origin. You can also go online for sources of vegan clothing and footwear (see Appendix B).

Cleaning Out Your Cabinets

Check your local health food store and retailers for cruelty-free beauty and personal products. Most will offer a selection of shampoos, conditioners, lotions, perfumes, and makeup that are free of animal ingredients and not tested on animals. These items tend to be a bit costly as they are often made with organic and better-quality ingredients. So begin by replacing one item at a time and don't put a crimp on your pocketbook!

Many health food stores offer shampoos, conditioners, and lotions for sale in bulk quantities, which makes these products even more affordable. You can even make your own natural household cleaners by mixing water with a little vinegar or lemon juice. This mixture can clean your windows, bathrooms, countertops—you name it— all natural and very cheap!

Staying the Course

Lifelong journeys begin with short, sure, and steady steps. Start with small changes at first, in your diet for instance, by giving up one animal food or group at a time. If it's something you aren't sure you can live without, search out substitutes to help fill the void so you won't feel deprived like you're on a "fad diet." The Internet and your local library can help you find a wide variety of information as well as recipes and cookbooks to inspire you.

You will likely have times when a craving hits you so hard you think you'll just have to go get some nonvegan food. Most everyone goes through these times. During these rough moments, remind yourself that you are making the right choice by going vegan and that it is good for you and the rest of the planet. And if you need more help, you've got it right now, in your hands. We provide you with further encouragement throughout the book. Keep turning pages, and know you're doing something great for yourself and for the world!

> **In a Nutshell**
>
> Check out www.veganchef.com for some of Chef Beverly Lynn Bennett's vegan recipes and menu ideas—from vegan soups to vegan desserts!

The Least You Need to Know

- ◆ Transition to a vegan lifestyle in your own way and at your own pace.

- ◆ Doing a little preparation, like going on a detoxifying cleanse, can help prepare your system for the nutritional changes you'll go through on your way to veganism.

- ◆ Eliminating one nonvegan aspect of your life at a time is often a gentle way of transitioning. For extra help, find alternatives for those nonvegan foods at the top of your craving list.

- ◆ Taking the transition one step at time, one day at a time, will help keep you from feeling overwhelmed by it all.

Part 2

Clearing Up the Misconceptions

There's a lot of confusion about what it means to be vegan, including how we can possibly survive without the animal foods we abstain from. If vegans had a dollar for every time we were asked questions such as "How can you get enough protein if you don't eat meat?" or "How can you get enough calcium if you don't drink milk?" quite a few vegan millionaires would be roaming the streets.

The chapters that follow provide you with the answers to those questions—and a whole lot more—for your own knowledge and to help you handle your next veg-curious encounter.

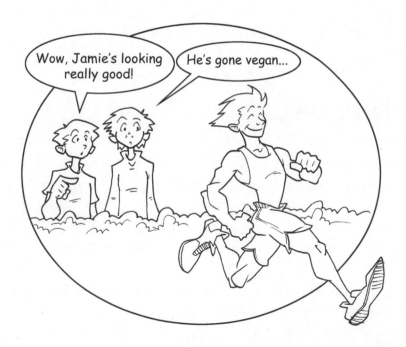

Chapter 5

But You Need Meat for Protein

In This Chapter

♦ Getting enough protein in your diet

♦ The importance of fiber

♦ All about beans, grains, and greens

♦ The many faces of soy

♦ A look at meat substitutes

How will you ever get enough protein without eating meat?

Without a doubt, when you're transitioning to a vegan diet, this will be one of the most commonly asked questions you'll hear. The veg-curious in your inner circle of friends and family and even complete strangers will ask you this question again and again. As you begin your journey toward eating vegan, you might even find this is an issue that's often on your own mind. Where *will* you get your protein, and are you sure you'll get enough of it without eating animal-based foods? You have no need to worry. The plant kingdom is full of protein-rich foods!

Protein: The Plants Have It!

How much protein does your body really need? It's recommended that 1 out of every 10 calories you take in should come from protein, and exactly how much that amounts to depends on your weight. The Recommended Daily Allowance (RDA) for protein is a little less than ½ gram per each pound you weigh. But most Americans consume 4 to 8 times their daily requirement of protein, which translates to 15 to 20 percent of their caloric intake coming from protein. For vegans, roughly 10 to 12 percent of their calories come from protein.

> **Hot Potato**
>
> High-protein diets are all the rage right now, but such diets have consequences. For one thing, taking in too much protein messes with your calcium absorption, which in turn increases your risk of kidney disease and osteoporosis. (We touch more on the body's calcium requirements and absorption capabilities in Chapter 6.)

> **Vegan 101**
>
> Essential amino acids—histidine, isoleucine, leucine, lysine, methionine, phenylalanine, threonine, tryptophan, and valine—also known as EAAs, are our bodies' key protein-building blocks. They must come from dietary sources.

Boneless Benefits

Proteins help our bodies build and maintain muscles, bones, hormones, enzymes, and many other body tissues. Proteins are made of building blocks—22 amino acids to be exact—and combinations of these amino acids form the proteins that exist in all living creatures. Our bodies make 13 of the amino acids; the other 9, referred to as *essential amino acids*, must be supplied by dietary sources. Our bodies use these essential amino acids to aid in synthesizing our own amino acids.

Most people assume that animal protein is superior to the protein found in plant foods and is full of essential amino acids as well. In reality, all the amino acids in animal foods derive from the vegetation the particular animal consumed, whether it be the grain fed to cows and chickens or the plankton, algae, or kelp the swordfish swallowed. Plant-based foods are the source of all the essential amino acids, and they also have significant amounts of protein. For instance, asparagus, broccoli, and tofu are all around 40 percent protein as a percentage of calories. Watercress weighs in at a whopping 83 percent!

It's a common misconception that you need to combine plant proteins at each meal or in each dish to make them form "complete proteins" or proteins that contain all the essential amino acids. This is not necessary, and even the American Dietetic Association agrees that eating a diet rich in a wide variety of fruits, vegetables, and grains will provide you with *all* your amino acids and protein needs *and* vitamins and minerals to boot! Plus, plant-based foods are cholesterol-free and low in calories and fats, unlike animal-based equivalents.

Soybeans contain all nine essential amino acids, making them a perfect food for our bodies. No wonder there are so many wonderful soy-based products out there, including tofu, tempeh, mock meats, nondairy ice creams, soy milk, and a vast assortment of vegan cheeses, yogurts, sour creams, and other dairy-free alternatives.

Moving Through the Works

Our bodies can better and more easily utilize plant-based protein sources than meat-based sources because they are built for them. Human saliva contains a carbohydrate-digesting enzyme, referred to as *salivary amylase*, which is responsible for the digestion of starches. Animal-based protein contains very small amounts of carbs. So if you consume as many animal-based products as the average American, your colon and elimination time can become a lot like the game *Tetris*. You keep consuming large quantities of food, which keeps getting compacted down, but you only eliminate part of it at a time. You may feel bloated or gassy, develop indigestion or digestive problems, and eventually put on weight.

The amount of fiber in foods affects digestion time and efficiency. Because proteins are generally not digested until they're in the small intestine, sometimes having the slow digestion of plant material is beneficial. Your body can draw out more of the nutrients and put them into use.

When you begin to shift toward an all-vegan diet, you may experience a few digestion problems at first, especially when consuming beans or cruciferous vegetables like cabbages or cauliflower. This will greatly improve as you consume these types of foods more, as your body will begin to produce enzymes that will help you process them. Cooking your vegetables and beans thoroughly may also improve digestibility. Try eating any bothersome foods in small quantities at first, and vary your selections. Also, be sure to chew your food thoroughly because chewing really kick-starts the whole digestive process into action.

Down with Fat, Up with Fiber

The medical community has widely accepted that if you want to reduce your risk of chronic disease, you should consume a diet low in fat, high in fiber, and full of fruits and vegetables. Plant foods are generally low in fat and high in fiber, so they meet all the criteria.

Depending on your level of health, your daily diet should include no more than 10 to 20 percent fat. If you need to make major alterations to your cholesterol levels, it's best to consume an even lower-fat diet of between 5 to 10 percent fat for several weeks or more or until your cholesterol levels take a serious nosedive. Pay attention to your consumption of tropical oils, because they are very high in saturated fat. Stick with olive, flax, hemp, pumpkin, and sesame oils for flavor with added health benefits.

You need 25 to 30 grams of fiber in your diet per day for proper colon function. Fiber comes from cellulose, which makes up the cell structure of plants. Dietary fiber is best described as the parts of vegetation that can't be broken down by digestive enzymes. There is no dietary fiber found in animal products, so they tend to accumulate in the colon, stubbornly refusing to be moved along.

In contrast, all the fiber in fruits and veggies cleans your pipes. It acts just like a brush. That's why so many people go on juice or raw food cleanses, because they are so good for your system, providing all the proper nutrients and detoxing benefits to boot. Fiber will keep you running like you should. Plus, a diet low in fat and high in fiber will have you shedding extra pounds and looking good!

Not all fiber is created equal. Fiber can be broken up into two categories: soluble and insoluble. When mixed with water or other liquid, soluble fiber turns into a gel that contains fatty acids and other nutrients your body can easily absorb and utilize. In contrast, insoluble fiber passes through your digestive tract mostly intact, as it does not easily dissolve in water. Each type of fiber has its own benefits, so be sure to include sources of each in your daily diet.

> **In a Nutshell**
>
> Soluble fiber found in flax seed, barley, oats, beans, apples, oranges, and carrots helps lower cholesterol levels and helps diabetics regulate blood sugar levels. Insoluble fiber found in corn, wheat, cruciferous vegetables, green beans, and the skins of many fruits and vegetables aids in digestion, elimination regularity, toxin removal, and system balancing.

On the Outs

The fiber in plant foods, often known as "roughage," helps keep your bowels moving regularly like they should and helps prevent painful constipation. Fiber provides bulk and binds with fats and toxins in your system, which are quickly eliminated by fiber's cleansing action. Most important, fiber keeps bile from recirculating in your system. Bile is formed from the cholesterol in your body, so you want to eliminate it instead of having it absorb into your bloodstream and affect your cholesterol levels.

High-fiber diets help with your natural elimination process. They also help you maintain a proper weight, as high-fiber foods are quite filling. They also require more chewing, which gets the digestion process off to a good head-start. Adding water into the mix will give you a feeling of fullness and satisfy your hunger even faster.

It's best to include as many sources of fresh raw fruits and veggies in your daily diet as possible. The RDA is at least 5 a day, but vegans often

> **In a Nutshell**
>
> Drinking a lot of filtered water—8 to 10 glasses per day—is highly recommended when you're increasing your fiber intake. It prevents constipation as fiber absorbs water, toxins, and bile from your system and flushes them away.

consume more servings than that in one meal alone. Raw food's transit time, or total time from digestion to elimination, is around 24 hours. Cooked foods take much longer—roughly two to four times as long—to work their way through your 29 feet of intestines. Foods in their raw state are easily broken down on a nutrient level, hastening their utilization and processing. (We discuss the benefits of eating foods in their simple raw state in greater detail in Chapter 11.)

Diamonds in the Rough

Plants provide us with so much, nutrition-wise: proteins, carbohydrates, sugars, fats, phytochemicals, vitamins, minerals, and on and on. You know they're low fat and have beneficial fiber. But plants can also meet all your nutrition needs as well. Where will you get your protein as a vegan? Oh, the choices you have!

If you're going to look to the plant kingdom for protein, you'll be amazed at what you'll find. Protein abounds in plant foods. Beans have it; grains do, too. And you can find lots of protein in most nuts, seeds, and veggies—especially green leafy ones. Veggies are such powerhouses that even if you ate only one of these types of foods as the majority of your daily diet, you would easily meet and exceed your RDA for protein. But it's recommended and much more exciting to eat a variety of plant foods to have a well-balanced diet. They don't say "Variety is the spice of life" for nothing!

Know Beans About It

It's recommended that you get 3 to 4 grams protein for every 100 calories you consume. Legumes such as beans, lentils, and peas deliver those numbers very easily. Most provide 12 to 15 grams protein per 1 cup serving, which is easy for a vegan to consume in a bowl of bean and veggie chili or split-pea soup.

In a Nutshell			
Want to know how many grams (g) protein various legumes have (per 1 cup serving)?			
Legume	Protein	Legume	Protein
black beans	15 g	peas (fresh)	9 g
chickpeas	14.5 g	soybeans	28.5 g
lentils	18 g	split peas	16.5 g
navy beans	16 g		

Legumes are also excellent sources of iron, zinc, calcium, phosphorus, potassium, vitamins A and B, and trace minerals. In addition, most are complex carbohydrates, low in fat and calories and high in fiber. Soybeans are one of the most commonly consumed forms of bean proteins for vegans (we discuss them a little later in the chapter).

The fiber in beans helps you feel full faster, so they help control your appetite, which comes in handy if you're trying to drop a few pounds. Some people experience digestion problems when they start adding large amounts of beans to their diets for the first time. If this happens to you, don't drop beans altogether; just cut back a bit. Try eating a smaller portion at one meal until your system adjusts. Then, as your symptoms subside, increase your serving size, and feel free to include them at more than one meal.

A Grain of Truth

What are grains exactly? It's easiest to describe them as the seed heads of grasslike plants. Sometimes they're also referred to as "cereal crops." We have used and cultivated grains throughout the centuries, and some have become more popular and widely used than others. Cultural and regional conditions often determine a particular grain's predominance in the daily diet. Mediterranean diets favor pastas, corn, and wheat while Eastern European diets center on spelt, wheat, and barley, which all add heartiness to the dishes they're cooked in. Most Asian diets are predominantly rice-based, whether it be in whole-grain or noodle form.

Grains are amazing. They contain complex carbohydrates, protein, vitamins B and E, phosphorus, potassium—and more—all of which are good sources of fuel to provide long-lasting energy for the body.

But what exactly do we mean by *grains?* Foods such as brown rice, corn, wheat, spelt, quinoa, amaranth, barley, bulgur, couscous, millet, pastas, and even those rice blends that you find in bulk bins or boxes on your local store shelves qualify as grains. With all these choices, you can imagine how easy it is to incorporate several servings of grains into your daily diet. For example, you can find 4 to 8 grams protein in 2 slices whole-grain bread or 1 cup cooked grains. You can find up to 10 grams protein in 2 ounces cooked pasta (that's before you add your favorite sauce or topping).

It's best to consume whole grains for optimal nutrition and health benefits. These are your best choice for getting the most vitamins and fiber benefits. Whole grains have all the germ and bran intact, which provide your body with vital fiber. Germ and bran are usually stripped away during the bleaching process, resulting in a whiter-looking (and less nutritious) flour.

> **CAUTION**
>
> **Hot Potato**
>
> When selecting grains, avoid products with words like *bleached, white, enriched,* or *bromated* in the ingredient list. These words means that vital fiber has been removed from the grains. Instead, look for terms like *whole grain, stone ground,* and *whole wheat* to ensure you will get all the grainy goodness nature intended.

Lean, Mean, and Green

Leafy green veggies such as lettuce, spinach, Swiss chard, collards, kale, and cabbage contain so many good-for-you things! They contain calcium, protein, iodine, magnesium, iron, plenty of fiber, complex carbohydrates, and vitamins A, B, C, E, and K. To get 3 to 4 grams protein, you would need to consume 3 to 4 cups raw spinach, kale, or lettuce, or 1 cup cooked collards, cabbage, or spinach.

All these veggies are delicious eaten raw, steamed, or sautéed; cooked into soups or stews; used to encase fillings; or added to dishes. If you munch on them as a salad, your saliva's digestive enzymes will immediately start breaking down the leaves into nutrients. Plus, all that chewing will give you a feeling of fullness faster and satisfy

> ### In a Nutshell
>
> In the South, many people love the "pot liquor" that results from cooking greens. They use this vitamin-rich broth in sauces, for cooking grains, or for making soups. Some people like to drink it, but it's especially good if you soak it up by dipping bits of cornbread or bread into it!

your appetite. So dig into a fresh, crisp salad full of a variety of greens, veggies, and even some beans, whether you wish to eat well or just drop a few pounds!

To preserve as much dietary fiber and nutrients as possible when cooking leafy green veggies, it is best to quickly sauté or stir-fry them until crisp-tender or just wilted. Or cook them into soups, stews, or with a lot of water and aromatic herbs until desired tenderness.

Soy—Oh Boy!

Ah, the magnificent soybean! We have the great Benjamin Franklin and a few other agriculture pioneers to thank for soy reaching the shores of America when it did. After learning about the amazing "cheese" made from soybeans on a visit to Paris, Franklin had several soybean plants sent to Pennsylvania farmers. Franklin himself was a vegetarian (for at least part of his life) as well as a writer, inventor, and statesman. He convinced farmers to grow soybeans as crops, which were then used to make the soybean cheese, better known to us as tofu, in addition to soy sauce and vermicellilike soy noodles.

> ### In a Nutshell
>
> The oldest soyfoods company in America, Quong Hop, started in 1906 in San Francisco. It's still in business today, known as Soy Deli, makers of tofu- and tempeh-based products.

Asian cultures are the true masters of the soybean, though. They have been enjoying it for centuries in everything from beverages to main dishes to desserts. They soak and grind soybeans into a refreshing soy milk beverage and eat fresh-picked green soybeans as a popular snack. Pieces of tofu or tempeh often find their way into appetizers like spring rolls, which are rolled in yuba, the dried skin that is removed during the process of making soy milk. *Miso*, which is a fermented soybean paste, is a popular condiment Asians use to flavor sauces and soups. They also use tofu and tempeh to make an array of interesting alternatives to meat and dairy products (see the following sections for more on tofu and tempeh).

The medical community has touted soy as a miracle food and has conducted numerous studies to analyze soy's nutrient content and confirm its positive effects on our health and well-being. It's a great source of *phytosterols*, which reduce blood cholesterol levels, and *phytoestrogens*, which reduce the risks of estrogen-related cancers, prostate cancer, osteoporosis, menstrual and menopausal symptoms, and cardiovascular disease.

Tofu to Ya!

You may have stumbled across tofu in your grocery store. You know, those white blocks submerged in liquid, in plastic or aseptic containers. It does look a little curious, floating there in that liquid, but don't be put off by tofu's appearance.

> **Vegan 101**
>
> **Miso** is the name given to a pastelike condiment made entirely from soybeans or in combination with other beans or grains like chickpeas, barley, or rice. Miso ranges from sweet, mild, and mellow with a light beige color, to strong and rich with earthy red tones that sometimes appear black.

We have Asia to thank for this miracle food. More than 2,000 years ago, Chinese culinary masters figured out how to process the simple soybean in such a way as to increase its digestibility and nearly double its protein content. This process is very similar to that of cheese-making, but instead of starting with cow's milk, it starts with soaked and cooked soybeans that are then ground to make soy milk. A coagulant is added to the soy milk and then the magic happens, turning this noble bean into a custardlike mass.

There are basically two types of tofu, regular and silken. Regular tofu is made very much like cheese. After the coagulant is added, the solids or curds are separated from the liquid or whey. The accumulated curds are then packed into molds, pressed, and left to drain to the desired consistency and texture. This separating of the curds and whey could explain why tofu is also referred to as *bean curd*. Depending on how much water is removed, the tofu is labeled as either soft, firm, or extra-firm.

Silken tofu, on the other hand, is made a lot like yogurt, and the solids and whey are not separated. In fact, some manufacturers pour the soy milk and coagulant directly into aseptic packaging. The tofu firms up inside the packaging and does not require refrigeration until that package is opened. Silken tofu is also available in soft, firm, and extra-firm varieties. It has a

> **In a Nutshell**
>
> In China, tofu has been nicknamed "the meat without bones" because of its versatility in creating so many meatlike replacement products.

softer, creamier texture, making it better suited for puréeing for use in sauces, soups, smoothies, and dairy-free desserts like vegan cheesecake.

On the commercial level, common tofu coagulants include the following:

◆ Calcium sulfate, commonly known as gypsum

◆ Calcium chloride, commonly known as Epsom salts

◆ Magnesium chloride, a salt derived from the sea

◆ Nigari, a sea salt in its natural state and one of the oldest-used coagulants

At home, if you want to curdle or coagulate soy milk and help separate the solids from the liquids in the production of homemade tofu, use lemon juice or vinegar.

Tofu has a spongelike texture that puts some people off at first, but keep in mind that, like a sponge, it can take on a lot of flavor from whatever surrounds it and it has an endless array of uses in your vegan kitchen. (Need some ideas? We discuss substitutions and recipe ideas in Parts 5 and 6, respectively.)

Tempeh: Not Just a Place in Arizona

Tempeh's roots start in Indonesia, not the Arizona desert. There folks developed and introduced a fermentation technique to the tofu-making process that resulted in something totally different, texture- and flavor-wise. Tempeh is made with soybeans alone or in combination with other beans or grains such as lentils, rice, millet, quinoa, or barley. In a procedure similar to that of making blue-veined dairy cheeses like Roquefort, a special mold is injected into the soybean mixture and left to ferment. The mold binds the mixture together, and the result is a thick slab with veins running through it. The veins are mostly white but sometimes you'll see gray, brown, and black veins, too.

> **In a Nutshell**
>
> Many people who have a problem digesting soy products such as tofu and soy milk don't experience the same symptoms with tempeh. This is mainly the result of increased digestibility arising from the fermentation process.

The fermentation process gives the tempeh a richer, almost mushroomlike flavor. For those of you who think you'll miss beef when eating vegan, give tempeh a try. It can be fried, sautéed, or baked or added to sauces, stews, or stir-fried dishes. Steaming it makes it swell in size and soak in additional flavorings, like its spongelike cousin tofu does.

TVP (No, Not a Paper Product)

We're talking about *TVP*, not *TP*. TVP is textured vegetable protein, which is actually considered one of the least heavily processed "second-generation" forms of soy protein. It is made from defatted soybean meal that is cut into chunks or small flakes that are then dried.

Cooks use TVP to extend meat in many schools and government-funded institutions because it is economical and high in protein. It makes a perfect substitute for ground hamburger in burgers, chilies, sauces, and veggie loafs. You can find it in packages and in the bulk section of your grocery store.

Soy Many Choices

One of the latest snack trends in the United States is edamame, or fresh, immature, and still-green soybeans. You can find them fresh for a limited time and in the freezer section of your grocery store almost any time of the year. You can boil them in their pods, seasoning them with salt, and then pop them out of their pods directly into your mouth. Soy nuts made from split soybeans that are then roasted and often seasoned are also available in most snack aisles. These goodies pack a whopping 34 grams protein in a ½-cup serving.

You can purchase the fully matured soybeans in the regular beige variety, as well as the black ones that come canned or dried. The black bean paste commonly used to flavor many Asian dishes is made from fermented black soybeans and seasonings.

You can also find many mock meat products in the refrigerator and freezer sections of your local grocery and health food stores. You will be amazed by the wide selection of products that range from veggie hot dogs, sliced luncheon meats, sausages, ground-meat replacements, to the ever-popular mock turkey products used during the winter holiday season. Most grocery stores carry soy protein powders, soy-based nondairy ice creams, and soy-based beverages and desserts.

It might take a bit of experimenting to discover which products you like best because they all vary in terms of flavor, consistency, and nutrition. If you don't care for a particular brand, don't be put off; just try another until you find one that suits your own personal taste. (In Parts 5 and 6, respectively, we discuss specifics in regard to using substitutions and give you some recipe ideas.)

No Bones About It: Other Natural Vegan Treats

We have the Buddhist monks, with their strict vegetarian, nearly vegan lifestyle, to thank for developing so many mock meat products. Not only did they come up with some amazing soy-based substitutes, but their culinary expertise and wisdom also helped to develop even more amazing foods from what some would consider nothing. They developed techniques for turning grains into everything from beverages to savory items to desserts. They transformed little morsels of humble nuts, seeds, and mushrooms that many just passed by or overlooked into culinary creations that produced intricate layers of flavor and texture while providing a hearty and filling meal that satisfied the palate.

Versatile Seitan

One of the most amazing culinary developments the monks made is definitely the development of seitan. Somehow, these wise disciples figured out how to rinse the starch out of wheat flour and leave only the gluten part, which then underwent amazing transformations. In an elaborate and timely process, they mixed together wheat flour and water, kneaded it to develop the gluten structure in the flour, drained off the water, and then rinsed it. They repeated this procedure until all the starch and bran had rinsed away and all that remained was the gluten part of the flour. They then simmered it in either water or a flavorful broth so the grain swelled in size and became infused with flavor.

From this point, it can be adapted to make many products that resemble the taste and texture of most meats, including beef, chicken, and seafood. For example, you can simmer small morsels in soups, sauces, or stocks. You can develop its chewy texture by baking it in loaves or small pieces.

Not only is the versatile seitan delicious, but it's also quite nutritious. A 2½-ounce serving contains no cholesterol or fat, has only 70 calories, and delivers 12 grams protein. That's not bad for a little flour!

In a Nutshell
For a treat, try simmering seitan in water; then cut it into fingerlike sticks, place it in a casserole dish, cover with your favorite barbecue sauce, and bake for 20 to 30 minutes or until seitan is a bit puffy and has a bit of brown around the edges. It's yummy as part of a down-home meal with black-eyed peas, brown rice, cooked greens, and cornbread!

Some Chinese restaurants, particularly vegetarian ones, use mock meats, many of which are soy and gluten based, in their menu items. If you see some of these "meats" on the menu, be a little adventurous and try one. This can be a great way to introduce yourself to gluten before attempting your own such concoctions at home. The all-vegan Lotus Garden restaurant here in vegan-friendly Eugene, Oregon, features many soy- and gluten-based mock meats in their many menu selections. They even make terrific batter-dipped and fried pieces of seitan that resemble those infamous fast-food chicken nuggets—only lighter in taste and crispier!

Vital wheat gluten, also referred to as instant gluten flour, is available in the baking and bulk bin aisles of most grocery and health food stores. Boxed products are also available, such as vegan chef Ron Pickarski's Seitan Quick Mix, which require only a little water and a few minutes to make a batch of homemade seitan.

> **Hot Potato**
>
> Although quite yummy, seitan does have one drawback: because it is made from pure wheat gluten, it is not suitable for those who suffer from celiac disease and wheat or gluten allergies.

Fungus Among Us

Many cultures throughout history have used mushrooms for food, medicine, and spiritual purposes. Considered fungi, mushrooms grow on organic material, preferring nutrient-rich soils and decaying tree limbs for their host homes. They grow wild as they see fit, even if we have managed to cultivate a few varieties, and their earthy aroma and flavor tantalize the senses. They come in thousands of varieties, but most of us only have access to a few types all year around, the most common being white button, shiitake, crimini, and portobello. Some areas have better access to mushrooms with more exotic and somewhat enigmatic names like porcini, morel, chantrel, truffle, oyster, lobster, enoki, and wood ear, just to name a few.

Mushrooms contain 70 to 90 percent digestible vegetable protein, a substantial amount of B vitamins, selenium, copper, and some other trace minerals. They are low in calories (1 cup raw mushrooms has about 20 calories), low in fat, high in dietary fiber, and cholesterol free. Moreover, researchers have discovered that mushrooms contain antibacterial and other medicinal qualities, including antitumor compounds called triterpenoids.

CAUTION

Hot Potato _____

Unless you are an expert on wild mushrooms, you shouldn't just pick and eat any ol' mushroom you find growing in your yard or in the woods. Some of them can be extremely poisonous!

You can purchase mushrooms fresh, frozen, canned, dried, and even in the supplement form. Their rich, almost "beefy" flavor and chewy texture work well as a meat substitute. You can marinate and grill whole portobello caps and enjoy them as burgers or mushroom "steaks." You can also slice or chop mushrooms and add them to veggie chilies, tomato sauces, or stews. The flavor and texture fools your palate into thinking it's meat, which is perfect for those who may be new to the veggie way of eating.

Just Nuts About It

Nuts and seeds are one of the earliest and simplest protein sources available. Many species enjoy these savory morsels as they grow abundantly in thousands of varieties and hang from trees within easy grasp. Just like a piece of ripe fruit, there's nothing like picking a handful of nuts fresh from a tree, cracking them open, and enjoying them in their natural, raw state. It's best to eat nuts and seeds raw to get the most of their many benefits, but many people enjoy the more developed flavors of dry-roasted nuts.

Nuts and seeds are important protein sources for raw foodists, vegans, and vegetarians alike. They are high in protein; most contain 3 to 8 grams protein in a small, ¼-cup serving. They also contain calcium, zinc, selenium, vitamin E, and other antioxidants and provide phytochemicals that help with mineral absorption.

Nuts and seeds do contain high amounts of fat and calories because they are such nutrient-dense foods, but fortunately, most of the fats are unsaturated. In addition, many nuts and seeds contain significant amounts of *essential fatty acids*, which help reduce blood cholesterol levels and prevent and fight disease. These fatty acids are also found in dark green leafy vegetables, grains, soybeans, broccoli, and sea vegetables. The vital oils found in nuts and seeds require a bit of special treatment to preserve them and prevent rancidity, so be sure to refrigerate or freeze nuts and seeds you have at home.

You can chomp on a handful of nuts for a quick and easy snack that will provide you with concentrated energy and help get you over the hump until your next meal. They are often ground into nut and seed butters, such as peanut, almond, or cashew butters and sesame *tahini*. They are available freshly ground, salted, unsalted, raw, and in roasted varieties to suit all tastes. As with nuts, keep nut butters in your refrigerator to preserve their freshness.

Vegan 101 _____

Essential fatty acids, better known as EFAs, are made of alpha-linoleic acid and linoleic acid, which are necessary for the formation and maintenance of cells. These fatty acids are commonly referred to as omega-3 and omega-6 fatty acids respectively, and they compete for dominance within your body. Having a greater proportion of omega-6 can increase your risk for chronic diseases, as it cancels out the beneficial effects of omega-3 acids.

Tahini is a thick paste or butter made from ground sesame seeds. It is often used in Middle Eastern cuisine and features prominently in hummus, baba ghanouj, soups, salad dressings, and many other dishes.

Surely you must have had your share of peanut butter and jelly sandwiches, but have you ever tried a cashew or almond butter sandwich topped with raisins, chopped fruit, or seeds? Delicious! Ground nuts and seeds can even add protein, texture, flavor, and binding qualities to veggie burgers, loaves, cutlets, and baked goods.

The Least You Need to Know

- It's easy to get enough protein on a vegan diet. Many plant foods are loaded with it.

- Fiber is essential for keeping your system moving and working efficiently. Be sure to regularly consume sources of both soluble and insoluble fiber.

- Legumes, green leafy vegetables, and whole grains are fundamental parts of a good vegan diet.

- The soybean is a versatile and nutritious food that can be prepared in a wide variety of ways.

- Vegans and others who are wanting to move toward a plant-based diet can easily find many healthful and nutritious meat substitutes.

Chapter 6

But You Need Dairy for Calcium

In This Chapter

- Considering calcium concerns
- The advantages of avoiding cow's milk
- Plant-based milk substitutes
- The truth about dairy cheese
- The wonderful world of nondairy cheeses

Where will you get your calcium now that you aren't eating cheese and drinking milk?

In addition to the often-asked questions regarding protein, you'll most likely hear this question, as well as other versions of it, as people learn you're going vegan. What many people don't realize, however, is that it's relatively easy to meet your calcium requirements while consuming a completely plant-based diet.

What the Other Animals Do

Calcium is one of Earth's most common minerals. It's also the one most abundant in our body. How does it get in us? Plants absorb calcium into their cells, then they pass that calcium on to us when we eat them. We access the plants' calcium when we eat calcium-rich foods or ingest them as either human or animal breast milk that has become fortified with the mother's dietary calcium. But consuming plant-based dietary sources of calcium is much easier and supplies much larger amounts of absorbable calcium.

Not Past the Age of Two

In general, most creatures that nurse their young do not breast-feed beyond the age of 2; therefore, the need for milk no longer exists past that age. This is the case for humans as well, and by the time we reach the age of 4, most of us have lost the ability to digest lactose. Lactose, which we touched on briefly in Chapter 3, is a type of sugar that is present in all animal breast milks, including human. As we age, our gastrointestinal tract matures and reduces our need for lactose as weaning is completed. When lactose isn't digested properly, it reaches our intestines, where bacteria attack it and try to break it down. During the "attack," acids and gases are produced; these are what cause the many painful symptoms associated with lactose intolerance.

CAUTION

Hot Potato

Cow's milk can contain growth hormones and antibiotics that are given to dairy cows to increase their milk production and alleviate conditions like infected udders. All these substances are then passed on to those who consume dairy products. Some have been linked to various forms of cancer and disease, food allergies, growth abnormalities, and birth defects.

Not Your Mama's Milk

It makes sense for our young to consume their mother's breast milk; after all, that's why we produce it in the first place. Most breast milk contains colostrum, which supplies newborns with all the vitamins, nutrients, and antibodies they need for the early developmental stages of life. It seems only logical that if you're going to consume any milk, it should be early in life and it should be human milk, as it contains the right kind of colostrum specific for your body.

Humans are the only species on the planet who consume the milk of another species and who continue to drink milk after weaning. So what's wrong with cow's milk and its colostrum for us humans? Cow's milk's main function is to take a young calf and "beef it up" to several hundred pounds in its first year of life. If you consume cow's milk instead of breast milk, it generally affects your size and development. This can also explain the increased obesity of toddlers in this country who consume dairy products; our size and the amount of fat in our cells is determined early in life.

It's interesting to note that mature cows don't need to consume milk to produce lots of calcium-rich milk. In the wild, they would eat a diet based on grasses and vegetation. Similarly, humans don't need to drink cow's milk to get calcium or produce milk for their own babies, either. Consuming plant-based forms of calcium to stay healthy and help produce our own milk, as the cows do, is the ideal way of getting it straight from the source, instead of secondhand.

Calcium Concerns

Our bodies use calcium to maintain strong bones and teeth, send nerve impulses, metabolize iron, regulate our heartbeats and other muscle contractions, and reduce the risk of chronic diseases. Yes, you should be concerned about whether or not you are getting enough calcium from dietary sources, but you should also be aware of your body's ability to absorb and utilize the calcium from those sources.

It's also important to hold on to the natural calcium already present in your bones and then take in dietary sources of calcium to make up for the losses that also occur naturally as you age. What you eat directly affects your calcium loss and the strength of your skeleton. Be sure to choose low-fat forms of plant-based protein, watch your salt intake, limit your caffeine to 2 cups of coffee a day, quit smoking, and get plenty of exercise outdoors. It's believed that if you avoid these calcium-depleters and also consume an average level of calcium in your diet, you can maintain strong, healthy bones.

The people of India and their cultural diet are a great example of the pitfalls of following a dairy-rich diet. There they follow a mostly vegetarian diet, but most of their native dishes contain large amounts of yogurt, milk, cheese, and ghee (clarified butter). As a result, Indians have high incidences of diseases associated with high-cholesterol and high-fat diets such as cancer, especially prostate and breast cancer. Heart disease is also on the rise, expecting to reach 2 million annually by 2010. Indians also have the highest number of diabetics worldwide and alarming amounts of iron deficiencies.

Sources and Absorbability

What are some calcium-rich foods, and how much of their calcium are we capable of absorbing and holding on to? You can find plenty of calcium in leafy green vegetables, and 40 to 60 percent is absorbable by our body. It was once believed that the *oxalates* in certain plant foods messed with our body's ability to absorb calcium by binding with it and forcing it through the elimination process, but the latest research proves otherwise.

> **Vegan 101**
>
> **Oxalates** are organic acids that occur naturally in leafy greens, berries, nuts, black tea, and other foods.

For proper calcium absorption, you need to consume food sources that contain types of calcium that are easily digested, assimilated, and absorbed. Keep a watchful eye on your protein, sodium, and other mineral intakes, as they all affect this process. Especially important to note is the special relationship between magnesium and calcium. These "bosom buddies" rely on each other, and both need to be present for proper absorption. Usually it's in a 2:1 ratio, with two parts calcium to one part magnesium.

Because of the calcium-magnesium ratio in dairy products, our bodies do not properly absorb the calcium they contain. Excess stores of calcium accumulate in our blood and urine and can cause kidney problems or failure or cause kidney stones and gallstones. Some greens, like spinach, contain oxalic acid, which may also cause a problem for those who are susceptible to kidney stones and gallstones. If you're sensitive, you might want to limit your consumption of certain leafy greens to several times a week. Also, drinking plenty of water can help prevent the formation of stones by diluting the concentration of oxalic acid and dissolved minerals in the urine.

The presence of vitamin D also affects calcium's absorption capabilities. The body easily absorbs vitamin D with just 15 minutes of exposure to sunshine per day. Vitamin D is produced within the body when the sun hits your skin. The sun triggers ergosterol, which is transformed into vitamin D, which helps us absorb calcium from the foods we consume directly into our bloodstream. Vitamin D is stored in the liver, and many believe that what you're exposed to in an average summer can be stored within your body and used throughout the winter. The liver is capable of storing up to a 3-year supply of vitamin D at one time.

Today, many foods are fortified with calcium, magnesium, and vitamin D. Check your grocery and health food store shelves for fortified soy-based products, cereals and grain products, boxed mixes and food items, and orange juices and other beverages.

With all these choices, it is virtually impossible to have a calcium deficiency if you consume a well-balanced vegan diet.

You do need to keep an eye on these fortification levels, however, as overly excessive amounts of calcium and vitamin D in the diet often lead to health concerns and problems, as previously discussed. You will absorb more calcium if you spread out your food choices throughout your meals and throughout the day.

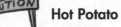

Hot Potato

There's no vitamin D naturally present in milk; it's added later as a supplement. Calcium is added back into cow's milk during the production process, because some of it is destroyed during pasteurization.

Comparing Food Sources

The U.S. RDA for calcium is between 800 and 1,200 milligrams, depending on your protein intake, but many feel that that number is too high. The World Health Organization (WHO) recommends between 400 and 500 milligrams calcium daily—half of the U.S. RDA. Plant-based sources of calcium are generally more absorbable than animal sources because we can digest the plant-based foods easier and break them down and utilize the nutrients better.

Proteins also have a negative effect on calcium stores because amino acids contain sulfur, which in turn affects the body's pH balance. Plant-based proteins tend to have lower concentrations of sulfur-based amino acids and are more alkaline in nature. Meat, on the other hand, is very acidic, and the body reacts to rebalance itself by leeching alkaline calcium out of the bones to neutralize the acid. For every 1 gram protein in your diet, you can expect 1 milligram calcium to be lost or eliminated in your urine.

Through his research, Dr. T. Colin Campbell of the famous China Project (see Chapter 3) has determined that even though most Chinese consume no dairy products in their daily diets, *osteoporosis* is uncommon in China even though they consume only half the amount of calcium consumed by Americans. Instead, they obtain all their dietary calcium from plant-based sources.

Ironically, osteoporosis is highest in those countries that consume the highest amount of calcium from animal-based sources. Because the high concentration of acidic protein in animal-based sources causes the body to lose more calcium than it consumes, a vegan diet will actually reduce your chances of developing osteoporosis.

Vegan 101

Osteoporosis is a bone-thinning disease that can rob you of 30 to 40 percent of your bone tissue. Calcium passes from the bones, filters through the kidneys, and is then eliminated in the urine. Factors like excess salt, animal protein, and high-protein dairy products in your diet cause rapid calcium losses and increase your chances of developing osteoporosis. Women in the United States take note, as osteoporosis affects 1 in 4 women in North America.

Plant-Based Powerhouses

Many plant-based foods are rich in calcium (and many are also excellent sources of protein; see Chapter 5). In the leafy green vegetable category, you have many choices, including spinach, collards, kale, Swiss chard, lettuces, rhubarb, mustard and turnip greens, and even broccoli.

Vegan 101

Quinoa (pronounced *keen-wah*) is an ancient grain that has made a comeback in recent years. Its popularity is due in part to the fact that 1 cup cooked quinoa contains as much calcium as an entire quart of dairy milk!

Soy foods have naturally occurring calcium and are also often enriched to further increase the calcium amount. Calcium-rich soy products include soy milk, nondairy cheeses, tofu, okara, tempeh, and veggie burgers and other mock meats, just to name a few. In cereals and grains, calcium can be found in *quinoa*, amaranth, corn, wheat, and brown rice. And you might be surprised to learn that many sea vegetables, nuts, seeds, dried fruits, and even blackstrap molasses all contain significant amounts of calcium.

Here's a small sampling of vegan foods that are high in calcium:

1 cup hijiki	648 milligrams
1 cup tofu	516 milligrams
1 cup cooked collard greens	358 milligrams
1½ cups calcium-fortified oatmeal	326 milligrams
1 cup calcium-fortified orange juice	270 milligrams
10 medium figs	270 milligrams

1 cup cooked spinach	244 milligrams
1 cup cooked white beans	160 milligrams

The Disadvantages of Cow's Milk

Even though cows eat a low-fat plant-based diet naturally, their bodies transform the polyunsaturated fatty acids they consume into saturated fats contained in their milk to help their young quickly "beef up" in size. As a result, cow's milk and most dairy products in general are high in fat, especially high concentrations of saturated fat and trans-fatty acids. These types of fats are associated with increased risks of chronic disease and obesity and higher mortality rates. High-fat dairy products, such as whole cow's milk, butter, and cheese, also contain larger amounts of pesticide residues and other environmental contaminants than their low-fat vegan counterparts.

> **In a Nutshell**
>
> The Dairy Council dropped its popular slogan, "Milk: it does a body good" after a lawsuit brought by the Physicians Committee for Responsible Medicine (PCRM; see Chapter 3) alleged that milk actually contributes to disease and does not indeed do a body good.

Allergen Alert

More than 80 percent of children throughout the world are lactose intolerant and have problems digesting dairy products. In fact, most people around the world are lactose intolerant. More than half the children in the United States are allergic to milk. Besides being allergic to lactose, many find themselves allergic to *casein*, which is one of the types of proteins found in cow's milk. Many further suffer from colic, which has been linked to consumption of cow's milk.

An allergic reaction to dairy can cause a wide variety of symptoms, including diarrhea, constipation, respiratory problems, muscle and abdominal pain, colitis, depression and irritability, skin rashes, and chronic fatigue. Diligent label-reading is your best defense. If you suffer from such allergies, avoid products with the following words on the ingredient label: *whey*, *milk solids*, *calcium caseinate*, *sodium caseinate*, *sodium lactylate*, and *lactalbumin*. You should take food allergies very seriously because in some instances, they can be life threatening.

Kick Your Cold

Dairy products also produce excess mucus in your system. This leads to such problems as sinusitis, nasal stuffiness, and runny nose, which in turn leads to colds and increased ear infections, asthma, and sinus infections. Plant-based substitutes for cow's milk, such as those made from a soy or rice base, are associated with fewer allergies. We strongly advise those who suffer from chronic colds or dairy allergies to drop the dairy from their diet to relieve their symptoms. Many see positive results within a few weeks after making dietary changes.

Finding Plant-Based Milk Substitutes

Our bodies don't have a physical need for milk after a certain age, but there's no doubt that the use of dairy products has had an impact on our cuisine. We have acquired tastes for rich and flavorful foods and creamy textures.

In a Nutshell
See Part 5 for more information on using substitutions. Then, if you like, turn to Part 6 for recipe ideas!

But just because you shun dairy doesn't mean you have to give up creaminess and satisfaction. Many plant-based substitutes to cow's milk exist. Creamy, milklike beverages are made from soybeans, rice, grains, and nuts such as almonds and cashews. Nondairy milks are also low in fat and good sources of complex carbohydrates.

Soy Milk

Soy milk is made from cooked ground soybeans and is rich in iron, calcium, and phosphorus. You can easily make it at home or purchase it premade in assorted sizes, in aseptic packaging making them shelf-stable, or in the refrigerated section next to their dairy counterparts. Soy milk comes in sweetened or unsweetened varieties and in a wide assortment of sizes and flavors, such as plain, vanilla, chocolate, carob, coffee, and eggnog.

Because it is made from soybeans, soy milk has a good deal of fiber. In a 1-cup serving of soy milk, you receive 9 grams protein, 4½ grams fat, and ½ gram saturated fat. Soy milk is also high in soy isoflavones, the beneficial phytoestrogens that have so many positive effects on our bodies. Some brands are also fortified with extra calcium and vitamin D, making soy milk even more nutritious.

Vegan 101

The U.S. Food and Drug Administration (FDA) defines **milk,** in its Standards of Identity, as "the lacteal secretions from mammals." That's why, in 2002, the National Milk Producers Federation asked the FDA to prevent soy and other nondairy beverage producers from using the word *milk* to describe their products. As a result, in the United States, you will often see these products labeled as "beverages" or "drinks," although there are exceptions.

Rice Milk

Rice milk can also be homemade or purchased commercially, and it's usually made from fermented rice alone or in combination with soy milk or other grains. It has a sweeter flavor than soy milk and is a high-quality source of carbohydrates and B vitamins. Compared to cow's milk, rice milk is lower in calories, fat, protein, and calcium. Rice milk only has 1 gram protein, 2 grams fat, and no saturated fat per serving.

You can also purchase rice milk in sweetened or unsweetened, light, enriched, and combination varieties. Rice milks are also available in a wide assortment of flavors such as plain, vanilla, chocolate, and carob. You will find it available in aseptic packages, in convenient juice boxes, in quart or half-gallon sizes, and also in some refrigerated sections next to their dairy counterparts.

Other Milk Substitutes

Those who follow a raw foods diet often make nut and seed milks. They use only raw nuts or seeds and water, fruit juices, or Rejuvelac, which is basically the water that results from soaking and rinsing sprouts. You can also find commercially pre-made nut milks in aseptic packages in most grocery and health food stores. These would no longer be considered "raw" due to the heating involved in their production processes, but they're still delicious and nutritious nonetheless.

Try Pacific Foods' almond and hazelnut milks in both plain and vanilla versions as a change of pace in your coffee or tea. These nut milks each deliver 2 grams protein, around 3 grams fat, and no saturated fat per serving.

Also on your grocery or health food store shelves, you will find oat milk, a combination of rice and soy milks from Eden Foods, as well as Pacific's multigrain milk made from a mixture of amaranth, barley, brown rice, oats, soybeans, and triticale. Per serving, these blends and grain-based milks deliver between 4 to 7 grams protein, around 2½ grams fat, and no saturated fat.

Cheese: Melting Through the Layers

Cheese is, hands-down, the most popular of all dairy products. And it comes in so many varieties, from cow's milk, goat's milk, sheep's milk, and don't forget the ever-popular buffalo mozzarella made from—you guessed it—water buffalo milk! In the 1970s, the average American consumed close to 11 pounds of cheese per year, and in 2005, that figure is up to more than 30 pounds per year per person. Since cheese is essentially concentrated milk, it also comes with higher concentrations of fat, calories, sodium, cholesterol, and agricultural contaminants.

For some, cheese is one of the hardest things to give up when going vegan, but it doesn't have to be. Just check out the refrigerated case at your local grocery or health food store, and you'll find a wide array of vegan soft and hard cheese, Parmesan-style cheese, and even cream cheese alternatives, made mostly from soybeans.

CAUTION

Hot Potato

One pound of cheese contains 10 times the amounts of hormones and antibiotics (used in factory farming) as the milk from which it came.

Cholesterol and Sodium Levels

Cholesterol, as previously mentioned, is produced by the body and also found in animal-based foods. One cup whole milk contains 10 milligrams of cholesterol, and cheese made from a high concentration of milk has a larger proportional amount of cholesterol.

Here's an example of the kind of cholesterol numbers you can expect to find in a 1-cup serving of some popular cheese products, according to the U.S. Department of Agriculture (USDA):

Cottage cheese	32 milligrams
Parmesan cheese	64 milligrams
Ricotta cheese	125 milligrams
Cheddar cheese	240 milligrams

Salt is used in cheese-making to add flavor, to ripen, and to cure the cheese. The exact amount of sodium in cheese depends on the variety and processing methods. But as with cholesterol and fat, there's also a higher sodium content in cheese compared to other dairy products. Processed cheeses, cheese foods, and cheese spreads contain more sodium than naturally aged cheeses; cottage cheese's sodium content falls somewhere between the two types.

More Fat Than Protein

In your average hunk of cheese, it's estimated that 65 to 75 percent of the calories come from fat. The current RDAs for dairy products recommend 2 to 3 servings a day, which can add up to 20 to 40 grams of fat alone. Most Americans don't follow the recommended serving sizes when it comes to eating cheese. An average serving constitutes 1 cup cottage cheese or 1½ ounces of sliced or shredded cheese, which equals about 3 tablespoons. Most cheese-lover's pizzas on the market have several times that amount on each slice of pie.

Cheese is also a very concentrated source of protein. Because the carbohydrates are removed during the milk pasteurization process, most of what is left are proteins. About 80 percent of milk and cheese is made up of the protein casein. Casein plays a major role in cheese-making, as it is used to bind the other milk proteins together, giving the cheese structure. It also gives it a stretchy, gooey quality when melted. These qualities are why even some otherwise nondairy cheese manufacturers still use casein in their products, making them unsuitable for vegans.

Cheese-making also uses coagulants to bind or give structure to the cheese. These coagulants can come from plant- or animal-based sources, and *rennet* is the most commonly used. What's wrong with rennet? For one thing, it comes from the digestive systems of pigs and other mammals. Inexplicably, a few nondairy cheese-makers also coagulate their products with rennet, so be on the lookout. Vegans need to read labels carefully to avoid these products, so don't assume a product is vegan just because it is labeled as nondairy.

The Pains of Lactose Intolerance

Many who are lactose intolerant are better able to digest cheese and yogurt because of the friendly bacteria and enzymes that are added in their production processes. However, the lactose that's still present may cause some to experience constipation, abdominal pain, digestion problems, and migraine headaches. It is still recommended that lactose-intolerant folks limit their servings to only 1 or 2 per day or to eliminate dairy products altogether. Over time, continuing to suffer the lactose-related irritation to your system will weaken your immunity and digestion processes.

Substitutes in Your Grocer's Dairy Case

More Americans are turning to nondairy and animal-free food products, and the retail industry is responding to the demand. You can find soy milk, rice milks, soybased cheeses, and dairy-free alternatives on the shelves of most grocery and health food stores. The products that come shelf-stable in aseptic packages work well for those on the go, as they enable you to keep your pantry stocked with vegan options to be opened when needed and are great for traveling. Most nondairy milks come in juice-box, quart, and half-gallon sizes to suit all needs and family sizes.

You can also find many products in the refrigerated case. Among them are nondairy cream substitutes in pint and half-pint sizes, for use in coffee and other beverages, and nondairy milks in quart and half-gallon sizes. You may even be fortunate enough to have various flavor options, including eggnog and other holiday or seasonal selections.

For those who truly miss their cheese and find it the hardest to give up, have no fear: you don't have to do without. You can make or buy your own dairy-free substitutes. Most people like melted cheese on their pizza, and vegan versions of nondairy cheeses, found at most stores, can do the job. You can also make and drizzle a vegan cheese sauce on your pizza for a different change of pace. (See Chapter 20 for Vegan Cheezy Sauce, a versatile sauce to help those suffering from cheese cravings.)

Hot Potato _____

Read product labels carefully and thoroughly to avoid dairy-based ingredients, as most vegans become lactose intolerant rather quickly after giving up the dairy products. Watch out for words such as *rennet, casein, whey, calcium caseinate, sodium caseinate, sodium lactylate,* and *lactalbumin* on ingredient labels. Otherwise, you may be in for some lactose intolerance symptoms of your own.

In a Nutshell

Most dairy-alternative products come with expiration dates on their packages, but it is best to keep refrigerated products for only 7 to 10 days after opening, to avoid any unwanted bacterial growth or unpleasantness for your digestion.

Not all prepackaged brands of vegan cheese are the same. Some are good, and some may seem just *bad* when you compare them to the dairy products you're used to. Do a little experimenting to see what you like best. Some are strongly flavored and others are mild, and some have softer or firmer textures than others, making some more suitable for slicing and shredding. Types, flavors, and availability will vary depending on where you live. You might be able to find sliced, block, and even Parmesan styles in shaker bottles. Some health foods stores even make their own homemade vegan cheeses.

Cheesy Nutritional Yeast

Nutritional yeast is high in supplemented B_{12} and has a nutty, cheesy, almost poultry-like flavor. Vegans should look for Red Star vegetarian formula because it's most readily available and comes in small and large flakes as well as in a powder. It's an inactive type of yeast, not meant to be confused with the kind of yeast used to make beer or bread.

Nutritional yeast is also gluten-free as it is grown on a molasses medium. You will find that it is used often to make nondairy cheese recipes because of the nutty, slightly salty flavor that it imparts. There's really nothing quite like it!

The Least You Need to Know

- Thanks, in part, to the many plant foods high in calcium, it's easy to get enough calcium in a well-rounded vegan diet.

- By avoiding dairy milk, you will also be avoiding a lot of fat, agricultural adulterants, inferior calcium, and lactose intolerance.

- Soy milk, rice milk, and nut milks are all delicious and healthful alternatives to cow's milk.

- Dairy cheese is a concentrated form of dairy milk and contains concentrated forms of cholesterol and fat as well.

- You can find many nondairy cheese alternatives on the market. Keep experimenting until you find one you like.

Chapter 7

But Carbohydrates Make You Fat

In This Chapter

- ◆ A look at the carb craze
- ◆ The differences among carbs
- ◆ Eating whole grain goodness
- ◆ The dangers of a low-carb diet

During the past few years, the United States has seen a dramatic increase in the popularity of diets that espouse a low-carb, high-protein approach to weight loss. Each claims that by dramatically decreasing one's carbohydrate intake, while increasing protein consumption and not worrying much about fat intake, a person can lose weight. Unfortunately for many people, these trendy, low-carb diets all seem to boil down to eating lots of meat and dairy and not getting enough fiber, fruits, and veggies. Is this a reasonable and healthy road to weight loss or just another dead end on the road to good health and fitness?

The Highs and Lows of Carbs

People following these diet plans have to obsess over their intake of carbs, and a good recollection of high school math really comes in handy with all the calculating and figuring that's necessary. Interestingly, most people really aren't even sure what carbohydrates are or what they do.

Carbohydrates provide the basic energy needed to fuel our bodies. Plants make carbohydrates from the carbon, hydrogen, and oxygen that they take in during their cycle of life. Carbohydrates usually come in the form of starches and sugars and are found in fruits, vegetables, nuts, seeds, and grains.

Carbohydrates are essential for providing energy to every part of our bodies, from our cells to our muscles, so they are certainly an important part of our diet. If we limit our carbs without being aware of what they are and why we need them, we could be doing our brain and body wrong, big time. Carbohydrates are an absolute necessity for brain function, so if you like your brain activity to be quick and responsive, you'll find carbs to be quite useful.

" " Golden Apple _____

The American Heart Association doesn't recommend high-protein diets for weight loss. Some of these diets restrict healthful foods that provide essential nutrients and don't provide the variety of foods needed to adequately meet nutritional needs. People who stay on these diets very long may not get enough vitamins and minerals and face other potential health risks.

—American Heart Association Recommendation, 2002

A lot of misinformation is floating around regarding carbohydrates these days. While proponents of low-carb diets are slamming carbohydrates and getting a lot of media attention, they are also causing people a lot of confusion regarding the differences between complex, simple, and refined carbohydrates. Consuming more complex carbohydrates, limiting your simple carbohydrates, and restricting or eliminating refined carbohydrates should make up the basis of a well-balanced diet for anyone—veg-heads and meat-heads alike—especially those who suffer from chronic diseases.

Of note to diabetics, modern medicine is siding with the veg-heads because it turns out that excess meat-based proteins seem to affect insulin levels more than complex carbohydrates do. Studies have also shown that following low-carb diets should not become lifestyle choices, as these diets open the door to numerous health problems that may not be reversible without expensive surgeries, medications, and drastic changes. Not coincidentally, heart disease and various forms of cancer do seem to be plaguing some of the more vocal supporters of these types of diets.

Carbs: Complex, Simple, and Refined

Complex, simple, and refined carbohydrates really are miles apart, and it's quite easy to distinguish the good from the bad. They each have a role in our lives, and how big a role each plays in your daily diet seems to be the key to the size of your waistline.

Carbohydrates are made of sugars and starches. *Complex carbohydrates* are starches in their whole forms, such as in whole grains and flours, beans, and fresh and frozen vegetables. *Simple carbohydrates* are found in fresh, frozen, and dried fruits; a few vegetables; and commonly used sweeteners such as unrefined sugar cane, maple syrup, and brown rice syrup. *Refined carbohydrates* are usually what we would refer to as highly processed or prepackaged foods. They contribute very little in terms of nutritional value to your daily diet.

Complex carbohydrates provide your body with dietary fiber to aid in digestion, keep you regular, and lower your risk of chronic disease. Whole grains like brown rice and quinoa, unrefined flours, corn, pasta, beans, root vegetables, and green leafy vegetables will all provide you with high concentrations of complex carbohydrates. You will benefit greatly from centering your daily diet around foods like these.

Simple carbohydrates, found in fruits like berries, citrus fruits, apples, cherries, dates, melons, peaches, and plums, and nature's sweeteners like agave, sugar cane, maple syrup, provide you with quick energy and help satisfy your sweet tooth with a better choice than a piece of candy. Enjoy these carbs more sparingly than the complex variety, but enjoy them nevertheless, especially fruits, as they are loaded with vitamins, enzymes, fiber, and lots of other good stuff!

Refined carbohydrates are abundant in prepackaged foods such as snacks, candies and confections, cookies, cakes, and other baked goods that are made with ingredients like white sugar, white flour, high-fructose corn syrup, hydrogenated oils, and lots of artificial colorings and flavorings. You should consume these foods only occasionally or not at all because

Hot Potato

Many vitamins, minerals, phytochemicals, fiber, protein, and beneficial essential fatty acids are removed during the refining and manufacturing process.

they are empty calories that can lead to weight gain, cause fluctuations in blood sugar levels, and provide you with very little on a nutritional level.

Carbs and Our Society

To say that our society seems to be carb-obsessed lately is an understatement. Wildly popular diets like the Atkins Diet, the South Beach Diet, and the Zone all follow the same basic path to shedding the pounds: reducing carbohydrate consumption while increasing protein (usually in the form of animal protein, a.k.a. meat and dairy) intake.

In a Nutshell
In January 2004, it was reported that 9 percent of all Americans were on a low-carb diet. That's more than 25 million people.

Even their proponents admit that these diets are only temporary fixes for quick weight loss and should not become a way of life, yet the term *low-carb lifestyle* keeps popping up again and again. In reality, a low-carb lifestyle makes about as much sense as a low-water or low-air lifestyle. Carbohydrates are *that* essential to our diets.

You can't turn on a television, listen to the radio, or open a newspaper or magazine these days without being bombarded by ads and articles about "low-carb" this and "Atkins-friendly" that. Obviously, this was not always the case. Dr. Robert Atkins started the whole "carb craze" in 1972 with the release of his book *The Diet Revolution*, in which he first espoused his now-famous "low-carb, high-protein" mantra.

Dr. Atkins followed his own diet for 39 years, until his death in 2003. In February 2004, *The Wall Street Journal* ran an article about a medical examiner's report that reportedly showed Atkins had a history of heart problems, including congestive heart failure and hypertension. The article went on to say that at the time of his death, Dr. Atkins stood at 6 feet tall and weighed 258 pounds, which is considered obese by any standard. This can't be encouraging for anyone who is considering following this way of eating for any length of time.

Diet Craze, or Just Crazy?

The Atkins, Zone, South Beach, and other low-carb diets push high-protein portions mostly in the form of meat, eggs, and dairy—and along with them come artery-clogging fats. Conversely, carbohydrates are practically demonized and avoided at all costs.

These diets call for limiting the intake of sugar (itself a type of carbohydrate), which in actuality is not a bad thing, but they take it a step further by limiting one's choice of fruits and veggies because they contain sugars. In the process, all the beneficial vitamins, minerals, enzymes, and essential fiber that those fruits and veggies contain are also limited.

All this, they believe, will make you a shining example of good health and cause you to lose tremendous amounts of weight without ever having to exercise. It's all the foods' fault that you are fat, they say, not that you possibly made bad food choices when going back for that third piece of fatty meat or cheese—both of which you are encouraged to keep enjoying to your heart's (dis)content, by the way.

Golden Apple

Dr. Atkins advocated substituting simple carbohydrates with high-fat, high animal-protein foods such as bacon, sausage, butter, steak, pork rinds and brie. I would love to be able to tell you that these are healthy foods, but they are not. Telling people what they want to believe is part of the reason that the Atkins diet has become so popular.

—Dr. Dean Ornish, *Journal of the American Dietetic Association,* April 2004

As we discussed in Chapter 5, too much protein in your diet can lead to numerous health problems, the most life-threatening being heart disease and various forms of cancer, but that's not the only problem with these diets. Proponents want you to believe that if you base your diet around lots of animal protein and dairy products, with seemingly unlimited intake of fats, you will actually lose weight as long as you give up all your breads and pasta. What they usually don't tell you, at least not in the many TV ads or articles, is *why* you'll lose weight by eating this way.

The reason for your weight loss is that your body is sent into *ketosis*, which is the physical state where your system is fooled into burning stored fats instead of sugars. Carbohydrates and fats are the body's two main forms of energy, and when you extremely limit your carbohydrate intake, your body then switches to burning deposited fats. Carbohydrates are usually burned and put to use immediately, while fats are usually stored up in deposits for later use.

In ketosis, everything is turned topsy-turvy. When your body burns fat as its main source of energy, toxic ketones are released into your system. Ketones are strong acids that are harmful to your body; they build up in your blood and urine. In high levels, ketones are poisonous to body tissue. Ketones are the reason why some people on these types of diets have such foul-smelling breath.

Tipping the Scales in Your Favor

For those who want to lose a few pounds, whether it be with a high-protein and low-carb approach or the reverse, begin by increasing your plant-based food options. The produce section of your grocery or natural foods store is the best place to start when you're looking for good sources of carbohydrates.

The biggest and smallest animals all chomp down on a little raw vegetation from time to time, often for the fiber benefits alone, and they are definitely more tuned in to their proper natural processes than we humans are. Eating a big carrot or leafy green salad will definitely fill you up faster, whether it be from the digestive enzymes released or the high fiber content. This means less food passing by your lips, and ultimately, less ending up on your hips.

Refining Our Way of Life

After the world wars, the powers-that-be got it in their heads that everything had to be pristine white to instill a sense of cleanliness in the minds and hearts of those in the United States. Whitewash covered every part of society, from uniforms and clothing, to architectural structures, to modern conveniences and appliances, right down to the foods we eat. Across the board, white was right, and brown caused a frown.

Hot Potato

During the bleaching process that turns beige-colored, unrefined cane or beet sugar into white sugar, all the good nutritional components are stripped away. Among them are the molasses and the vitamins and minerals that were present. The only things left are refined carbohydrates and empty calories.

Manufacturers of grains and sugars also began bleaching and polishing their foods to make them appear better and healthier to consumers, in addition to giving them a slightly longer shelf life. In the process, they stripped items such as flour, rice, and sugar of their vital nutrients, fiber, and bran, all of which made these foods beneficial in some way to our diet. No nutritional benefits were added during all this bleaching and refining, only negatives.

We *need* bran, fiber, and other naturally present nutrients. Our insides are color-blind and don't care if a product is white or brown in color, just that it is wholesome and gives us the fuel we need to keep us up and running like a well-oiled machine.

When you're choosing dry goods for your pantry, pick those that appear in shades of brown, not white. Select brown rice instead of white, whole-wheat or oat flour instead of bleached and bromated, and evaporated or unbleached cane juice instead of bleached white sugar. Buy whole grains such as whole-wheat couscous, quinoa, millet, brown rice, and so on.

When purchasing grain or rice blends, be sure the words *brown rice* or another whole grain appears on the label either instead of or before white rice. Whole-grain pastas, for example, are made from whole-wheat flour, and sometimes even brown rice, corn, quinoa, and vegetables. You can find them next to their white-flour counterparts on grocery shelves. You might even be able to find them at a savings in the bulk section of many stores as well.

> **In a Nutshell**
>
> For some good recommendations of delicious and nutritious vegan food items to help stock your pantry, refrigerator, and freezer, turn to Part 3.

The Least You Need to Know

- Eating a low-carb, high-fat, and high-protein diet can be detrimental to your health, especially when the diet becomes a way of life.

- When choosing carbohydrates like grains and sugars, always look for whole or unrefined varieties.

- Complex carbs should be the basis of a well-rounded vegan diet. Simple carbs should be enjoyed more sparingly, and refined carbs should be rarely used or avoided altogether.

Chapter 8

Vegans: You're All Weak and Sickly

In This Chapter

- A look at vegan athletes
- Getting fit and trim, the vegan way
- Fueling your body with the right stuff
- The conflicting world of dieting
- The slow burn of carbs

For one reason or another, people sometimes have the impression that vegans and others on plant-based diets are frail, too thin, weak, or sickly. This couldn't be further from the truth, although vegans *are* much more likely to be more fit and trim than their nonvegan counterparts. Vegan athletes abound and excel in the sports world, and some of our greatest athletes have followed a completely plant-based diet.

Be confident in knowing that going and eating vegan does do a body good, and your physique will *not* suffer from your new way of eating. In fact, it will almost certainly improve. Remember, small steps taken in the right direction can have a positive impact on your journey to good health and happiness. Each of the changes you're making in your lifestyle will have an effect on your quality of life now and down the road.

Veganism: It Does a Body Good

The American Dietetics Association and the Dietitians of Canada have stated many times that a well-balanced vegan diet is appropriate for all stages of life, from pregnancy, the early stages of infancy on into childhood, through the growth spurts of adolescence, and on into adulthood. Vegan diets provide nutritional benefits in abundance. This translates into a body that is a lean, mean, vegan machine.

> **Golden Apple**
>
> My best year of track competition was the first year I ate a vegan diet. Moreover, by continuing to eat a vegan diet, my weight is under control, I like the way I look ... I enjoy eating more, and I feel great.
>
> —Carl Lewis, winner of nine Olympic gold medals

As previously mentioned, vegan diets are lower in fat than other kinds of vegetarian and animal-based diets. Plant foods are fiber-rich and often lower in calories, which assists in weight loss. Evidence exists that, due to their low-fat and high-carbohydrate diet, vegans have higher metabolic rates than people who consume animal-based foods.

A higher metabolic rate means you're burning calories faster, which is good for weight loss. As you age, your basal metabolic rate (BMR) steadily decreases. When you're young and strong, your BMR is very high. Then, as you get older, you lose lean body mass, which in turn slows down our BMR. The more lean body tissue you have, the higher your BMR. The more "fatty" body tissue you possess, the lower your BMR. You can raise your metabolic rate by getting regular vigorous exercise and consuming a healthy vegan diet.

Worth the Weight?

On average, vegans have lower incidences of obesity and tend to be leaner and trimmer. Most people who try a vegan diet for any length of time generally experience some weight loss, whether it be just water weight initially or some serious poundage. When going vegan full-throttle, it's not uncommon to lose a significant amount of weight, especially as you rid your system of excess fat stores and cholesterol you may have accumulated. Vegans are also well equipped for avoiding yo-yo weight fluctuations and usually consistently maintain their ideal weight.

Carbohydrates and simple sugars are the main sources of fuel for our bodies, and these are not found in meat. Providing your body with the proper fuel will give you endless amounts of energy and cause you to burn more calories. As a rule, plant-based foods are usually low in salt, saturated fats, and calories, which make them perfect for those who are crunching their dietary intake numbers.

There are exceptions to every rule. Here those exceptions are convenience junk foods, some chocolate, and a few tropical foods like coconut and palm oils. These foods contain higher concentrations of fat, so limit your consumption. If you only consume foods that are low in fat and high in fiber, you will be off to a good start for supplying your body with the optimal fuel it needs.

> **Golden Apple**
>
> Since becoming vegan, my running has improved considerably. Vegan food is ideal: high carbohydrate, low fat and plenty of vitamins and iron. I'm proud that I run without exploiting animals in any way.
>
> —Sally Eastall, marathon runner

The Skinny

A vegan diet can help you reach and maintain your optimum weight. A plant-based diet is full of fiber from plant vegetation and whole-grain sources that help flush out toxins, keep foods digesting properly, and make elimination time faster and more efficient. Veggies are also low in calories. Beans and green and yellow vegetables, like zucchini and summer squashes, celery, greens, peppers, onions, and carrots, all are perfect low-calorie munching foods. If you want to drop a few pounds, stick with your vegan diet. You can easily expect to have double the weight loss than someone following a low-fat animal-based diet.

Eating well is important when it comes to weight loss, but physical activity and vigorous exercise are also a must. Exercise boosts your metabolism and controls your appetite. Putting your body into a fast-paced mode during exercise triggers your body's "fight or flight" response. As a result, your digestion processes and appetite go into a holding pattern for a while to help your body handle the increased workload. Exercising an hour before eating will help you satisfy your hunger with much less food and burn more calories to boot.

Being a vegan is not about being on some trendy new diet; it is a lifestyle. It encompasses a way to think about the world and your relationship to it, as well as a moral code to make life choices by. It's not only the most cruelty-free way to nourish ourselves, but it's also the healthiest. That's an indisputable fact. Veganism as a way of life and a way to approach eating is meant to sustain us for the long haul. Although it certainly is growing in popularity around the world, it is not just the latest fad diet or "in thing" to do. A vegan diet is sound nutrition, not a fad.

The Buff

Vegans tend to have more lean muscle on their bodies and better overall muscle tone in general. You don't need to eat animal protein to put on muscle. Look at the elephant, one of the largest and strongest creatures in the animal kingdom. It eats an all plant-based diet full of roughage and fiber. It simply strips the leaves off the branches and chows down. Some think we vegans survive on eating "leaves and twigs," as some foods, especially trail mix, appear this way to some. But maybe we *would* all eat more leaves and twigs if we thought it would help us grow to be as strong and healthy as elephants are!

Vegans Fit and Famous

It is a common misconception that you need animal-based protein to meet your protein needs and that you need extra amounts of protein if you're an athlete or lead a physically demanding lifestyle. But doctors have discovered that you really don't utilize proteins any more rapidly while at work or play than you do at rest.

CAUTION

Hot Potato

Don't go overboard with protein, because too much protein can do more harm than good and lead to poor health (see Chapter 5).

Meat and dairy products are high-fat forms of protein, and though high-fat foods do provide you with energy, just as high-sugar foods do, they don't give you sustained energy. Rather, your uplifting feeling fades quickly, leaving you feeling sluggish and "out of it." Grab a carrot, a handful of nuts, or some broccoli instead. Plant-based proteins amply support muscle development and endurance during physical exertion and activity.

The Yale Medical Journal concluded that there is strong evidence that a meatless diet is conducive to endurance. Similarly, Dr. Ioteyko of the Academie de Medicine of Paris discovered that vegans and vegetarians averaged two to three times more stamina and recovered from exhaustion in one fifth of the time as meat-eaters.

Vegans have more endurance and stamina than most meat-eaters, and our high-carbohydrate diet has everything to do with it. Carbohydrates give a slow, steady burn and provide a constant energy source (fuel) for the body. That's why many athletes carb-load before a big race or competition. Lean sources of protein that are low in fat and high in fiber, like beans and other veggies, are like powder kegs for the body. And athletes know it!

Many well-known athletes know the benefits of a meatless diet. Check out a list of meatless athletes at veggie.org.

In a Nutshell

In a position paper on athletic performance and physical fitness, the American and Canadian Dietetic Association and Dietitians of Canada recommended that, for most athletes, 60 to 65 percent of total energy should come from carbohydrates. Those who compete in prolonged endurance events, or who exercise intensely on consecutive days, should increase their carbohydrate-based energy to 65 to 70 percent.

Finding Balance

No matter how or what you do or do not eat, the most important thing you can do to ensure your good health is to eat a well-balanced diet, one that is full of fruits, vegetables, grains, healthful fats, lean proteins, and complex carbohydrates, with plenty of water and other liquids. What you put into your body, you do get out of it. Good, wholesome foods will result in your whole being—body, mind, and soul—functioning in a happy, healthy way.

Fantastic Fruits and Veggies

Fruits and veggies are the good stuff your body needs. They can easily supply all your nutritional needs—and do it far better than animal-based foods. The phytochemicals alone are enough to give you an arsenal of beneficial nutrients to prevent and treat disease. Most plant life contains many different phytochemicals that work in symbiotic relationships within foods. Cooking increases the availability of some phytochemicals, while it diminishes others. So be sure to enjoy both fresh, raw produce and cooked culinary creations to get the most nutritional benefits you can.

Generally, the more vivid the colors a fruit or veggie possesses, the more phytochemicals it contains. It's best to eat a wide variety of fruits and veggies in a rainbow of colors to ensure you are getting enough sources of the mighty phytochemicals in your diet.

Antioxidants are also found in all fruits and vegetables, and to ensure that you get as many as possible, try to eat foods from every color of the rainbow: reds, yellows, oranges, greens, blues, and purples. Strolling through a well-stocked produce department will make this all very easy, as you should find a wide assortment of colors and textures to choose from there.

When purchasing fruits and veggies, it is very important to buy organic rather than conventionally grown veggies where possible. Organic foods actually seem to be more vibrant in color, more fragrant, and more delicious-tasting than their nonorganic counterparts. Also, by consuming organic produce, you are limiting your exposure to pesticides, fungicides, and other environmental contaminants that could affect your health and counteract the positive nutritional effects.

In a Nutshell

Many people feel they don't have time to chop. One solution to this is to buy pre-washed lettuces or greens in bags or precut fruits or veggies. If it will make your life easier or be the only way to ensure that you will incorporate them into your diet, these convenience foods can really come in handy. Use them quickly, as fruits and veggies become more perishable as more surfaces are cut and exposed to air and light.

Amazing Grains

There's nothing like a little grain to fill out your meals and satisfy your appetite. Whole-grain foods like barley, brown rice, amaranth, quinoa, bulgur, corn, millet, triticale, buckwheat groats, oats, and wheat are all smart choices for your body. They provide you with protein, carbohydrates, fiber, and an endless supply of energy with their slow burn. You will receive a good deal of vital vitamins and minerals from whole grains, in addition to *lignans* and other phytoestrogens, antioxidants, and other disease-preventing nutrients that cannot be found in supplements and can only be found in actual food sources.

Three often-overlooked grains are amaranth, millet, and quinoa. These powerhouse grains pack a wallop, so you should incorporate them into your diet as much as possible.

Vegan 101

Lignans are a variety of phytoestrogen, similar to isoflavones, that help regulate estrogen production in the human body. Lignans have been shown to have cancer-fighting properties that can help inhibit or prevent the growth of breast, colon, and prostate cancers.

Amaranth is a very tiny grain; you will find about a quarter million of them in 1 pound. But don't let its diminutive size fool you; a ½-cup serving will supply you with 18 percent of your daily requirements of calcium, 28 percent of your protein, 55 percent of your iron, and 60 percent of your dietary fiber. It's also high in lysine, cysteine, and methionine, which are essential amino acids needed for cell and brain maintenance.

You may only be familiar with millet as that little yellow grain in bird seed, but cultures throughout the world have been enjoying millet for centuries, making this grain third in consumption behind rice and wheat. Millet comes in thousands of varieties and in an array of colors from shades of white and gray to red and yellow. Millet is rich in magnesium, manganese, phosphorus, potassium, calcium, iron, and vitamins A and B. Most noteworthy are millet's heart-healthy benefits: its concentrations of niacin lower high cholesterol levels, its magnesium lowers high blood pressure levels and reduces risks of heart attacks, and its phosphorus can develop and repair damage to body tissue.

Quinoa, often referred to as the "gold of the Aztecs," is an ancient grain, first used by the Aztecs and Incas. It, too, comes in a wide variety of colors from yellow, orange, red, pink, purple, and black. Many foodies and medical professionals are also calling it a "supergrain" because it contains all nine essential amino acids in addition to being high in protein, calcium, magnesium, manganese, phosphorus, iron, copper, and B vitamins. In fact, 1 cup quinoa contains more calcium than 1 quart milk—100 percent absorbable and useable by your body—and twice the protein of rice and barley.

In a Nutshell	
In ½ cup dry quinoa, you'll find …	
11 grams protein	5 grams fiber
51 milligrams calcium	629 milligrams potassium
179 milligrams magnesium	7.9 milligrams iron
2.8 milligrams zinc	42 micrograms folic acid

The National Academy of Sciences considers amaranth and quinoa two of the best sources of vegetable protein. These two sources have a superior amino acid balance over cow's milk or soy-based products.

The Least You Need to Know

- Many bodybuilders and athletes have achieved fame and fortune by fueling their bodies with a completely plant-based diet.

- Eating a well-balanced vegan diet is a great way to shed excess pounds and maintain your optimum weight level.

- Carbohydrates burn slowly and provide your body with the steady source of sustained energy needed for physical exertion.

- Avoid fad diets, and instead turn to time-tested and true weight loss methods.

Part 3

A Vegan Survival Guide

On the ever-popular survival reality shows that flood our television screens, the contestants are left to their own resources to feed themselves, and they sometimes go hungry. What they need is an educated vegan, preferably a raw foodist, to show them all the wonderful plant foods that surround them!

Plants are definitely where it is, nutritionally. They give you a strong and healthy body, provide plenty of energy and endurance, and keep you mentally quick and alert. Eating vegan definitely gives you an advantage to help you win the game. After reading the following chapters, you'll have a leg up on the ins and outs of vegan nutrition, whether you're a child, young adult, pregnant, or in the prime of life. All you need to win at the game of life is right here!

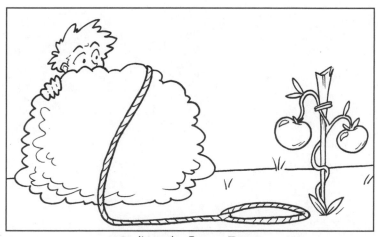

Stalking the Jersey Tomato

Chapter 9

Nourishing Yourself

In This Chapter

◆ Following dietary guidelines

◆ The building of the Food Pyramid

◆ A look at the Standard American Diet

◆ Climbing the meatless pyramid

◆ Meeting all your vegan nutritional needs

You may not have been much of a chef or short-order cook in your pre-vegan days, but if you truly want to embrace your new vegan lifestyle, you're going to need to roll up your sleeves and get cooking. Check out your pantry, refrigerator, and freezer for supplies and inspiration. Sometimes wandering in the market or cleaning out your cabinets can really spark some culinary creativity that results in a fabulous vegan meal.

In later parts of this book, we guide you through the process of stocking your pantry with vegan goods (Part 4) and provide you with suggestions on how to use some of the vegan alternatives you might not have used—or even heard of—before (Part 5). Then in Part 6, we provide you with some vegan recipes you can add to your repertoire to help you through your transition into eating vegan, as well as a few dishes to impress the veg-curious or veg-skeptical in your life.

The Formation of Food Guidelines

The idea of using formal or semi-formal dietary guidelines has been around for quite some time now, but it wasn't really widely used until the last century. Having recommended daily intake guidelines to follow for specific types of foods makes it easier for some people to be sure they're getting enough of what they need. Several dietary guidelines exist, from pyramids to food groups, and are widely used by carnivores and vegans alike. We look at a few of them, and a bit of their histories, in this chapter.

Congress created the United States Department of Agriculture (USDA) in 1862, and from the get-go, concerns existed over conflicts of interest. The USDA became the overseer of farmers' crops and the regulator of the nation's food supply levels. It was also in charge of educating the public on all things agricultural, including instructing and giving advice on what they considered proper nutrition via their own recommended food guidelines. The combination of these two roles meant that the USDA essentially controlled both the supply of and the demand for the nation's food.

The USDA soon found itself coming under the influence of heavy-hitting special interest groups like the meat and dairy industries. The first public food guidelines were published in 1916, and since their very beginning, their nutritional accuracy has come under scrutiny.

In the 1950s, the Basic Four Food Groups began their climb to fame and comprised the bulk of what most schoolchildren learned about proper nutrition for more than 30 years. The Four Food Groups, which were made up of meat and other protein sources, milk and dairy products, grains, and fruits and vegetables, became the first of the food guidelines to give serving recommendations. We were told to eat in this manner:

In a Nutshell

Food industry special-interest groups greatly influenced the Basic Four Food Groups serving suggestions. Included among these was the National Dairy Council, which produced a vast amount of its own Four Food Groups promotional literature, including posters and other "educational materials" that were used in classrooms.

2 servings per day of milk and dairy products

2 servings per day of meat, fish, poultry, eggs, dry beans, and nuts

4 servings per day of fruits and vegetables

4 servings per day of grain products

The New Four Food Groups

In 1991, the Physicians Committee for Responsible Medicine (PCRM) was hard at work developing an alternative to the Basic Four Food Groups. PCRM thought the USDA's food guidelines should better reflect what had become widely considered as the most healthful way for people to eat: a diet low in fat and cholesterol and high in veggies and whole grains. The New Four Food Groups provided a healthier, meatless alternative. The New Four Food Groups were and continue to be:

   5 or more servings per day of whole grains

   3 or more servings per day of vegetables

   3 or more servings per day of fruit

   2 or more servings per day of legumes

The New Four Food Groups dietary approach was intended to be a low-fat, zero-cholesterol, completely vegan way of meeting the daily nutritional requirements of the average adult. Several weeks before the USDA had planned to launch its Eating Right Pyramid, PCRM approached it about substituting the old Four Food Groups with their New Four Food Groups. They rejected the idea.

Golden Apple

The old four food groups serve to misinform consumers about some aspects of nutrition. Two of the four food groups—meats and dairy products—are clearly not necessary for health and, in fact, may be detrimental to health. ... Populations with the lowest rates of heart disease, colon and breast cancer, and obesity consume very little meat or no meat at all.

—From a 1991 PCRM report recommending the New Four Food Groups

Building a Pyramid

The Senate Committee on Nutrition and Human Needs published Dietary Goals for the United States in 1977 that totally supported a plant-based diet. In it, the committee recommended lowering cholesterol levels by limiting the amount of fats in the diet, especially saturated fats, and consuming generous amounts of fruits, vegetables, and whole grains. But after the meat and dairy industries complained and flexed their political muscle, the committee had to revise the report to be more accommodating to those industries.

In 1988, the USDA began to develop what they called the "Eating Right Pyramid" as a replacement for the old Four Food Groups. This new food guide stressed the importance of plant-based foods by placing them at the foundation of the pyramid (the group with the largest number of servings per day) and relegating meat and dairy products to a small section at the top of the pyramid (with the least number of servings per day). For the first time in USDA history, meat and dairy would no longer take center stage in the recommended food guidelines.

Just weeks before the scheduled release date, the National Cattlemen's Association teamed up with the National Milk Producers Federation and other pro-industry groups to oppose the Eating Right Pyramid. A few weeks later, amidst protest from various health and medical groups, the USDA scrapped the Eating Right Pyramid, citing that children would find it "confusing." A year later, they released the current Food Guide Pyramid, after it had undergone 33 changes, many of which were demanded by special-interest groups.

The Shape of the Pyramid

Five major food groups that are supposed to supply you with all your nutritional needs on a daily basis make up the Food Guide Pyramid. At the very top of the pyramid are fats, oil, and sweets—indulgences to consume sparingly. A supersize order of french fries or a couple doughnuts could easily exceed your daily allotment of fat and sweets.

In a Nutshell
Want to shed a few pounds or eat a more heart-healthy diet in general? Choosing lean sources of protein such as beans instead of bacon and cholesterol-free soy milk instead of whole milk products is a step in the right direction.

Next is the animal-based foods level, or the milk and meat groups, which should really be called the calcium and protein level. The foods in these two groups are meant to deliver iron, zinc, vital B vitamins, calcium, and protein. The Pyramid recommends 2 to 3 servings of each a day from legumes, nuts, fish, poultry, and meat for the protein sources and various dairy products for the calcium requirement.

We have previously discussed how our bodies better utilize and more easily absorb plant-based sources of calcium compared to their dairy counterparts. Based on that information, this section of the pyramid should be altered to include other calcium sources. It is also ironic that the smallest section of the pyramid is made up of fats, which even the USDA says should be limited, while the next tier recommends animal-based foods high in fats, especially saturated fats.

The next and largest levels of the pyramid are encouraging for vegans and vegetarians alike, as the foods all come from plant-based sources. To provide you with vitamins, minerals, and plenty of fiber are the fruits and vegetables groups, which share equal billing on the next level. The USDA recommends getting roughly 2 to 4 sources of fruits and 3 to 5 servings of veggies per day.

Finally, at the base of the pyramid is the grain group, made of breads, grains, rice, cereals, pasta, and so on. It's recommended that you get 6 to 11 servings per day of these nutritional powerhouses that supply you with protein, calcium, carbohydrates, vitamins, and minerals.

What's a Serving, Anyway?

So what does all this mean in practical terms? After doing the math and adding up your recommended numbers of daily servings, it may sound like the recommendations mean a lot of food, but it's really not because of what's considered a "serving size." For example, an apple or a banana would be 1 serving of fruit. A big carrot, ½ cup chopped vegetables, or 1 cup leafy greens are all you need to get 1 serving of veggies. A slice of bread or ½ cup cooked rice or pasta is considered 1 serving of grains.

Two to three ounces, which is considered the average serving size in the meat/protein group, would be equal to the average single hamburger patty, 2 eggs, 1 cup cooked beans, or ¼ cup peanut butter. A cup of milk or yogurt, 2 to 3 ounces cheese, or 1½ cups ice cream would constitute a serving from the milk group. As you can see, keeping the amount of dietary fat and cholesterol under control can be difficult following the USDA guidelines.

The Standard American Diet: SAD

Even though the United States leads the world in the amount and quality of its food supply, many people don't fully appreciate it or use it to their best health advantage. Instead of being a nation of healthy and well-nourished individuals in great physical shape, a growing number of Americans are actually overweight, deficient in nutrients, and prone to disease—often all at the same time. When you list the dietary factors that increase the risks of cancer, heart disease, stroke, diabetes, gastrointestinal and digestive disorders, and other chronic and degenerative diseases, the standard American diet has them all.

The Standard American Diet (SAD) has evolved in time from meaning nutritious homemade meals prepared with love, into nutritionally inferior meals of convenience designed to fit hectic lives and schedules. As a result, most Americans have to rely on quick fixes and fast foods for many of their daily meals, and those types of menus usually don't feature the wisest and most nutritious options.

The SAD diet tends to be highly processed and very high in fat, calories, and animal-based ingredients like cholesterol. At the same time, they're also low in crucial dietary fiber, complex carbohydrates, and sources of vitamin and nutrient-rich fruits and vegetables. Often, a slice of tomato or lettuce leaf are the only fresh vegetables some people get in their fast-food diet, and even then, the tomato slice is usually buried under a fried all-beef patty, gobs of cheese, and oil-laden sauces. It's not easy for the body to find nutrients hidden in all the fat and empty calories.

According to the U.S. Census Bureau's Statistical Abstract (1999) on the American diet, the average consumption of major food commodities per person, per year included:

> **CAUTION**
>
> **Hot Potato**
>
> In 1990, chances of getting cancer were 1 in 33; today it's estimated as 1 in 3. The American Heart Association claims that 53 million Americans suffer from cardiovascular disease, which includes arteriosclerosis, strokes, and high blood pressure.

580 pounds dairy products

54 pounds sugar

150 pounds wheat

111 pounds red meat

66 pounds fats and oils

53 gallons soft drinks

39 gallons alcohol

29 pounds ice cream

24 gallons coffee

In the course of the past 50 years or so, America went from elaborate homemade spreads that included tossed green salads, entrées accompanied by two or more side dishes, freshly baked bread, and even a dessert, to the total epicurean opposite of so-called "fun meals" and meals in a box. One major contributing factor would be a little thing called advertising. Any given corporation has spent billions of dollars to shape minds and target all ages with whatever message it wants to spread. Many people give in to these messages, buy their products, learn to love them and feel they need them, and don't see the harmful dietary drawbacks.

To truly see if products or foods are good for you and provide you with actual sound nutrition often requires taking a step back, analyzing products, and reading labels. Often, fast-food businesses don't have the nutritional information available for you to easily access, and food companies use slick advertising and doubletalk to mislead you about the nutritional content of their products. Using common sense when making food choices for yourself and your family will help guide you through the quagmire of advertising mumbo-jumbo.

Golden Apple

There are 4,000 heart attacks every single day in this country. The traditional four food groups and the eating patterns they prescribed have led to cancer and heart disease in epidemic numbers, and have killed more people than any other factor in America. More than automobile accidents, more than tobacco, more than all the wars of this century combined.

—Dr. Neal Barnard, M.D., in his book *Food for Life*

A Look at Other Cultural Diets

The striking fact is that cultures that eat the reverse of the standard American diet—or diets that are low in fat, high in complex carbohydrates and fiber, and plant-based—have lower incidences of cancer and coronary artery disease (CAD). What's even sadder is that countries whose populations can afford to eat the healthiest disease-preventing foods often don't. The United States has spent more money on cancer research than any country in the world, yet the American diet contributes to the very diseases they are spending money to prevent.

Those cultures that have adopted a more "westernized" way of eating have all experienced elevations of many forms of chronic and degenerative diseases. Many countries are becoming aware of the connection between diet and disease and are trying to establish healthier dietary guidelines to help turn around the health of their people before it's too late and epidemics take hold.

Many of the cultures that have the longest and oldest recorded histories have traditional diets based on plant-based foods. Three significant geographical regions, Asia, Latin America, and the Mediterranean, will be the focus of our discussion. Food pyramids have even been developed for these cultures, as their way of eating is enjoyed by a diverse world population. The nutrient composition of the traditional rural Asian diet is very similar to both the Latin American and Mediterranean diets, in that they are largely plant-based and their pyramids recommend that meat be consumed no more than once a month and then in only very small amounts.

> ### In a Nutshell
>
> According to Dr. T. Colin Campbell, people eating plant-based and dairy-free Asian diets experience low rates of osteoporosis. Western nations who get most of their calcium from dairy products have much higher rates of osteoporosis.

In these three traditional diets, fruits and vegetables were, for the most part, locally grown or gathered, seasonally fresh, and often consumed minimally processed or even raw. They also have heavily starch-based diets that feature beans, nuts, potatoes, rice, corn, wheat, and other grains that are all also locally cultivated, thus preserving more of their nutrients.

These cultures also avoid or limit their use of dairy-based products, yet they don't have the calcium deficiencies or problems with osteoporosis plaguing the United States. Those who follow their more traditional diets also experience better overall health and maintain proper body weights. When they adopt a more SAD way of eating, their health, figure, and well-being often go right up in a puff of smoke with their char-broiled burger.

Vegetarians and the Pyramid

Despite all of big business's efforts to promote an animal-based diet, the medical community has come to the aid of the veg-heads. In fact, both the American Dietetic Association and Dietitians of Canada take the position that appropriately planned vegetarian diets are healthful and nutritionally adequate and provide health benefits in the prevention and treatment of certain diseases. There you have it: the dietitians—the professionals we turn to for nutritional advice—favor plant-based diets.

So how exactly would you fulfill your dietary needs as a vegetarian, according to the food pyramid's recommendations? Well, for breakfast you could have a bowl of oatmeal made with milk or soy milk and topped with fruit plus a glass of juice. Then for lunch, have a bowl of vegetable soup or chili and a veggie burrito rolled in a corn or whole-wheat tortilla or a veggie burger on a whole-grain bun. For dinner you might have a tossed salad, some stir-fried vegetables over brown rice or pasta with your choice of sauce, and maybe another side dish. You may have a few snacks here and there throughout the day such as a piece of fruit, a handful of nuts or crackers, and maybe a little dessert.

How would this measure up in terms of servings? Breakfast easily supplies 2 servings of fruits, 1 serving of grains, 1 serving of calcium or milk, and 1 full serving of protein with the oatmeal and milk combination. Your lunch could supply you with 3 to 4 servings of vegetables, 2 or more servings of grains, and with any luck, 1 or more servings of protein from lean plant-based sources. Your dinner, depending on the variety of ingredients, could include 4 or more servings of vegetables, 2 or more servings of grains, 1 or more servings of protein, and depending on the sauce, 1 or more servings from the milk and fats groups. Add in those mid-morning or after-dinner treats, and you could easily meet all the recommended pyramid requirements without even trying.

The Vegan Food Pyramid

Overall, vegans have the best diet of all—full of vitamins, minerals, essential amino acids—and they can easily fulfill all their dietary requirements. Eating plenty of fruits, vegetables, and grains from every color in the rainbow will well provide you with many phytochemical-rich foods and give your body the building blocks it needs for good health.

A well-balanced vegan diet is generally lower in fat, cholesterol, and calories than the SAD and vegetarian diets. A diet that is lower in calories makes you more resistant to various forms of cancer, can reduce the signs of aging, and can lower your risk of developing diabetes. And by not eating an animal-based diet, you lower your risk for both high cholesterol and excess saturated fat, which can lead to many health woes from obesity to heart disease. Your body's ability to digest foods properly is the key to it all: how many vitamins and minerals you are able to utilize for various body parts and functions; how much energy you receive from carbohydrates, proteins, sugars, starches, and fats; and whether you burn them immediately or they go into reserves or fat storages.

> **CAUTION**
>
> **Hot Potato** _____
>
> A person on the Standard American Diet holds 8 meals' worth of undigested food and waste material in his or her colon at any given time, while the person on a high-fiber diet holds only 3!

Just like the other food pyramids, we can break a vegan diet down into five major food groups and view it as a pyramid. At the top are fats, oils, sugars, and enriched or fortified foods. The next level is made of high-calcium milk and dairy alternatives like leafy greens and nuts, along with high-protein meat alternatives like legumes and soy-based products. Generous servings of fruits and vegetables, either fresh, frozen, canned, or dried, make up the large middle section of the pyramid. And as with all food pyramids, a good variety of grain-, cereal-, and bread-based foods makes up the largest base level.

In a Nutshell

Many nutritionists, dieticians, and doctors recommend that you consume several small meals throughout the day instead of only 3 large meals a day every 5 to 6 hours. They believe this would help to better regulate your blood sugar levels, thereby helping prevent mood swings and fatigue. Ever notice that depriving yourself of your afternoon snack sometimes results in your turning into Godzilla, stomping around and biting off your co-workers' heads for the slightest reason? That could be the result of a mood swing stemming from low blood sugar.

Vegan Nutritional Needs: The Basics

It's been a long and winding road for vegans, but finally, in the last few decades, research and modern medicine have acknowledged the nutritional soundness and advantages of a completely plant-based diet. The evidence has shown time and time again that a well-balanced vegan diet positively sustains people of all ages and backgrounds and that it greatly reduces risks of the major diseases that are plaguing our global village. Also, it has been shown that those who suffer from malnutrition, obesity, and disease can use a vegan diet to reverse, prevent, and reduce suffering associated with those ailments.

CAUTION

Hot Potato _____

Limit your consumption of alcohol and caffeine products such as coffee, soda, and black tea to occasional use only. Instead, drink water and other liquids such as fruit or vegetable juices and green and herbal teas to help flush your system; keep you hydrated; and provide you with phytochemicals, vitamins, and minerals.

So how do you go about making sure you'll meet all your nutritional needs? Start by eating a wide variety of foods from each of the vegan food groups. Keep your consumption of sweets, fats, and refined foods to a minimum, as they are usually just empty calories with no real nutrient value. These types of foods will fill you up but will not provide you with the sustained energy you need.

Physical activity and exercise are as important to your quality of health and body frame as proper diet, so you need the right fuel to keep you energized and moving as you should be. Also, get plenty of fresh air and sunshine, and stay properly hydrated as well. You should drink about ½ gallon of filtered water and other liquids per day.

A Well-Balanced Vegan Diet

Eating healthily as a vegan is actually pretty simple. Just approach it with a little common sense and apply what you know about proper nutrition to your everyday food choices.

You can start by reducing your intake of fats by making wise food choices like limiting or eliminating fried or other fatty foods. Be sure, however, to include regular sources of good fats, such as the beneficial omega-3, omega-6, and omega-9 fatty acids found in some vegetable oils like safflower, sunflower, flax, and soybean as well as in seeds and nuts like pumpkin, hemp, sesame, and walnuts.

Consume 2 to 3 servings of protein-rich foods like beans, soy, greens, and other veggies each day. Many of these foods also contain significant amounts of calcium. Vegans can easily fulfill their RDA for calcium by eating green vegetables, grains, soy products, and other calcium-rich foods (see Chapter 6 for a refresher).

Vegans who actually eat a good variety of real foods and don't try to survive solely on convenience meals and processed foods can easily consume 8 or more servings of fruits and veggies every day. This meets and exceeds the recommended daily amounts. The recommendation of 6 to 11 servings of grains is easily met throughout the day as well.

Zeroing In on the Right Foods

If you focus on consuming a good variety of fruits, vegetables, and grains throughout the day, without worrying too much about serving sizes or quantities, you will have no problem meeting or exceeding the recommended serving amounts. As they say, variety is the spice of life, and it gets pretty boring eating the same foods day in and day out, so be sure to shake up your life and taste buds a little by eating a smorgasbord of delicious plant foods!

It's best to begin by basing your diet on vegetable food sources first, especially fresh veggies, as they have more of their live enzymes intact. In a pinch, frozen and canned sources can also serve you well. Then, begin fulfilling your remaining calorie and nutrient requirements with fruits, grains, and starch-based food sources. Daily caloric requirements differ from person to person and depend on various factors, but the average American takes in about 2,200 calories per day.

It's recommended that you consume about 4 cups, or 1 quart, of vegetables per day. In the USDA's *2005 Dietary Guidelines for Americans*, it breaks up the vegetable group into five subgroups and recommends that you include the following in your diet each week:

   3 cups per week of dark green or leafy vegetables

   2 cups per week of orange-colored vegetables

   3 cups per week of legumes

   3 cups per week of starches

   6½ cups per week of other vegetables

Vegans can easily meet those numbers, as those types of veggies make up the majority of most well-rounded vegan diets.

Fruits are like nature's desserts and are excellent sources of natural sugar to satisfy the cravings of those of you with an active sweet tooth. Reach for a piece of fruit instead of that next piece of candy; you'll get antioxidants, vitamins, minerals, and fiber instead of empty calories and mood swings after your blood sugar spikes and crashes after processing all the refined sugar.

Make whole grains, breads, and pastas a part of most of your meals. These foods form the base of the pyramid and thus should form the foundation of your menu selections as well. Grains and starches are nutrient-dense foods that provide you with slow-burning fuel for sustained energy. Consume whole-grain and stone-ground grains instead of white, polished, or nutrient-stripped versions.

Not only is eating a balanced vegan diet a wonderfully healthful and nutritionally complete way to eat, but it's also a good way to drop a few excess pounds. As you know, veggies are low in calories and high in fiber, and simple whole grains such as rice and quinoa are also low in calories and fat; high in fiber, calcium, and protein; and contain lots of other good stuff your body needs. Eating lots of whole grains and veggies can help make you feel full faster, which means you consume less food and maybe drop a few pounds, if that's what you're aiming to do. And think how healthy you'll become in the process!

> **CAUTION** **Hot Potato** _____
>
> When whole grains are processed or refined, much of their nutrients are stripped away and only a few of them are added back in during any subsequent fortification. As refined carbohydrates, they release sugars rapidly into your system, which raises your insulin and triglyceride levels and negatively impacts your health. Consume these refined and processed foods as secondary grain group selections or as only occasional food choices.

The Least You Need to Know

- ◆ Following proper dietary guidelines can be a useful tool in being sure your diet isn't lacking in essential nutritional elements.

- ◆ The Standard American Diet (SAD) lacks many healthful components that are found in a diet based on plant foods.

- ◆ Vegans and vegetarians can easily take a pyramid-style approach to monitoring their daily meatless dietary intake.

- ◆ Regularly partaking in a wide variety of foods from each of the vegan food groups will ensure that you meet all your nutritional needs.

- ◆ Keep your consumption of sweets, fats, and refined foods to a minimum, and eat as many veggies as you like!

10

Seeking Supplementation

In This Chapter

- Getting your vitamins and minerals from food
- Keeping an eye on key nutrients
- Monitoring your need for supplements
- A look at the vitamin B_{12} issue
- Finding sources for vegan supplements

If you eat a well-balanced vegan diet, you should have no problems getting the vitamins, minerals, and other vital nutrients your body needs to be healthy and happy. Getting all those good things straight from food sources is the most beneficial way to get them, but at times you might want to take a supplement of one sort or another, whether it be a basic daily multivitamin or something more specialized, just to play it safe. In this chapter, we look at some of the issues surrounding supplementation you should know about as you embark on your voyage into veganism.

Mining for Nutrients

Phytochemicals, which are found only in plant foods, help treat and prevent many health disorders, including cancer. Plant-based foods also contain high concentrations of vitamins and minerals. When seeking beneficial sources of nutrients in your diet, look first to foods as the primary sources. Supplements are just that, and they should remain as such. They are not as good or as usable by your body as those that come from food sources. Supplements should be used only in addition to, and not in place of, proper nutrition and a nutrient-rich diet. Many people rely too heavily on multivitamins and should really go straight to the food sources to get the best nutrients.

Vegan diets are abundant in vitamins, which are found in all of the vegan food groups. Fruits and vegetables have vitamins A and C. Grains, veggies, legumes, and sea vegetables contain B vitamins. You can easily obtain vitamin D by spending a few minutes in the sunshine, but you can also get it from some herbs and fruits. Vitamins E, F, H, and K—yes there are more letters in the vitamin alphabet than you may have known about—are found in many fruits, vegetables, grains, nuts, seeds, and plant-based oils.

We find minerals, too, in nearly all plant-based foods. Calcium, copper, chromium, iron, magnesium, potassium, *selenium*, iodine, and zinc appear in all colored vegetables, leafy green vegetables, grains, mushrooms, legumes, soy foods, nutritional yeast, and sea vegetables. Many fruit juices, breads, grains, and soy-based products are also fortified with various vitamins and minerals these days.

Vegan 101

Selenium is a rare mineral, closely related to sulfur, with a distinctive red-gray metallic appearance. It is an essential mineral for mammals and higher plants—in small amounts; it is toxic in larger amounts. Selenium helps stimulate metabolism and protect against the oxidizing effects of free radicals. These days, most selenium is produced and obtained as a by-product of the copper refining process.

Many plant-based foods overlap in food group membership and contain multiple nutritional benefits. For instance, beans, grains, and greens are each full of protein, carbs, calcium, B vitamins, and many other key nutrients your body puts to great use for many different functions. Nature does some amazing things, and combining many different types of nutritional benefits into a single food source is on that list. Consuming these types of foods as often as possible will give you a leg up on your quest for good health.

There's no reason your vegan diet shouldn't provide you with all your vitamin and mineral needs, as long as you try to keep it varied on a daily and weekly basis. And that's really the best way to approach your dietary needs, on a weekly basis, as it fits most people's lifestyles and gives you the opportunity to do a little home cookin'.

Good Health Doesn't Come from a Bottle

Other animals don't need to take pills to meet their nutritional needs, and when we eat an optimal diet rich in all the good stuff we need, neither do we. The importance of eating a well-balanced diet simply can't be stressed enough, whether you are vegan or not. You only get one body, and although it will certainly go through many changes over time, it is strictly one per customer. You owe it to yourself, inside and out, to take the best care of your body you possibly can. Putting in good foods will keep you up and running at optimum capacity.

It's best to start with the natural and whole forms of foods to supply all your nutritional needs. A vegan diet is rich in vital nutrients. In fact, a vegan diet contains higher amounts of vitamins A, C, E, and B, especially folate and biotin, and also more copper, iron, magnesium, manganese, and potassium than most omnivorous and many vegetarian diets.

Specific nutritional needs can vary from person to person, however, and also from day to day, depending on how one manages to feed himself throughout the course of any given day. So if you think you will fall short of fulfilling any of your daily requirements from food sources alone, you may want to think about taking a supplement like a multivitamin or a specific nutrient.

Keep in mind, though, that a healthy and fit body doesn't come from a bottle, at least not for the long haul. Advertisers for diet supplements would have you believe otherwise, with their claims of salvation-in-a-bottle—for a small fee. Many "diet miracle workers" have convinced many people to pop pills instead of taking matters into their own hands nutritionally. But don't be fooled. If you want health and vitality, you have to go for it and continue to work at it. Life's richest rewards taste the sweetest when a little sweat and hard work go into achieving them.

Foods: Your First and Best Sources

What should be your first line of defense in protecting your body and safeguarding your health against imbalances and ill health? Good clean living, as they say, with plenty of fresh air, clean water, and sunshine, vitalizes your spirit and body. Physical activity and exercise are necessary to keep your body moving and running properly, so don't skip out on it. Then, be sure to nourish yourself properly and adequately. Begin by eating right in the first place, and then turn to supplements as a backup.

Be sure to eat plenty of fruits and veggies every day, as well as a couple servings of whole grains as either breads, starches, or as part of your meal selections. Try to eat green leafy salads or obvious protein-rich foods like soy or other legumes to be sure you cover your calcium, iron, and protein needs.

Eating fruits and vegetables provides you with an array of phytochemicals. In fact, you get hundreds of them in a simple carrot—hundreds of different compounds, all arranged in a nice, neat sequence, just as nature intended, and usually in the correct form for another part of nature (your body) to utilize to its fullest potential. Certain compounds or substances seem to be present together because they work better that way, even if we don't always see the connection or correlation. That's why it's best to consume actual foods to try to obtain as many phytochemicals as you can, if solely for the antioxidant benefits alone.

Medical science has figured out how to isolate and identify certain vitamins, minerals, and nutrients, but it doesn't understand everything that's a part of our natural world yet. So it doesn't hurt to give yourself a little insurance and cover your bases in both areas. Eat right as often as you can and take a multivitamin, and any other supplements, sensibly and as you see fit, as a way of safe-guarding your good health and ensuring the best life possible.

Key Nutrients to Watch

Nutrient deficiencies not only occur in third-world countries where there isn't enough food to eat, but also in the United States, where many follow a Standard American Diet (see Chapter 9). Many Americans live on a diet full of empty calories, fat, sugar, sodium, and cholesterol and get very little needed beneficial nutrients.

What key nutrients should you be concerned with? You know fruits and veggies contain tons of vitamins and minerals. You get essential amino acids and fatty acids from leafy green plants, legumes, nuts, and seeds. Then there's protein and calcium, which hopefully are no longer of concern to you now that you know good vegan food sources of both, like green leafy vegetables and beans. But did you know that these same types of foods provide you with iron, zinc, and selenium as well? Even so, why do you need to be concerned about these nutrients?

Ironing Out Your Iron

You need to get plenty of iron for your blood. The level of iron in your blood plays an important function in the amount of oxygen that's fed to your cells, as well as the carbon dioxide that's released and eliminated from your body. Iron is an essential part of hemoglobin, the oxygen-carrying component of your blood. This "precious" metal, iron, is found in two forms: heme iron, which comes from animal-based sources, and non-heme iron, which comes from both plant- and animal-based sources. Athletes, pregnant and menstruating women, and children need to be the most concerned about the amount of iron in their diets and be sure to have iron-rich blood.

From nation to nation, across all corners of the globe, iron deficiencies are a major nutritional concern. How do iron deficiencies occur? The main causes are quite obvious:

♦ Blood loss from heavy menstruation or hemorrhaging

♦ Growth spurts, in the case of infants, children, and even pregnant women

♦ Strenuous exercising and excessive sweating, of concern to athletes

♦ Inadequate dietary intake

Hot Potato

Cooking your food in a cast-iron skillet supplies your body with some additional iron because your food absorbs some iron from the pan during the cooking process. Beware though, because the same can be said of aluminum and aluminum cookware. Ingestion of aluminum has been linked to Alzheimer's disease, so avoid cooking in aluminum.

In a Nutshell

Did you know that vitamin C affects your absorption of iron? Eating vitamin C–rich foods with iron-rich foods increases your absorbability of iron several times over. So add a little colored pepper or orange, or have a little citrus vinaigrette on your next leafy green salad to increase the amount of iron your body receives.

An iron deficiency that goes unchecked often results in iron deficiency anemia. You have little control over the other factors that effect iron, but you certainly can have control over your own diet, which you can directly and quickly impact.

Getting Zinc in Sync (Selenium, Too)

Your body and immune system need adequate levels of zinc and selenium to keep you on your toes and fighting off disease and infections. A few Brazil nuts, each containing around 70 micrograms selenium, can easily supply your daily needs.

Getting your zinc balance right can be a bit tricky. Getting daily doses less than 100 milligrams can enhance or boost your immune system, while doses more than 100 milligrams will often depress your immune system. Add to that the fact that phylates, a form of phosphorus found in whole grains and legumes, bind with zinc, which interferes with its absorption. The amount of calcium in your diet can affect your body's ability to absorb zinc, too. Supplements with high levels of calcium, iron, and copper, can also interfere with zinc absorption and balance in your body.

Vegan 101

Bioavailability is the proportionate amount or level of a certain nutrient contained within a specific food that is actually used or utilized by the body.

But the culinary techniques you employ can help you increase the *bioavailability* of zinc. Try roasting or sprouting sunflower seeds or cashews to increase the amount of zinc. Soak beans prior to cooking, or use fermented foods like tempeh or sauerkraut, to help increase your absorbability of zinc. Remember that the next time you are munching down on a vegan tempeh Reuben sandwich!

Is B_{12} an Issue?

One vitamin seems to come into question time and time again for vegans and vegetarians, and that's vitamin B_{12}. Our bodies need it in very small amounts for healthy blood cells and proper nerve functioning.

Vitamin B_{12} is actually made by bacteria and other microorganisms in nature. The bacteria attach themselves to a host and work their way into its system. B_{12} is not naturally produced by plants or animals directly, but plants and animals often find themselves as its hosts.

It's a good thing the human body can amply store vitamin B_{12}. We can store up to a 3- to 5-year supply in our livers, and the Recommended Daily Allowance for adults is a mere 2.4 micrograms per day. Keeping this in mind, you generally only need to worry about your intake of B_{12} on a weekly, rather than daily, basis.

Although it does not reflect mainstream thinking, some doctors and nutritionists believe your body can actually fulfill all its vitamin B_{12} needs on its own. They reason that you already have the bacteria swimming around in your intestines, liver, and even saliva, which can perhaps be reabsorbed internally without ever having to worry about getting any extra into your diets. Still, this is just a theory, and it's better to play it safe and have a good supplemented source of vitamin B_{12} in your diet each week.

B_{12} Origins

Vitamin B_{12} is prevalent in nature in the soil, which is how we once got all we needed naturally: by eating foods fresh from the soil with a little bit of dirt still on them and then perhaps licking our fingers clean. And before toothbrushes, dentists, and modern personal hygiene became a part of our daily lives, the B_{12} bacteria would get stuck between our teeth and grow, as our mouths were warm and welcoming hosts.

Vitamin B_{12} is present in many meat products, but how did the animals get it in the first place? Most of the animals that end up on American dinner plates consume a (mostly) plant-based diet themselves. When they graze on grasses or ingest traces of soil, manure, or other contaminants, the beneficial B_{12} bacteria gets in their systems. The animals' livers then process the bacteria to absorb the vitamin B_{12}.

> **In a Nutshell**
>
> Dr. Frey Ellis and Dr. T. A. B. Sanders, both British hematologists and natural hygiene pioneers, along with Dr. E. Lester Smith, the discoverer of vitamin B_{12}, showed in their studies in the 1960s that vegans have generous levels of vitamin B_{12}, even without supplementation.

Much of the traces of B_{12} found in meat products were produced within the gastrointestinal tracts of the animals and not exactly within the cut of filet mignon itself. Without going into all the gory details, the slaughtering process is what really helps disperse the B_{12} onto the meat. Fortunately for vegans, there are many better ways to get vitamin B_{12}!

Plant-Based Food Sources

Plant-based foods are far better sources of B_{12}, as they contain zero cholesterol and are lower in fat than animal-based sources. Because vitamin B_{12} is from bacteria in the soil, you can easily get a reliable source from your own freshly and organically grown foods. Simply give your foods a gentle rinsing in water, if needed, and you'll reap the benefits of clinging B_{12}. Eating foods in their raw state also preserves more of the naturally occurring B_{12}.

But you don't need to rely on dirt particles alone for your B_{12}. Vitamin B_{12} is fortified into so many vegan-friendly foods, including orange juice, grains, breads, nutritional yeast, cereals, sea vegetables, and many other soy-based products. A cup of fortified soy milk or orange juice can contain between 1 to 2 micrograms B_{12}—well meeting your daily needs. With an adequately planned, well-balanced vegan diet, you shouldn't have to worry about being deficient in B_{12}.

Stock up on these food sources of B_{12}:

◆ Fortified fruit juices

◆ Fortified soy milk and soy-based products

◆ Fermented soy-based products such as tempeh, miso, shoyu, and tamari

◆ Enriched grains, cereals, and starch-based products

◆ Nutritional yeast (1 tablespoon nutritional yeast supplies 4 micrograms—more than you need)

Just because it's easy to get enough vitamin B_{12} while being vegan, don't get careless about it. Deficiencies in vitamin B_{12} can cause serious problems, including increased risk of stroke, heart disease, and Alzheimer's. Stay on your toes, and be sure to regularly include good sources of B_{12} in your diet!

Supplemental Sources of B_{12}

There's much talk about how the processing of foods affects their B_{12} levels. As a result, some people feel you shouldn't count on foods as reliable sources, but that goes against the law and logic of nature. Foods are always the best way to feed your body and should be the first option you choose to achieve good health. But there's nothing wrong with having a little insurance now and again, which is why supplements come in so handy. Including some sort of B_{12} supplement certainly won't hurt, and you only need to think about it a couple times a week.

Vitamin B_{12} is naturally made of the mineral cobalt and nitrogen amines and is also commonly referred to as cobalamin. But on most fortified foods and supplements, you will see the word *cyanocobalamin*, which is the synthetic form of B_{12}. When choosing supplementation, look for sublingual (absorbed beneath the tongue) form, which is the quickest and best-absorbed form.

Be careful when purchasing B_{12} supplements in tablet form, as most capsules tend to have a gelatin base, particularly lower-quality brands. Follow the manufacturer's suggestion for dosage; most supplements come in 500 to 1,000 microgram doses, which makes it easy to meet your needs.

In a Nutshell
Red Star Vegetarian Formula Nutritional Yeast is the most widely available form of nutritional yeast in the United States, and it's a deliciously convenient vegan source of vitamin B_{12}. A natural bacterial fermentation process not involving any animal products produces the B_{12} used in this nutritional yeast. Nutritional yeast also contains amino acids, important minerals, and folic acid.

Do You Need to Take Supplements?

Read labels to be sure you're receiving the proper dosages of nutrients and not falling under or over recommended dosages. Sometimes more is not better, especially when it comes to taking supplements. Taking too much of some nutrients can actually cause you harm and even do irreversible damage.

Taking excessive amounts of iron and vitamins A, B_6, and D can be toxic, so keep this in mind when choosing a multivitamin. You should choose the one that best suits your needs … but how do you know which one to pick? First, analyze your diet. You know it's important to eat well, but do you actually do it? How well you eat determines whether you need a multivitamin with mega-doses of nutrients or one with levels that provide you with around 100 percent of your RDAs for certain nutrients.

If your diet is generally full of lots of servings of fruits, veggies, and grains on a daily basis, maybe you only need a multivitamin with the basics: vitamins A, B, C, D, E, and so on, with levels that are below or bring you up to 100 percent of your RDAs. With an adequate diet, you also receive many nutrients, and you don't want to put your levels over the top or at a point where they actually start doing you harm instead of good. If, on the other hand, you tend to not eat as well as you should more often than you would like to admit, think about taking a supplement with slightly higher doses. But remember, it isn't wise to rely on supplements as your main sources of needed nutrients, so you really should be getting your eating habits in order. You owe it to yourself!

There will be times when you may want to take a specialized or single nutrient-type supplement. For instance, if you are feeling a little sluggish, you may not be getting enough B vitamins. They are the real movers and shakers in your body, fueling many functions and adding luster to your hair, skin, and nails. During times of stress, your body can require even more B vitamins. If this applies to you, you may want to take a B vitamin complex supplement every once in a while or at those times when you feel you are especially in need of them. You'll definitely feel a boost in your energy levels.

Hot Potato

Beware: excessive amounts of vitamin C can have a laxative effect. Some people even intentionally use vitamin C, in doses of 5,000 milligrams per day and more, as a natural laxative.

Most are familiar with taking a little extra vitamin C to build up your immune system and fight off colds. But be careful: taking too much vitamin C at one time can cause stomach upset, especially when taken on an empty stomach. If this is the case for you, look for "buffered vitamin C" as it should be gentler on your system.

In recent years, it's come to be known that taking a little extra vitamin C and E can actually help reduce the signs of aging and fight off many chronic diseases and cancer. Especially significant are their effects on preventing and treating skin cancer. Topical applications have had some amazing results for basal cell carcinoma victims. As it turns out, vitamin C is toxic to melanoma and causes it to dry out, leading to scabbing and eventually scarring over.

One of the best and most inexpensive forms of supplemented vitamin C is the crystalline form of ascorbic acid, available at health food stores. A mere ¼ teaspoon mixed into a glass of water provides 1 gram (1,000 milligrams) of pure vitamin C, and you don't have to worry about the fillers that accompany vitamin C in its pill form, whether you're a vegan or not.

Finding Vegan-Friendly Supplements

As a vegan, taking a supplement isn't as simple as running down to the corner drugstore. For one thing, *gelatin*—that gelling agent often used to make the outer coating of many supplements—is animal-derived. If you see the phrase "gel-cap," you will have to do a bit of investigating to see if it's a gelatin- or veggie-based gel. Some brands do say "vegi-cap" or "suitable for vegans or vegetarians" on their packaging if the gelling agent used is from plant sources. If it doesn't say what the capsule is made of, it's best to assume it's made of gelatin and avoid it, just to be on the safe side. If you have an option of buying it in different pill forms, avoid capsules and look for tablets instead, as they are usually gelatin-free.

Also beware of supplements containing vitamin D_3. In pill form, vitamin D_3 is only derived from animal sources. Have no fear, though: you can get all the vegan D_3 you need, free of charge, by being out in the sun for 15 minutes or less. If you see vitamin D_3 among the vitamins listed on your multivitamin, perhaps as "cholecalciferol," it isn't vegan. Supplemented vitamin D_2, though, *is* vegan.

Vegan 101

Gelatin or *gelatine* is a gelling agent made from boiling the connective tissues and skins of animals. It is used in the manufacturing of many products used for consumption and personal use, including foods, beverages, beauty products, pills, and even photographic film.

You might be able to find some brands of vegan supplements in different drugstore and retail chains. But for the most part, you may have to search the shelves of your local health food store when first looking for vegan supplements.

A word of caution: supplements can be expensive, but you do usually get what you pay for. Look for natural sources, not synthetic ingredients, as many are truly substandard and full of fillers or unnecessary or even harmful ingredients. Choose supplements produced from food sources if you have this as an option, as they are much better in terms of bioavailability. These are relatively new to the market but have been popping up more and more in the last decade.

Some popular vegan supplement manufacturers include Solgar, Twin Lab, VegLife, Deva, Freeda, New Chapter, Nature's Plus, and Herb Pharm, just to name a few. After you find vegan brands you like, you can search out other sources and do a bit of shopping around and comparing prices. The Internet is a great tool for purchasing vegan supplements at a savings. Check out Appendix B for some good websites where you can begin your search.

The Least You Need to Know

- It's a good idea to take a vitamin B_{12} supplement on at least a weekly basis.

- In addition to the nutrients naturally present in fruits and vegetables, many packaged food items are also fortified with additional vitamins and minerals.

- Get as many nutrients as possible directly from their food sources primarily, and use supplementation only as a backup.

◆ Iron, zinc, and selenium are three very important dietary minerals, so watch your levels to be sure you're getting the right amount.

◆ Finding good sources of vegan supplements isn't difficult, but it requires a little thought and research beforehand. The web can be a big help.

11

Raw Foodists: Raw and Uncut

In This Chapter

- ◆ Reexamining cooked foods
- ◆ Juicing and dehydrating raw foods
- ◆ Growing your own sprouts
- ◆ Preserving live enzymes
- ◆ Reaping the benefits of raw foods

Have you ever seen a pack of lions sitting around a fire roasting their prey? Or a rabbit boiling a carrot before eating it? Humans are the only creatures to take fire and harness it for use in food preparation. Cooking makes food more digestible and more enjoyable, and when it comes to meat, it also helps reduce the possibility of food-borne illnesses.

But is regularly subjecting our food to extremely high temperatures beneficial to our long-term health? Many people feel the answer to that question is a resounding "no," and in this chapter, we take a look at some of the issues surrounding cooked foods and some of the raw vegan alternatives.

The Cooking Crock

Sometimes keeping things simple is the best way to approach life. We humans can really make eating too complicated, compared to our fellow members of the animal kingdom. They know to eat all their foods in a simple and raw manner. That's fortunate for them because they're able to avoid all the drawbacks of cooked foods. The notion that you must cook your food before eating it really is a crock—pun intended.

Many studies have shown that cooking meat in particular causes big problems in terms of health. Cancer-causing chemicals known as *heterocyclic amines* are of major concern. These carcinogens are formed when the natural sugars (which cause carmelization on the outer surface), amino acids, and creatine present in the meat are exposed to high cooking temperatures. Fortunately, this isn't a concern when you're roasting a pepper or other veggies.

CAUTION

Hot Potato _____

Digestive leukocytosis, or an increase in the number of white blood cells in the blood, can occur soon after eating cooked foods but does not happen when eating raw foods. In 1930, Dr. Paul Kouchakoff at the Institute of Clinical Chemistry in Switzerland was studying the effects of eating on the immune system. He noted this strange phenomenon and attributed it to the body's viewing the cooked food as an invader and sending in white blood cell "reinforcements" to defend against it.

Raw foodists—those who only eat foods in their natural, uncooked state—believe eating raw foods is truly the best way to nourish our bodies. When we eat foods just as they come from the ground, raw and uncooked, our bodies can retain and utilize vitamins and nutrients better. Eating raw also leaves all the beneficial fiber intact, which is good for the GI tract and colon.

The Cold, Raw Facts

Fortunately, eating raw and vegan does come quite naturally for us humans. There's no denying the desirability of a freshly picked apple or cluster of fresh grapes. Go with your cravings for fresh produce, and you could reap some great rewards. It's a good idea to try to fit in as many sources of raw fresh fruits and vegetables as possible every day.

Eating an all raw or mostly raw foods diet is nothing new. Many great thinkers who were ahead of their time ate this way, including Hippocrates, who used a raw diet to provide relief from disease and cancer to the people of his day. It makes sense that eating fresh, whole, raw foods can improve your overall health in many ways, giving you increased energy, better skin tone, mental clarity, loss of excess weight, and reduced and reversed symptoms of disease.

So what exactly would you eat if you wanted to consume a raw vegan diet? You would eat the same as most vegans, enjoying all fruits, vegetables, sprouts, nuts, seeds, grains, sea vegetables, and other organic/natural foods that have not been cooked or overly processed. Raw foodists do sprout, germinate, dehydrate, pulverize, and chop their foods, but they do not expose them to high temperatures or excessive processing.

Heavily processed foods that have been canned, bottled, or prepackaged are out of the question for those on a raw diet. Usually these types of foods have been heated to high temperatures or pasteurized or contain additives, preservatives, artificial colorings and flavorings, and refined sugar. These foods are often not considered raw, and many raw foodists avoid them.

"Alive" Brings Life

A common philosophy shared by many raw foodists is that from life comes life, or that eating raw foods with all their vital enzymes and nutrients intact and alive has an incredibly healthful effect on the consumer.

Raw foods that have been freshly picked are at the height of their nutritional value, as vitamins and minerals found in plant foods are most absorbable and available to your body in their uncooked state. The live enzymes provide energy to your cells and assist in the digestion and absorption of food sources. When you heat foods, you destroy or diminish many vital vitamins, minerals, and enzymes. Eating raw foods is also less stressful on your body in terms of digestion.

The more raw foods you eat, the stronger your body becomes. Your immune system also becomes stronger, making you better equipped to fight off allergies, illness, and disease. Raw foods also help cleanse your body of toxins and mucus, which helps your inner workings run better, provides you with more energy, and improves your breathing and overall appearance.

It may seem a little intimidating at first to think of yourself adopting an all raw diet. That's why most people begin it in small steps. Your body will also adjust better that way, especially as you detoxify yourself of all the years of bad eating habits, such as overconsuming sugars and fats. Just make whatever changes feel comfortable to you, and try to approach it one meal at a time.

In a Nutshell

Include at least one source of raw fruits, vegetables, or nuts in each meal. An apple or banana for breakfast, a salad with lunch or dinner, and a crunchy snack of some raw sunflower seeds or nuts helps you incorporate more raw foods into your diet without much effort. Before you know it, your raw food intake can soon exceed the cooked with a little effort and thought.

Preserving "Live" Enzymes

Those who eat as true raw foodists do not cook their foods. If they do expose food items to high temperatures in some way during the preparation process, they are cautious to not exceed 115 degrees Fahrenheit. Temperatures hotter than 105 degrees Fahrenheit alter vital enzymes, and temperatures hotter than 115 degrees Fahrenheit kill them.

When foods are heated, free radicals are created. The free radicals bombard your cells, altering, destroying, and infecting them with disease, especially cancer. How do you fight free radicals? With plenty of antioxidants found in raw plant foods. Consume as many as you can in your diet to win the battle of good health.

Your body naturally makes enough enzymes to operate your brain, heart, lungs, kidneys, organs, and all your other muscles and tissues. These enzymes are the sparks that get your motor running. Enzymes fall into two categories: metabolic and digestive. The body uses special digestive enzymes to break down the foods you eat. Foods in their raw state contain exactly the right enzymes your body needs to break down the food to be immediately metabolized as essential fatty acids, amino acids in the form of proteins, and glucose or sugars in the form of complex carbohydrates.

In a Nutshell

Plant foods that are concentrated calorie sources—such as avocados, bananas, mangoes, and other fruits—are high in enzymes that can also help keep illness at bay.

Digestive enzymes are found in many fruits, especially those from tropical locales. Pineapple contains bromelain and papaya contains papain, both of which help digest proteins. They also have anti-inflammatory and cancer-combating properties. It's best to consume them in their fresh fruit forms, but some people opt for supplements in pill form, which you can find in most pharmacies and natural foods stores.

Cooking destroys or depletes most of food's naturally occurring enzymes. As a result, the body pulls enzymes from other areas within itself to pick up the slack in digestion. This endless cycle of take, take, take when eating mostly cooked foods wears down your system and opens the door for disease to invade you. If you can manage to eat 50 to 75 percent of your daily intake of foods in their raw state, you can help your body keep up with processing and eliminating the cooked foods you eat.

A Few Things to Chew On

Are you curious as to what your daily diet would consist of if you choose to eat a raw or mostly raw vegan diet? Wonder no more: most raw foodists like to begin each day by eating fruit. Eating fruit in the morning helps cleanse your system. Often undigested foods or waste still remains in your system from the day before, and eating an apple with all its fiber will whisk it all away. This is actually quite a smart way for everyone to start off his or her day.

How about a smoothie or glass of fresh juice, made with several servings of fruit, for breakfast? Maybe add a few dates, cashews, or seeds to your smoothie for a boost in flavor and nutrition. Got you thinking, or making you thirsty?

You could eat some soaked grains or nuts early in the day. Ever hear of muesli? Europeans have enjoyed it for a long time. It's a mixture of whole grains, dried fruits, and nuts that are soaked in your nondairy milk of choice and eaten like a porridge or breakfast cereal. To make some yourself, soak all the ingredients and then enjoy it with a little creamy nut milk poured over the top. Delicious! And it provides you with great sources of complex carbohydrates and protein to provide you with a constant supply of slow-burning energy throughout the day.

Figuring out what to eat for the rest of the day isn't too hard either. Munch on raw fruits and veggies, or get creative with your ingredients. You can spoon down some raw soup, or you might dive into a crisp and crunchy tossed

> **In a Nutshell**
>
> You can make a raw veggie burrito by mixing veggies with a raw dressing or sauce and then rolling them up in a crisp lettuce or cabbage leaf!

salad, with lots of veggies cut in all different shapes and sizes, nuts or sprouts scattered over the top, and topped with a tantalizing raw dressing.

Pull out the heavy equipment such as a dehydrator or food processor, and you can create some gourmet appetizers, snacks, loaves, pâtés, desserts, and on and on as far as your imagination and creativity will take you. Eating raw is tantalizing and revitalizing and certainly not bland and boring!

The Joys of Juicing

No one knows when humans may have first discovered the joys of juicing. References to the enjoyment of fruit nectars, juices, and fermented beverages exist throughout the literature and artifacts of many ancient cultures, including Babylonian, Egyptian, Greek, Roman, Hindu, and Buddhist. After all, wine, which is nothing more than fermented grape juice, is often referred to as the "drink of the gods."

Dr. Norman Walker was a pioneer in the medical field commonly referred to as juice therapy. You're probably familiar with the saying "physician, heal thyself," and that is precisely what Dr. Walker did. Born in 1867 and plagued with illness early in his life, he cured himself with a diet of raw foods and fresh juices. He went on to live to the ripe old age of 118 years old.

Dr. Walker was the author of many books, including *Fresh Vegetable and Fruit Juices*, *The Vegetarian Guide to Diet and Salad*, *The Natural Way to Vibrant Health*, and *Become Younger*. He helped provide treatment to thousands throughout his 70-year career, which lasted until 1984. He even used a raw juice diet to help cure many people of cancer, including Jay "The Juiceman" Kordich. The Juiceman continues to spread the juicing message to millions of people through his infomercials demonstrating his own brand of juicer.

We also have Dr. Walker to thank for inventing the first modern juicer. In 1934, he developed the Norwalk Hydraulic Press Juicer, which made it possible for people to efficiently turn fresh produce into healthy vibrant juice. His juicer is still on the market and is considered among the finest because it processes without overoxidizing and preserves all the food's vital nutrients. The Norwalk Hydraulic Press Juicer works by finely cutting and grating fruits and vegetables and then squeezing out the juice via a hydraulic press.

In a Nutshell

The Champion juicer was introduced in 1954 and was the first masticating (grating) type of juicer. It remains one of the most popular brands.

You can find many different brands of juicers available on the market. Most of them fall into four categories:

◆ Juice presses, such as a manual hand press or the Norwalk Juicer.

◆ Twin-gear presses, which have two gears that shred the food between the gears and then squeeze out the juice.

◆ Masticating juicers, such as the Champion, that work by first grating, then masticating into finer pulp, and finally pressing out the juice.

◆ Centrifugal ejection juicers that use centrifugal force, or rotation at high speeds, to force the foods against a cutting screen that separates juice from solids.

The Norwalk Hydraulic Press Juicer allows for the least oxidation or destruction of enzymes. The centrifugal-type juicers mix in tremendous amounts of oxygen during the juicing process, so you must drink juices made in these juicers immediately to retain most of the nutrients. Juicers vary in price, so analyze your needs and anticipated usage to help you determine which juicer will best suit your needs.

Juicing is an easy way to help you get enough servings of fruits and vegetables each day. Juicing veggies also separates the pulp solids from the liquid nutrients, and not having to process the fiber enables easier and faster digestion. The enzymes that were just alive a minute ago in the fresh fruits and veggies are still active when you ingest them. This means added nutrition, increased energy, and rejuvenation of each of your body's cells, organs, and tissues.

> ### In a Nutshell
>
> Wheat grass is one of the most popular juiced items. You can find it in juice bars and even special wheat grass bars. This vibrant green nectar is full of live enzymes and rich in chlorophyll. It will cleanse your system, boost your immune system, and improve the condition of your hair and skin. Who doesn't want to look more vibrant? Buy yourself some fresh produce, get juicing, and start creating a new and healthier you!

When juicing, pretty much anything goes, so allow yourself to experiment. Feel free to combine fruits or vegetables to create your own blends. A mix of carrots and apples can make a good base, and add to it cucumbers, celery, or parsley to help cleanse your system. A clove of garlic boosts your immunity, fights off infections, or relieves the symptoms of a cold. Adding a little piece of ginger in the juicing process results in a spicy flavored beverage that will speed up your metabolism and help reduce any inflammation you may be experiencing.

Sprouting a New You

Tiny seeds germinate and sprout forth as new life and then go on to grow, each in their own individual ways, into plant life. The tiny sprouts contain increased levels of nutrients, especially concentrated levels of minerals and vitamins A, B, C, E, and K.

> **Vegan 101**
>
> **Enzyme inhibitors** are present in plants' seeds or nuts to aid in self-preservation. The enzyme inhibitors protect the seed so it will have a better chance to germinate and reach full maturity before being gobbled up. If ingested uncooked or unsprouted, enzyme inhibitors attempt to neutralize the other enzymes in your body, making digestion difficult.

> **In a Nutshell**
>
> Alfalfa sprouts have been available in most produce sections for years, but recently new strains of sprouts have hit the markets, including broccoli, red clover, spicy radish, and mixed sprouts made with a mixture of beans, grains, and seeds.

Sprouts are also one of the most significant sources of dietary live enzymes; they often contain 10 to 100 times more than the fully developed foods. The enzymes actually make the seed sprout in the first place. Sprouted foods are easier for your body to digest, as *enzyme inhibitors* are knocked down, starches are converted to simple carbohydrates, and proteins are broken down into amino acids.

You can sprout almost anything—anything that comes from a seed, that is! When it comes to sprouts, most people usually think of alfalfa sprouts, which adorn many healthy sandwiches, or mung bean sprouts, which are a staple in Asian cuisine and found on many a salad bar. But you can sprout other beans as well, such as lentils, peas, soybeans, black beans, or chickpeas. Grains such as wheat, rye, oats, corn, quinoa, and rice are made more digestible through sprouting. Don't forget nuts and seeds of sorts, from almonds and cashews to sunflower and chia seeds.

Sprouting is really quite easy. You can find special sprouting bags and jars in hardware stores, health food stores, and through online sources. You can also use a large jar, such as a Mason jar, which you may already have in your home. Then either use a piece of cheesecloth or mesh, with the ring lid or a rubber band over it to hold it in place over the mouth of the jar.

When you decide what you want to sprout, try to find some organic seeds. Pick through them and discard any debris that may be among the seeds. It doesn't take a lot of seeds to yield a quart of sprouts, and depending on what you sprout, you only need from 1 to 4 tablespoons of seeds per batch. Start small, and begin with more seeds next time if desired.

Start by soaking the seeds overnight in plenty of filtered water. After the seeds have soaked, secure the cheesecloth or mesh to the top of the jar, drain off the water, fill the jar with fresh water to rinse the seeds, and then drain. Rinse and drain your seeds at least twice a day during the sprouting process, and be sure to thoroughly drain off the excess water. Store the jar upside down in a bowl, at a 45-degree angle, in a well-ventilated place but away from direct sunlight.

Continue the rinsing and draining process until your sprouts fill the jar and grow little leaves. Now you are ready to put the jar in direct sunlight to develop the chlorophyll and turn the tender young leaves green. When that happens, you can begin to enjoy your sprouts! Store any unused sprouts in the refrigerator and enjoy for 2 to 3 days. You can also experiment with sprouting grains and legumes in the same way.

Hot Potato

Although we said you could sprout nearly anything, some things you shouldn't try to sprout. Never eat tomato or potato sprouts! They are both members of the nightshade family and contain an extremely toxic chemical called solanine. Sorghum sprouts could contain toxic levels of cynanide. In the 1990s, alfalfa sprouts caused a stir when several cases of E coli and salmonella were attributed to their consumption, which undoubtedly could be traced back to poor food handling and sanitation. All the more reason for you to grow your own sprouts!

Drying and Dehydrating

Sun drying and dehydrating are two popular uncooking techniques raw foodists and others use. Both are inexpensive ways to preserve excess produce as well as make some tasty simple or gourmet treats. Also, a large amount of the nutrients and enzymes remain in the food as long as they're dried or dehydrated at temperatures cooler than 105 degrees Fahrenheit. Basically, you just want to remove as much water from the food as you can, which will prevent bacteria or mold from developing. Always store your dried foods in an airtight container in a cool, dry, and preferably dark place. Air, moisture, and light all affect the quality of your dried foods.

> **In a Nutshell**
>
> When sun-drying or dehydrating, foods will dry faster if they're cut or sliced into smaller pieces. The longer you dry foods, the greater the nutrient loss and reduction in quality of the end product.

You can simply sun-dry pieces of fruits or vegetables by placing them in direct sunlight and turning them once in a while to help the drying process. Herbs can be bunched, tied into bouquets, hung upside down, and left to dry in a convenient, well-ventilated place.

Electric dehydrators have become more than just a way of preserving foods; they are now used to make gourmet raw cuisine and healthy snacks. Pulverized sprouted grains, nuts, or seeds, and some seasonings can be transformed into dehydrated crackers or flat breads. Fruit purées become instant fruit leathers. You can infuse foods and then dehydrate them for a slightly roasted flavor. Shoyu-flavored cashews and ginger-covered mango slices are both good.

The biggest advantage of using an electric dehydrator is that you can dry many items at one time—depending on the brand, dehydrators usually have 5 to 10 racks. You can place thin slices or small pieces of foods on the drying racks, load them into the dehydrator, turn it on, and leave it to do its thing. Check on your food periodically to see how it's drying. Drying times vary from machine to machine and the size and moisture content of the items being dried.

Uncooked Cuisine Takes Off

Eating raw foods has gone from simply grazing on a piece of fruit or a carrot stick to one of the hottest—or make that the coolest—trends in food cuisine.

> **In a Nutshell**
>
> A food processor or simple vegetable peeler can turn fresh zucchini, carrots, or other vegetables into long, noodlelike strands. Make a sun-dried tomato sauce or herb pesto, toss it with vegetable "noodles," garnish or embellish it as you like, and you have a raw gourmet "pasta" dish!

You don't need to spend a lot of money to get started, either. Just work with what you already have in your kitchen. Pull out your knives, cutting board, peeler, grater, blender, and food processor. These tools can help you create some amazing raw vegan foods that can mimic many of the cooked foods you're used to.

If you love tinkering around with raw foods, you can expand your collection of culinary tools as you need and desire them. Juicers, spiral slicers, special sprouting jars, and dehydrators may one day find themselves on your list of must-have equipment. Then you can experiment with making your own dried fruits, treats, crackers, or interesting salads and entrées with your new slicing capabilities. These tools can really help spark your creativity!

For further information and inspiration, check the Internet for raw foods websites, cookbooks, potlucks, support groups, and restaurants. You can find raw foods restaurants all across the United States and throughout the world! They range from simple juice joints and deli-style places to casual and fine gourmet dining. Some raw restaurants have become hot spots with the media and public, such as Roxanne's and Juliano's RAW, both in California; Blossoming Lotus Cafe in Hawaii; Karyn's in Chicago; and Quintessence, which has several locations in New York. These restaurants have proven that eating raw is not bland and boring but exciting, nutritious, and delicious!

The Least You Need to Know

◆ Juicing and sprouting are excellent ways to give your body high concentrations of the nutritional benefits of raw veggies.

◆ Consuming your foods in their raw state preserves their vital nutrients, including vitamins and important enzymes.

◆ Eating too much cooked food has drawbacks, including digestion difficulties and wasted energy.

◆ Remove the moisture content from foods while retaining all their vitamins and live enzymes with dehydrating and sun-drying.

◆ Increasing the amount of raw foods in your daily dietary intake provides you with numerous health benefits.

Chapter 12

Oh Baby! and Bringing Up Baby

In This Chapter

◆ Understanding the safety of vegan pregnancies

◆ Looking at motherly nutritional needs

◆ Feeding vegan children

◆ Getting to the truth about vaccinations

◆ Considering breast-feeding issues

Ah, the joys of motherhood! To bring a new life into the world is a wonderful and amazing thing. The experience brings with it a wide range of emotions as both mother and child develop and grow. As a new vegan and a new mother, you will naturally be concerned about the physical changes your body will be going through. Be confident in knowing that a good vegan diet can easily ensure you a healthy and happy pregnancy, and you and your baby will grow and develop as you should.

Handling a Vegan Pregnancy

Being sure your nutritional needs are met is a concern of all expectant mothers, vegan or not. As a vegan, you can also expect friends, family members, and especially your own mother and mother-in-law to be concerned that your vegan diet may not be able to provide you and your growing baby with all the nutritional requirements during pregnancy.

Have no fear; a vegan diet can cover all the bases and then some! Just arm yourself with some good information; read all you can; and apply what you learn to eating as healthily as you can during this important time. It will soon be apparent to everyone that your vegan diet is having wonderfully positive effects on both mother-to-be and her growing child.

Vegan 101

Preeclampsia is a condition involving hypertension, retention of fluids, protein loss, and excessive weight gain during pregnancy. It occurs in at least 2 percent of all pregnancies in the United States.

Many medical studies have backed up the positive effects of a vegan diet during pregnancy. One of the largest involved The Farm, a vegan community in Summertown, Tennessee. In the study, researches gathered information from more than 775 pregnancies. They discovered that a vegan diet had no impact on infant birth weights (all were normal or above); most had relatively easy labor; and only 1 in 100 women delivered their babies by cesarean section, which is only a fraction of the national average of 1 in 4. Also, in the last 20 years, only one case of *preeclampsia* has been reported with the group participants.

The women at The Farm sustain themselves and their families on an all vegan diet, and they are living examples that it really is the optimal way for us to nourish ourselves, pregnant or not. So relax and know that if you eat a well-balanced vegan diet, you and your baby will be all the better for it!

Here's a short list of some of the great books out there for vegan mothers-to-be to help get you started:

♦ *Pregnancy, Children, and the Vegan Diet* by Dr. Michael Klaper (Gentle World, 1988)

♦ *Raising Vegetarian Children: A Guide to Good Health and Family Harmony* by Joannne Stepaniak and Vesanto Melina (McGraw-Hill, 2002)

♦ The *Vegetarian Mother and Baby Book* by Rose Elliot (Pantheon, 1996)

♦ *Raising Vegan Children in a Non-Vegan World* by Erin Pavlina (VegFamily, 2003)

If you're a vegan who eats all or mostly organic foods, you can also be confident in knowing that you and your baby will have less exposure to the antibiotics, hormones, pesticides, and other toxic chemicals commonly found in conventional produce and animal-based foods.

Mother-to-Be Nutritional Needs

When you discover that you're pregnant, you do need to be concerned about what you put into your body and what you expose yourself to because we know the life growing inside you feels secondhand effects. It is highly recommended that you quit smoking and stop drinking alcoholic or caffeinated beverages as soon as you discover you're pregnant as these can lead to pregnancy complications, birth defects, and health problems in newborns. Remember that everything you do or that affects you on a physical or emotional level also affects your baby. Keep this in mind when making lifestyle choices and decisions.

Now, more than ever, is a good time to analyze the way you eat and start making wise food choices. After all, as the saying goes, you are eating for two. You need to be sure the foods you're eating provide you with a legitimate benefit instead of being just empty calories to satisfy one of the many cravings you experience while pregnant.

> **In a Nutshell**
>
> Expect to gain between 20 and 35 pounds during a normal pregnancy. You may not gain a lot of weight at first, but you should expect to gain at least 1 pound per week during your second and third trimesters.

Eat a wide variety of foods, in every color of the rainbow, to be sure you're getting all the vital phytochemicals you need. Plant foods can more than adequately meet many of your increased needs for B vitamins, calcium, iron, zinc, and protein. You need to increase your daily intake of protein and calcium as your baby will be sharing in your intake as it grows and develops. Try adding additional servings of protein and calcium-rich foods to each of your meals.

While you're pregnant and lactating, you should try to consume at least 2,500 calories per day. This shouldn't be difficult, as your appetite usually increases after morning sickness lessens and goes away completely. Increase your servings from each of the food groups and be diligent to consume four or more servings of fruits, vegetables, and protein. More important, get six or more servings of whole grains and whole-grain-containing products. Such foods contain significant amounts of B vitamins, which help with proper fetus development; deficiencies can lead to birth defects.

In addition to eating right and getting some form of exercise, it is also recommended that pregnant women, vegan or otherwise, take proper supplements to be sure they're regularly meeting all their baby's needs as well as their own. As with all supplements, search out high-quality brands and be sure they have all-vegan ingredients. Remember, you get what you pay for, and you really want to do the best you can for your growing baby and give him or her all the advantages you can.

> **CAUTION**
>
> **Hot Potato** _____
>
> Nutrient deficiencies have been linked to many birth defects; pay close attention to your diet and take a vegan prenatal supplement. Increasing your folic acid intake before and during your pregnancy can reduce your baby's chances of spina bifida, anemia, and even cleft palates. Cystic fibrosis has been linked to deficiencies in selenium and essential fatty acids, and cerebral palsy has been linked to low levels of zinc and B_6. Low levels of iron can result in anemia for both mother and baby.

Whichever brand vegan supplement you choose, be sure it contains at least the noted amounts of the following:

30 milligrams iron

10 to 15 milligrams zinc

In a Nutshell

You can get vitamin D from a supplement or from 15 minutes of direct sunlight exposure daily.

---

500 to 600 milligrams calcium

600 micrograms folic acid (folate)

3 micrograms B_{12}

10 micrograms vitamin D

Also, be sure to include in your diet adequate sources of omega-3 essential fatty acids, which are important for the development and growth of your baby's brain. Foods such as flax seeds, pumpkin seeds, soybeans, grains, and green leafy vegetables supply you with loads of omega-3s. Peruse the shelves of most health food stores and retailers, and you'll also find several good vegan brands of prenatal supplements such as Freeda, Rainbow Light, Nature's Plus Source for Life, and Nature's Way.

Dietary Suggestions for Vegan Mothers

Yes, you are now eating for two, and your food intake requirement has increased, but that doesn't mean you should munch on any old thing—especially tons of junk food or fried foods full of saturated fats. These will put on the pounds needed to support the extra life growing inside you, but such foods do not provide the proper vitamins and minerals.

Eat as many fresh vegetables at every meal as you can because they are low in calories and fat and high in nutritional benefits. Limit your fruit eating a bit as it is higher in calories, but do not eliminate them from your diet. Eat fruit in the morning or as a snack for a nutritious energy boost. Fill your plate with a lot of complex carbohydrates such as whole grains, pasta, beans, soy-based foods, nuts, and seeds.

Try these suggestions for a typical day: start the day with a few saltines or whole-grain crackers if you are still suffering from morning sickness. Then have a piece of fruit such as a banana or apple. In an hour or so, after those foods have settled, you might have a bowl of oatmeal or granola with some soymilk and a little sprinkle of dried fruits, raisins, or nuts. Or consider a tofu and veggie scramble, with some hash-brown potatoes and a few slices of whole-grain toast. Both are breakfasts of champions that will help start you off on the right foot and give you enough energy and nutrition to meet your needs.

You might want some sort of a mid-morning snack to hold you over until your next meal. Try some trail mix or a few carrot sticks with a glass of juice. For lunch, you could have a taco salad made of assorted greens and veggies as well as a vegan soy and bean-based chili topped with salsa or guacamole and a little nutritional yeast. Maybe include a few tortilla chips on the side, preferably the baked and low-sodium variety.

After a few hours, you may be in need of a nibble or small snack to carry you until dinner. Depending on how you have eaten so far, maybe you would like a sandwich made with some crisp raw veggies and slices of mock meat, a nut butter and fruit spread sandwich on whole-grain bread, or even some hummus with pita bread and veggies as dippers.

CAUTION

Hot Potato

If you get the urge for an after-dinner treat, be sure you limit your binges of high-fat and high-calorie foods. Just because some pregnant women eat tons of ice cream and pickles doesn't mean you have to, too. Although, here's a little food for thought: most nondairy ice creams are much lower in fat than traditional milk-based ice creams.

Your dinner should be filling but not too heavy; otherwise, it could cause heartburn and indigestion, which are already common occurrences for pregnant women. Try a nutritious and satisfying evening meal of stir-fried veggies and tofu over rice or some pasta with a tomato or creamy sauce and veggies and maybe a tossed salad.

Bouncing Vegan Babies

If you're eating properly, there's absolutely no reason your vegan baby shouldn't be as healthy as any other young mother's child. Study after study has shown this to be true. Adequate nutrition is what's most important for good health for the mother and baby.

How do vegan babies measure up in terms of weight and size? The birth weights and lengths of vegan babies are relatively the same as, if not slightly higher than, those born to meat-eaters. Healthy, strong vegan babies abound, while low birth weights and pre-term births are on the rise in the United States and around the globe. Inadequate nutrition is most certainly to blame, but not so with the average baby born to a vegan mother!

In a Nutshell

If an expectant mother's in tip-top physical shape, she'll have an easier time during labor. It has also been shown that well-rested mothers have an easier time during labor, fewer complications, shorter delivery times, and fewer incidences of cesarean sections. It is recommended that you get at least 8 or more hours sleep per night, especially as the due date draws nearer. Try relaxation techniques, soothing music, and massage to ease your discomforts and increase your hours of sleep.

The Logical Dr. Spock

One of the most respected pediatricians and child-rearing experts was Dr. Benjamin Spock. He was the author of *Baby and Child Care*, first published in 1946 and currently in its eighth edition. Dr. Spock's book is America's second best-selling book after the Bible and has helped generations of parents address questions and concerns regarding pregnancy and child rearing.

Dr. Spock went vegan in the 1990s in an effort to improve his health, which it did, and he was so impressed that he began focusing his research on learning all he could about vegan nutrition. He caused quite a stir with the seventh edition of his famous book, issued after his death at the age of 94 in 1998. Why all the uproar? Because he advocated a vegan diet for kids!

He wanted to share with parents what he had learned himself while turning his own health around. He told parents that if their children were raised as vegans, they were less likely to be overweight and have less incidences of diabetes, heart disease, high blood pressure, and various forms of cancer. He felt compelled to share the information to help parents as he had always done throughout his illustrious career.

> **In a Nutshell**
>
> The name *Spock* is apparently synonymous with *meatless*. Dr. Benjamin Spock was a vegan, and popular *Star Trek* character Mr. Spock, as well as the actor who played him, Leonard Nimoy, are vegetarians. Some young mothers may be confused when Dr. Spock's name is mentioned as they may initially think of the super-intelligent Vulcan played by Nimoy.

Breast-Feeding Benefits

Nature has provided mammals with the most convenient and wholesome means to adequately feed their babies: breast milk. It is the perfect food, full of proteins, carbohydrates, and fats, which your baby needs to develop properly during the first stages of life. It is suggested that you breast-feed your baby up to at least the age of 2.

During the first several weeks after giving birth, a new mother's breast milk is rich in colostrum, which contains immune-boosting antibodies that help reduce a child's risks of allergies and illnesses. The mother's milk adjusts to the baby's and the mother's needs over time.

Because the new mother has to share all her nutritional intake with her baby, eating a vitamin-rich diet while breast-feeding is very important. Her body divides and sorts the nutrients from everything she consumes and passes a portion of them along to the baby through her breast milk.

Sometimes, breast-feeding doesn't come easy at first or seem natural to new mothers. It takes a bit of practice for the baby and mother to get things right. Correct angles for nursing, irritation, and supply-and-demand issues can cause concern and frustration. But keep at it and be patient—it is certainly well worth the effort in terms of health benefits to your child.

Breast-feeding also helps develop a bond between mother and child. The baby begins to recognize his or her mother by the touch, smell, and sound of her breathing and voice. This bonding process is vital to helping the mother address needs, concerns, and problems throughout the baby's growth and development.

Covering Your Baby's Nutritional Needs

The best way to be sure all your baby's nutritional bases are being covered is to concentrate on your own diet. Ultimately, what you eat and drink makes up your baby's diet as well, and in a more concentrated form. Put good things in, and your baby will get all the right things out.

Eat well-balanced meals on a regular basis, supplemented with healthy snacks throughout the day, and avoid empty calories and excessive amounts of fats and sugars. These will cause fluctuations in your blood sugar levels, energy levels, and overall mood. They will also affect your baby's digestion, energy, sleep cycle, and moods.

Breast-feeding is the cheapest, most natural, and optimal way to feed your baby. Unfortunately for some new mothers, it is not always an option. They may have low production levels, medical issues, or don't want to breast-feed; after all, it is a personal choice. Your other option is to feed your baby a fortified infant formula for up to the first 2 years of age.

> **Golden Apple**
>
> A pair of substantial mammary glands has the advantage over the two hemispheres of the most learned professor's brain in the art of compounding a nutritive fluid for infants.
>
> —Chief Justice Oliver Wendell Holmes (1809–1894)

> **In a Nutshell**
>
> Breast-feeding your baby in direct sunlight for 15 minutes is a great way for both you and baby to get your daily requirements of vitamin D, in addition to making you both feel rejuvenated and revitalized by the warmth of the sun's rays.

Finding a suitable fortified vegan infant formula can be next to impossible. You don't want to use just any old soy milk; you really want to look for a formula that contains the right fat content and is made with organic ingredients, along with added vitamins B_{12} and D, iron, zinc, calcium, and other vitamins and minerals. Unfortunately, most soy-based infant formulas are made with supplemented vitamin D_3 derived from animal sources such as lanolin and, thus, are not vegan or even vegetarian. Hopefully, infant formula makers will soon respond to consumer needs and demands by making a vegan formula.

So what is a vegan mother to do if she simply can't breast-feed? You have to make this decision for yourself. Baby's Only Organic is a powdered soy-based organic formula, but it does contain D_3. Nonetheless, it has become a popular brand among many non-breast-feeding vegan and vegetarian mothers due to the lack of a suitable alternative.

You can introduce supplemental (non-breast-milk or formula) foods such as creamy cereals, fruits, and veggies into your baby's diet sometime in the middle of his or her first year. Creamy rice cereals, fortified with iron, are often among the first soft foods given. Later, you can add other grains to the repertoire, followed by fruit and veggie purées and good sources of protein such as beans and creamy tofu.

The right time to begin adding supplemental foods to your child's diet depends on his or her rate of development, so check with your pediatrician before making any changes.

> **In a Nutshell**
>
> Some prepared organic vegan baby foods on the market can help fill the gap when you aren't able to cook something up yourself. Just take a look around and read some labels!

Raising Vegan Children

As a vegan parent, you may come under fire for choosing to raise your child vegan. Those who are under the impression that vegans are sickly and malnourished will be doubly concerned about the safety of your child, and they may say rude things or act inappropriately toward you. No one has the right to tell you how to raise your child, but it's best to try to patiently and honestly address their concerns as many misconceptions about vegans abound.

You will have to teach your child as you raise him or her about eating properly as a vegan, in addition to explaining *why* you don't eat like everyone else. Be honest with him, and try to explain things in ways he can understand at his particular age. Your conversations and explanations will evolve and develop as he grows older and understands more about life.

You owe it to your child to feed his body nutritionally, and talking with your child about the issues surrounding veganism will help develop his mind as well. It will also provide him with the means to handle questions from young friends, friends' well-intentioned parents, and other adults such as teachers and family members.

If you explain to your child why a certain food is beneficial when you are serving it, he will absorb the information and often pass the information along to others. A child's mind is amazingly quick and absorbs information from outside sources with little effort. Without even knowing it, you may be raising a young vegan advocate who is armed with knowledge!

Are Vegan Diets Adequate?

From the time you start to include supplemental foods or wean your child off breast milk or formula, you have to be concerned about what goes into his or her mouth and not just what goes into yours anymore. Just feed him like you do yourself, only in much smaller quantities.

Health experts agree that a varied, well-rounded diet that is free of meat, dairy, and eggs is the healthiest way for children, as well as adults, to eat. A vegan diet is more than adequate for children; it is far superior to those containing animal products.

> **CAUTION**
>
> **Hot Potato** _____
>
> Most children who follow the Standard American Diet get excessive amounts of saturated fats, salt, and sugar. Compound that with the fact that they get inadequate amounts of whole grains and fresh fruits and vegetables, and it's not surprising that juvenile diabetes and obesity are on the rise.

On average, vegan children eat more healthily than most of their nonvegan friends. After age 2, the standard American child's diet consists heavily of hot dogs, pepperoni pizzas, grilled cheese sandwiches, fried chicken, hamburgers, and french fries. Some children consume these foods at several meals throughout the day.

In contrast, a vegan child consumes several sources of fruits and vegetables, lean sources of protein, and complex carbohydrates from grains in his daily meals. These foods more often than not contain organic ingredients, and less GMOs, pesticides, and chemical fertilizer residue, as well as none of the growth hormones and antibiotics contained in animal-based products.

Dietary Suggestions for Youngsters

As a parent, be very conscious of what your children are eating. Start them off with a good breakfast and then sustain them with a nutritious lunch and filling dinner. Have healthy snacks such as fresh fruits, raw vegetables, nuts, dried fruits, granola bars, and whole-grain cereals around for them to munch on. Feeding them healthful foods teaches them good eating habits, which will serve them well throughout their lives.

Children are basically little versions of the grown-ups they will one day become. Their nutritional needs and nutrient concerns are the same as adults', just on a smaller scale. Throughout the day, they need to consume several servings of complex carbohydrates in the form of whole-grain breads, pasta, rice, or cereals, in addition to good sources of calcium, vitamin-rich fruits and vegetables, and protein-dense foods.

As children grow and start to exercise their independence, their tastes in activities, clothes, and foods will most likely change. Once-healthy eaters often become picky eaters. Foods they once loved and eagerly ate may become unappealing, unappetizing, and plain old icky to them. It's best not to fight them as it will only fuel the problem and may lead to others.

> **In a Nutshell**
>
> When feeding children, remember: their little stomachs get full quickly, so it's best to give them foods that have multiple nutritional benefits such as leafy greens, beans, nut butters, cruciferous vegetables, citrus, and whole grains.

Instead, ask your child what foods *he* would like to eat. This will make him feel that he has more control over his food choices and what he's eating. After you know what his current favorite foods are, you can then bargain with him to fill out the rest of his nutritional needs.

For instance, if your son is currently into eating peanut butter, encourage it. Just try to get him to pair it with a healthful jelly or fruit spread on whole-grain bread, and he will be getting a serving of fruit, protein, and depending on the size, one to two servings of whole grains. Or if he smears it on celery sticks, he'll get a serving of vegetables and protein. The servings and sources can add up quickly, and even though it may not be a varied diet for the time being, it can meet many of his nutritional needs with a little coaching and coaxing.

As with vegan adults, it doesn't hurt to give your child a supplement. That supplement doesn't have to be a mega-multivitamin if your child is a healthy eater and eats a variety of foods. Just be sure it's a vegan supplement that contains significant amounts of calcium, iron, zinc, B vitamins (especially B_{12}), and vitamin D.

> **In a Nutshell**
>
> Vegan children's supplements come in chewable pill forms, in liquid formulas, and recently, in candylike shapes such as gummy bears and lollipops. Look for vegan vitamins made by Freeda, VegLife, Kid Bears, Yummi Bears, Rhino, and Nature's Way in your local pharmacy or natural foods store.

Vaccinations: The Issues

For the vegan parent who wants to raise a child according to vegan ideals in every way possible, vaccines are an issue that needs to be considered. Vaccines are designed to help build up a child's immunity to various diseases, but a good deal of controversy surrounds their use, side effects, dangers, and efficiency. And they're not in the least bit vegan.

Vaccines are made using various animal ingredients. Most of the viruses used in vaccines are cultured on animal and human tissues, including embryos, cells, and organ tissues. Vaccines routinely contain things such as pus, urine, and serum from horses and calves—obviously none of which are consistent with a vegan lifestyle.

Vaccines also contain viruses, bacteria, and other substances intended to help bolster a child's immunity to diseases. Some vaccines even contain thimerosol, a mercury-based preservative, as well as aluminum, phenol, and formaldehyde. You're probably already aware of the many dangers of mercury, and phenol and formaldehyde are both known carcinogens. Many people are convinced that the mercury and other harmful substances in vaccines are responsible for many childhood health problems and disorders, including autism, and that the risks outweigh the potential benefits.

Many problems and complications are associated with vaccinations: pain and infection at the point of injection, respiratory problems, asthma, sudden infant death syndrome, convulsions, diabetes, autism, multiple sclerosis, meningitis, and various forms of cancer, not to mention chances of developing a toxic reaction or death as a result of the exposure to the live viruses contained within the vaccines. Often, an outbreak of an inoculated disease is traced back to the live viruses contained in the vaccines themselves.

Hot Potato

Many state laws require that a child be immunized before entering public school or that parents sign a waiver acknowledging that they have refused vaccination. It is very important to remember that no public or private school may deny entry to a child for not having been vaccinated.

But aren't vaccines essential for protecting children from disease? The track record for most of the major vaccines has been questionable at best. Government and medical sources have reported that up to 65 percent of all occurrences of diseases for which people are routinely vaccinated (such as measles and tetanus) occur in people who have already been vaccinated for them.

Many people feel that vaccines cause more harm than good. We recommend that you take some time and do your own research into the safety and efficacy of vaccines and the ingredients that they contain before you decide to expose your child to them.

It's up to you, the parent, as to what goes into your child's body. No one can force your child to be vaccinated against your wishes. You will encounter a lot of pressure to vaccinate from as soon as 24 hours after birth and at many other times in your child's development.

Be sure to become an educated parent and advocate for your child by researching each and every vaccination your doctor recommends. Always ask to see the package insert that comes with the vaccine. Read the warnings on the insert; research the issues surrounding vaccines on the Internet and at your local library; and then decide for yourself how to handle the vaccine issue.

The Least You Need to Know

- A vegan mother-to-be can more than adequately nourish herself and her growing baby during pregnancy; still, a supplement is recommended for peace of mind.

- Breast-feeding is the optimal way to nourish your baby, as breast milk provides everything your child needs to grow strong and healthy.

- Eating a well-rounded vegan diet, rich in whole grains, fruits, and veggies, is the healthiest way for a child to eat and is a big improvement over the Standard American Diet.

- Vaccines are loaded with nonvegan ingredients and potential health risks, and their effectiveness and safety are questionable at best.

Part 4

Veggin' It: Tips for Maintaining a Vegan Lifestyle

As you meander through your transition into the wonderful world of veganism, living a meatless and cruelty-free life should become easier and easier for you. To be armed with a little know-how helps, so in Part 4, we give you some tips for things such as handling the veg-curious you may encounter, surviving family gatherings and parties, cooking to impress others, and getting a vegan meal when dining out.

Going vegan often means getting rid of your old animal-based stuff and bringing in new plant-based replacements. You can do this at your own speed, a little at a time, or in one fell swoop in the form of a major spring cleaning. Don't worry, we give you some advice on shopping wisely to restock your cabinets, pantry, and closet.

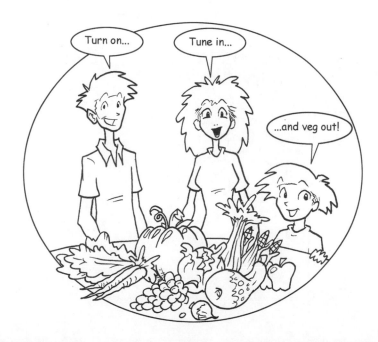

Chapter 13

Handling Family and Friends

In This Chapter

- ◆ Answering questions about veganism
- ◆ Being a good example
- ◆ Arming yourself with knowledge
- ◆ Getting through the rough spots
- ◆ Co-existing with nonvegans

Living as a vegan on a day-to-day basis, you will find that those around you have a lot of questions—and a lot of confusion—about what it means to be vegan. Being informed about the issues is really important in handling your veg-curious friends, family, or co-workers. Be ready to occasionally have to field some really silly, sometimes insensitive, and often personal questions about your vegan lifestyle. Be prepared to answer inquiries about what you eat and wear and how you live your life, and it will help if you can do so with a healthy, happy glow about you.

Questions and Answers

Grasping what vegan life is all about, and why, can be a bit tricky for some, and it will require some patience and understanding on your part as those around you deal with the changes you're going through.

Be ready for questions of all sorts and from all sides. Some questions may be strange or even bizarre, but try to answer them as honestly as you can and to the best of your ability. Try not to laugh, either, which can be hard, particularly when you get a real off-the-wall question like, "Don't plants feel pain, too?" or, "Can you eat animal crackers?" or, "You can eat fish, because fish isn't meat, right?" Some questions will be more serious in nature and more difficult to answer.

> **CAUTION**
>
> **Hot Potato**
>
> Before Vatican II put an end to it in the early 1960s, the Catholic Church had long prohibited the eating of meat on Fridays and certain holidays. Eating fish on those days was permitted, however, and this gave rise to the widespread belief that fish are somehow not meat. Many people you encounter will probably still share this belief, so don't be surprised!

More often than not, how you answer these questions will be just as important as what you actually say, in terms of what your inquirers take away from the conversation. The more you learn about the many issues surrounding vegan living and the more experienced you become, the more gracefully you will be able to answer questions about your lifestyle.

Being a Vegan Ambassador

When dealing with questions friends, family, and the veg-curious ask, you will inevitably find yourself in the position of answering on behalf of the entire vegan community when you try to explain why vegans think the way they do. It's like you become a vegan ambassador to the rest of the nonvegan world, but in reality, you're just one person explaining your particular view of the world.

The best way to deal with questions is with well-reasoned answers, and be sure to put your responses in terms that are easy to understand. For example, when asked about what a vegan is and why you think the way you do, you can say something like this:

> Well, I eat fruits, vegetables, and grains, and I don't eat anything that comes from animals, including meat, fish, dairy products, eggs, and honey. Why? Because I feel that no animal's life is less important than my own. I try to apply that thought to what I put on and in my body and to all other aspects of my life.

I'm just trying to make a difference for animals in whatever way I can. You can say I'm a big animal lover.

When asked to explain your choices about clothing and personal items, you can again keep it simple:

I like to wear man-made fabrics and natural fibers instead of items that come from animals, like leather, suede, wool, and even silk. There are some great nonanimal alternatives out there, and it makes me feel good to not involve animals in what I wear.

Expect that as you say this, they will be checking out your wardrobe choices from head to toe and will most likely comment on your footwear or your belt, particularly if those items look a little too leatherlike.

Of course, the reasons for being vegan are often personal and vary from person to person, so only you can explain what brought you to this way of approaching the world around you.

> **CAUTION** **Hot Potato**
>
> Putting people on the defensive is an easy way to get them to close their hearts and minds to what you're saying. If you can phrase what you're saying in a nonjudgmental way and not make the other person feel as if he is being challenged, you'll have a more receptive audience.

Avoiding the Shock Treatment

When talking about veganism with the veg-curious, you can have more of a positive impact on their overall view of what you're saying if you take it slow and don't shock them too much right off the bat. It's best to save those shocking and disturbing facts—and there are lots of them—for when you feel someone is ready to hear them.

There may be times when you'll be conflicted between hitting someone with the cold, hard facts they probably aren't in the mood to hear and holding your tongue until a more appropriate time when they may be more receptive. The longer you live as a vegan, you'll probably learn that lots of in-your-face preaching doesn't usually have the intended effect and that getting a little more creative in the way you spread the vegan message can have surprising results.

Alleviating Their Concerns

Many people have problems with or fears about veganism that stem from inaccurate perceptions of what it's really all about. Their misconceptions can come from many different areas, including the media, whose portrayals of vegetarians and vegans in various movies and TV shows has led some to believe that vegans and vegetarians are more than a bit strange, with their "really weird beliefs" and choice to "not eat properly."

It may help to inform people with such concerns about the sound nutrition and added health benefits of an all-plant-based vegan diet, as mentioned in Chapter 3. Personal stories of weight loss and your obvious robust appearance and healthy glow will help further illustrate your points.

It can also help to present them with examples of veg-heads, past and present, and their contributions to society. If you think it will help, name-drop vegan celebrities like Woody Harrelson, Alicia Silverstone, Brandy, Prince, Joaquin Phoenix, Alec Baldwin, and Moby, as well as some of the illustrious vegans and vegetarians throughout history we mentioned in Chapter 2. Knowing that someone they admire and respect is also a vegan may lessen their concern for your new vegan lifestyle and hasten their acceptance of it.

> **In a Nutshell**
>
> For a great list of famous vegans and vegetarians, and lots of other interesting stuff, go to www.famousveggie.com.

Certainly, not all people will be opposed to your new lifestyle and ways of thinking. Many will be curious and want to know more. You will undoubtedly have some great conversations with those who are really interested in what you're saying and want to learn more about it. These conversations can be very rewarding to everyone involved—and downright empowering. They can also go on for hours, as we can say from experience!

Knowledge Is Power

After going vegan, many feel so completely inspired and empowered by what they have learned that they're a little like a butterfly emerging from a cocoon. They feel like spreading their wings and flying all around to spread the good word about being vegan. For some, it's like being clued in to one of the big secrets of the universe, and they feel compelled to share their knowledge and acquired wisdom with others. The key is in knowing the right time, place, and method of doing so, and that will come with experience. (We'll talk about that more later in this chapter.)

Be both prepared and eager to engage in conversations about being a vegan. Being an informed vegan will really help you handle some of the opposition and comments that may come your way. If you're going to quote something, be sure you have your facts straight to avoid someone calling you out and exposing your mistake during an exchange or to prevent a conflict or altercation from arising in the first place.

Feeding the brain with knowledge tends to spark the imagination and get the creative and intellectual juices flowing more than ever. The more you learn, the more you'll want to keep learning. Being informed is the most important thing when debating any issue, and debates happen quite a bit when you're a vegan, particularly when you find yourself in the wrong circles or situations. Being prepared for inquiries, as well as insults, will keep feelings on both sides from being hurt and prevent you from being labeled as the "vegan troublemaker."

Checkin' Out the Library

Doing your own research and reading from as many different sources as possible will help shape your views as well as expand your knowledge base. Your local library is one of the easiest and most economical ways to educate yourself and open your mind to new concepts and to the world around you. Armed with nothing but a library card, you can gain access to stacks and stacks of books on all sorts of topics from animal rights to nutrition to how to make your own vegan soap. It's also a great way to check out books for content before purchasing to determine which ones are just what you need to fill out your own library at home.

> **In a Nutshell**
>
> If there's a book you really want to read and your local library doesn't own a copy, they might be able to special order it for you from a neighboring library for free. For that and any other issues or questions you may have about resources and how to obtain them, ask the friendly people at your local library.

Surfin' the Web

The Internet can really mean the difference between vegan isolation and vegan support. With a few mouse clicks, you can have a wealth of information at your fingertips on any subject imaginable. And there's no shortage of information about veganism on the web; that's for sure! Use it to find out the latest health information for vegans, get nutritional advice, pick up a few vegan recipes for dinner, or even shop for cruelty-free items and vegan baked goods. The web can be an incredibly useful tool for vegans, so be sure to make the most of it.

It's a good idea to find a good search engine you feel comfortable with, like the popular www.google.com, and take a moment to read the instructions, so to speak.

Knowing the proper ways to use a search engine, including the best ways to phrase your search queries, is one of the most important skills you can have. It can mean the difference between finding exactly what you're looking for and having it lost in a long list of unrelated search results.

The Internet can also make you feel less alone as you start your new life as a vegan. You can use your computer to find message boards and chat rooms that allow you to share your views and concerns with other like-minded people. Or use it to track down veg-friendly businesses, restaurants, organizations, or groups that may be of interest to you. In Appendix B, you'll find information on various online resources to locate vegan products, support, and information about global and local vegan and vegetarian communities and groups.

If you don't have a computer or if you have a computer without Internet access, have no fear. Your local library probably has some Internet-connected computers you can use free of charge, although there will most likely be some time restrictions on your use. And if you have a computer but can't afford to pay monthly Internet access fees, some providers allow you to connect to the net for free in exchange for having to view pop-up banners and other advertising.

Exemplify Sound Nutrition, Not Malnutrition

You may encounter some people who will think your going vegan is some sort of new trendy diet. After all, by going vegan, you will naturally lose weight and begin to look healthier and more robust after cleaning your system of animal-based products. Those around you who may want to lose a few pounds or get their health together a little more may look to you and your new way of eating with renewed curiosity. So be sure you are living and eating as a positive example, and try to be a good vegan role model.

After all, you want to show others that living and eating as a vegan is based on sound knowledge and nutrition, not on a whim or because you have an eating disorder or are plunging head-first into malnutrition. Be a positively glowing example of good vegan health—it's one of the best things you can do to influence those around you at home, at work, or at school to want to adopt a more vegan approach to eating.

Eat Your Fruits and Veggies

It's best to show people a healthy and happy vegan, so be sure you're taking good care of yourself by getting enough exercise and sleep. It's also important to eat a well-balanced diet, one composed of several delicious and nutritious meals throughout the day, full of fruits, vegetables, and whole grains. You also can work in an indulgence here or there if you see fit.

Eat right, and soon your body will start looking and feeling better and better. On an occasional basis, it's fine to have junk-food types of snacks around to indulge in a little and show other people that vegan versions do exist of many of their comfort foods and favorite foods of youth. But show them the wide variety of nutritious foods we have available to us, too. Let them know being a vegan is not at all boring and is actually quite an exciting and delicious way to eat.

> **Hot Potato**
>
> Having only a plate of onion rings and a soda when you're at lunch with friends *may* be vegan, but it certainly isn't healthful. Why not set a better example and encourage others to eat right themselves by having a veggie-packed salad with a bowl of soup or a slice of whole-grain bread?

The Protein Issue: Resolved

Expect to get a lot of questions about protein: where you get it, how you can do without meat and dairy sources of it, and more. Be prepared by familiarizing yourself with the facts. In your reply to protein questions, mention that plant foods are better sources of lean protein for your body, and are lower in fat and calories and higher in fiber and calcium, than meat and dairy sources. Then throw in that plant-based sources provide no cholesterol whatsoever to your diet. Be ready to mention plant-based protein-rich foods such as broccoli, leafy greens, beans, and grains, which are absolute nutrition powerhouses.

You could point out that fruits and veggies supply our bodies with all the vitamins, minerals, and key nutrients they need, while animal-based foods provide very few in comparison. You could also mention that animal foods often only pass on to us what the animals consumed in their own plant-based diets. If your questioners challenge the accuracy of any of your statements, be prepared to back them up with some of your newly acquired factoids and offer to direct them to where they can learn more for themselves.

Fit by Example

Besides living as a positive example of sound vegan nutrition by what you eat and what you say, it's important for your overall inner well-being to look healthy on the

In a Nutshell

Exercise can be as simple as taking a walk, preferably outdoors where you can also breathe fresh air into your lungs and be a part of nature instead of just watching a nature show on television. Riding a bike is also one of the best forms of exercise as it provides many different health benefits while being gentle and low impact.

outside as well. It is best for anyone to avoid being overweight or obese if he wants to fend off chronic disease and live a healthy and happy life. But making dietary changes isn't always enough for some people to maintain an optimal weight.

Remember, if you don't move it, you will lose it, and in this case "it" is a lean and trim figure. Getting off your butt and getting some regular cardiovascular exercise is good for getting your heart pumping, blood flowing, and taking excess inches off your hips or belly. Exercise is essential for staying in shape and truly being healthy, not just looking healthy.

Relationships Put to the Test

Upon becoming vegan, your personal relationships may become challenged, especially if those nearest and dearest to you don't seem to support your decision to go vegan. How you decide to handle this will greatly determine whether it will be an "us versus them" situation or an amicable one.

Some people feel threatened by the concept of veganism and vegetarianism and think that somehow your vegan lifestyle choices affect or challenge them directly. They may feel that their own personal lifestyle choices are being called into question. These perceptions can have a tremendous impact on your relationships and interactions.

Most vegans do not usually find themselves surrounded by only vegans or lucky enough to have been raised in a vegan family. So naturally, your circle of friends and family and those you encounter in your everyday life will be made up of those who may completely understand where your head is, those who will be slightly confused by your lifestyle but still accepting, and those who think you are nuts or going through some kind of "thing" and hope you'll eventually return to your senses.

Expect Some Opposition

Family members and especially well-intentioned parents who are unfamiliar with veganism and uninformed about all the health benefits of a vegan diet might put up some resistance to your new lifestyle. They may view you as being "difficult" or rebellious, or they may simply fear that you are embarking on a dangerous diet that will leave you lacking nutritionally. Some just won't understand why you can't just stop all this silliness and be "normal" like them. Many have also been influenced by a lifetime of negative, unflattering, and inaccurate portrayals of vegetarians and (more recently) vegans on TV and in the movies.

You should always feel confident and secure in your decision to become a vegan (or whatever your life choices), and don't let other people have an effect on you. Let your compassion for your fellow living creatures extend to those you deal with on a daily or personal basis. Try to have patience, compassion, and understanding, even for those who don't show it to you. Answer their questions as best and as tactfully as you can, and most important, live by positive example.

Needing a Little Extra Support

Joining a support group—such as a vegetarian, vegan, or animal rights organization—may also help with answers and support, especially if you face opposition from your friends and loved ones to your new vegan lifestyle. Many such groups exist, and with a little searching, you will hopefully be able to find one in your area to serve your needs.

Nowadays, because vegans don't usually live in the same geographic proximity as lots of other vegans, a bulk of the communication we have with one another is electronic in nature. The Internet really helps bring lots of vegans together!

> **In a Nutshell**
>
> To begin your search for a veg-related group, check your local newspaper, bulletin boards, and even your local natural food stores. Your best bet, though, is probably online. You can search the net for groups in your area and even join a virtual group online.

Finding Common Ground

If you encounter antagonism or a lack of support from those closest to you, don't let it get you down or discourage you. Try seeking out common ground. Having an open and honest conversation can often prove that opposing sides really aren't that far apart when it comes to many aspects of life. This can be as simple as stating that you both want the same things, to be happy and healthy, and that living this way does that for you.

Because veganism is a lot like a moral code we use to base our decisions and actions on, stemming from compassion, some vegans choose to compare their vegan views to the kind of belief systems that exist for religions. Putting it in that light can help others better understand the level of commitment you have toward being vegan. They probably wouldn't put someone down for his choice of religious denomination and most likely wouldn't want someone to do that to them, either. When they understand how deeply your vegan beliefs are rooted and they're not going to change your mind about it, they will hopefully back off.

Respect should ideally flow from both sides, and when it does, it can help to open lines of communication. Show respect and ask for the same in return. Live by positive example, and show patience and understanding when faced with diversity and opposition. Command respect in your demeanor and words, and you will most likely receive it. Having a sense of pride can be contagious. Those around you will pick up on your self-confidence and self-esteem, and hopefully you will have a positive effect on them as well.

The Least You Need to Know

- Being well informed about the issues surrounding being vegan is essential, so take advantage of educational resources available to you.

- Looking healthy and happy is one of the easiest ways to convince people that going vegan was the right decision for you, so be sure to take good care of yourself in every way.

- It's important to have understanding and patience when dealing with questions friends and family members have about the whys and hows of being vegan.

- If peaceful coexistence with some friends or family members just isn't possible and the negatives start to outweigh the positives, then taking time away from them might be warranted.

Dining, Vegan Style

In This Chapter

- Co-existing in the kitchen
- Holiday survival tips for vegans
- Eating out with friends and family
- Ordering up a vegan meal
- Avoiding problems at mealtime

Mealtime should help nourish the soul as well as the body, and when you go vegan, it can take on quite a few new aspects. For one, you'll now have to give quite a bit more thought to where and what you'll eat. Add other people to the mix, and it can take on another dimension completely. Most of us aren't lucky enough to be surrounded by friends, family members, and colleagues who share our vegan perspectives on eating, so it takes a little extra thought and effort to keep everything, including our relationships, working smoothly. And what about going out to eat now that you're vegan? This chapter will give you some tips that will hopefully make the world of vegan dining, both in and out, a little easier.

Communal Time, Not Battle Time

Dinnertime should never be battle time; it's bad for your digestion for one thing. Being aggravated can cause your stomach to get upset, which can lead to indigestion, loss of appetite, or worse, gobbling down your food without chewing properly just to quickly remove yourself from an unpleasant situation.

> **CAUTION**
>
> **Hot Potato**
>
> Talking about politics, religion, and moral beliefs—"hot button" topics to be avoided in most social situations—can be extremely touchy at meal times and family gatherings. Discussing veganism and its philosophy is best left for before, but ideally after, the meal.

Informing your dinner companions about the negative aspects of factory farming right as they're about to dig in to the meal before them will only lead to conflict. There's no doubt that they'll feel threatened by you and your dietary choices, which can lead to a lot of unpleasantness during mealtime. Save the arguing for later, and hopefully others will approach it that way as well.

"Can't You Just Pick It Off?"

As a vegan and dining with others, you'll likely hear one question over and over when nonvegan food is served: "Can't you just pick it off?" Or its sister, "There's barely any on there, can't you just eat around it?" Some take it a step further with "Can't you just eat it anyway? It's just a little." Well-intentioned mothers and other relatives often make these comments, but they probably don't realize that it makes most of us a bit nauseous just being in close proximity to the meat on *other* peoples' plates, let alone on our own. Just sigh to yourself, consider they just really haven't thought about the issue, and then try to find yourself something suitably vegan to eat.

Many people forget, or aren't aware to begin with, that being vegan goes beyond dietary choices. If they had thought about it for a minute, they might not have suggested it in the first place. They would probably never tell someone who is Jewish or Hindu to "pick off" an offending item or "eat it anyway," especially if it conflicted with their religious or moral code.

Using this example at the opportune time (*after* dinner) could be advantageous and illustrate your point in a simple manner they can understand and accept. You can also file the incident away for when you prepare some vegan delicacy you are eager for them to try. After all, what goes around, comes around; trying to force that pepperoni on me may result in tofu for you later!

Sharing the Space

We really feel for vegans in meat-eating households. It can really be tough at times and often makes the transitioning process even harder if you don't have any support for your newly adopted lifestyle or, worse, face open opposition to it. It's best if you take your meals and the preparation of them into your own hands. If you leave it up to the folks to try to make something up to your vegan standards, you may be eating a lot of iceberg lettuce salads.

As you get more into veganism, you'll have to substitute many of your basic necessities for vegan-friendly versions. Ask for a special space for your items, if need be. In the kitchen, it can be a big help to have your own cabinet, or part of the refrigerator or freezer, to stock all the foodstuffs for your vegan meals. You may also want to invest in your own utensils and cookware or designate already-existing items as exclusively your own. You will probably find it unappetizing (to say the least) to think that a piece of meat had previously been cooked in a pan that you now need to use to stir-fry your veggies.

Taking Control of Your Meal Preparation

Being sure you're eating a well-balanced diet and getting all the servings and nutrients necessary for fueling your body is important for everyone, not just vegans and vegetarians. Taking control of your meal preparation is the best way to ensure good health and proper nutrition as a vegan. And as mentioned in previous chapters, making a conscious effort to prepare well-balanced meals for yourself will help alleviate any health concerns your friends and family may have about your eating as a vegan.

Preparing your own meals also means there's less chance of cross-contamination or sabotage (adding animal products) of your vegan meals, which can happen. When you are first starting out eating as a vegan, you may have to watch out for Aunt Sally or Grandma trying to sneak a few bits of meat into your dish or a little chicken broth to "enhance" the rice. So stay on your toes! Leaving your meals up to others, when they don't thoroughly understand veganism and its confines, could lead to problems on multiple levels.

Hot Potato _____

Some vegans experience symptoms of lactose intolerance and nausea when they unintentionally consume animal products. The symptoms can hit suddenly and without much warning.

Some may think that preparing your own separate meals is a hassle, but it's certainly warranted and well worth it. After not consuming meat and dairy for some time, your body will start to adjust, and you may no longer be able to properly digest those types of foods when they are slipped by you unexpectedly.

Strutting Your Vegan Stuff

One of the best ways to sway your family toward accepting your new vegan lifestyle is to create some phenomenally delicious vegan food and entice them to try it. Make a salad vibrant with mixed greens, colorful and crunchy vegetables, and tossed with a tantalizing dressing. It will blow away the typical iceberg lettuce, shredded carrot, wedge of tomato combination found in most steakhouses!

> **In a Nutshell**
>
> If you need vegan recipe ideas, check out Part 6! We give you four chapters full of delicious vegan recipes. The Internet or the library are also good sources for recipes and cookbooks to help give you some inspiration. See Appendix B for some useful websites.

Make a pasta, grain, or main dish that is flavorful, eye-catching, and hearty enough to satisfy even the largest of appetites. Then, pull out all the stops by making a fabulous vegan dessert, whether it's as simple as some cherry-chocolate-chip nondairy ice cream and some vegan cookies or a homemade decadent vegan cake or pie.

You will find that most people are very curious about what vegans eat, and a good way to open up some eyes to the concept is by filling their stomachs with tasty and satisfying food. Some may be skeptical about your offerings at first, but don't let that put you off. You know it's good, and so what if they don't? They're the ones missing out, and that leaves more for you! Maybe they'll be more receptive to trying something new next time, so don't give up.

Taking time to learn how to cook and dedicating yourself to knowing how to whip up a wide variety of healthy and delicious vegan food is really helpful when it comes to eating right and being well nourished. It also gives you an advantage when it comes to dealing with meat-eaters at mealtime. As your culinary talents progress, you'll usually only need a very little coaxing for people to want to try your food.

With a little practice and patience, you will soon go from having one vegan dish in your repertoire to several, to preparing entire vegan meals for the whole family to enjoy. Start slow, and remember that although it's generally not a good idea to push your beliefs on others, turning them on to a little delicious food can, at times, be welcomed with much enthusiasm. Who knows, it might even help change some attitudes toward your being vegan!

Finally, preparing a whole vegan meal for all to enjoy should be a gradual progression, too, if you want to have it met with the least resistance from those who may not be exactly thrilled with veganism. Remember, slow, steady, and small steps will help things stick.

> **In a Nutshell**
>
> Asking the chief household meal-maker if you could take the burden off of her for one meal will usually be met with little or no resistance, and for some, it will be a welcomed break. Your willingness to do it all, including cleaning up the kitchen afterward, will usually be eagerly accepted.

Friends, Family, and Food

Most of us also have an active social life, and with it come invitations. Being vegan, some of those invitations will be for restaurants or events where you may no longer feel comfortable being, because what they offer either doesn't appeal to you, conflicts with your vegan beliefs, or can no longer accommodate your new dietary requirements. For example, the smells in restaurants and other gathering places where meat is served now probably leave a bad taste in your mouth instead of making your mouth water.

This may prove to be difficult when going out to eat with friends and family members. It will be easy to avoid these places on your own, but problems may arise from invitations from friends and family. Let your instincts and personal choices guide you, and hope that those around you will understand when something conflicts with your vegan values.

Handling Invitations

Most of us enjoy dining away from home. It can be an exciting change of pace, especially after having put in a long day at work or being overwhelmed by the chaos of everyday life. Anticipation of a wonderful meal, out with friends and family, can really get our juices flowing! But anticipation can turn to heavy-heartedness quickly when your friend invites you to come along and you no longer feel comfortable with the eatery or what they offer there.

What to do? If the circumstances conflict with your vegan values, explain to your pal fully and clearly why you no longer feel comfortable going along. Honesty is the best policy. Use tact, and remember that you are explaining your position, not making excuses for it. You have a right to your opinions and beliefs, just like anyone else. Stand strong, tall, and proud with your convictions. True loved ones should understand and support you.

Handling invitations to dine out can be a bit tricky. Your acceptance may be influenced by *who* is going but will definitely be influenced by *where* you will be going. In ideal situations, those inviting you along will consider your veganism and allow you to have input on picking a place to dine. Chances are they won't feel adventurous enough to try your favorite veggie place, but you never know. It has been known to happen. Being informed about your local eateries and their menus can be vital, if not crucial, in determining whether you will be dining on an entrée, à la carte, or only a salad.

To check the vegan friendliness of a restaurant, call ahead of time or ask fellow vegans or vegetarians for recommendations of veg-friendly places. Calling ahead can be particularly helpful if your dining companions insist on going to a certain meat-oriented place and you have decided to go along anyway. If the kitchen staff is worth their salt, they will be able to feed you something vegan, whether it be something already on the menu or something they have to create specially for you. Calling a day or even several hours in advance should be sufficient for most places to do this.

> **Hot Potato**
>
> Many vegans refuse to go to *any* restaurant that serves meat. Some vegans don't want to spend their money in restaurants or companies that support and profit from the meat industry, and others find that being in close proximity to meat, especially the smell of it cooking, is disturbing and unappetizing. Instead, these vegans support the restaurants that more closely embody their own vegan values.

Parties and Potlucks

Handling invitations to someone's house for dinner, a potluck, or other type of gathering is also cause for some contemplation. It's best to be honest with your host right away and address any concerns you may have. They may or may not know you are a vegan, much less what you do or do not eat. Try to stick to the basics: fully spell it out, but try to be tactful when inquiring about what they will be serving and what may be suitable or available for you.

Again, prior notice is best, as your host will probably appreciate not having to scramble at the last minute to see if she has something more than a salad or raw veggies to feed you. If you wait until the last minute, your host may have already tossed the salad with a nonvegan dressing or adorned it with cheese or bacon bits.

Offering to bring something of your own, with plenty to share, works well for potlucks or any occasion and is usually appreciated. Bringing your own dish can also be a great way to show off how delicious eating vegan food can be. Many vegans enjoy "wowing" people with their vegan culinary creations, especially delicious desserts, as they are often particularly appreciated and enjoyed.

Hosting Your Own Gathering

After attending one too many get-togethers where you are the odd vegan out, you may be inspired to host your own all-vegan shindig. This is the best way to showcase the benefits of being vegan and all the wonderful culinary possibilities the lifestyle has to offer. Depending on your culinary talents, start with something simple like having a few friends or family over for dinner. Then, if that goes well, try to tackle a holiday blowout with several vegan courses.

Go for your tried-and-true recipes first off, but if you get stuck for ideas, enlist the help of the recipes in Part 6, some vegan cookbooks, or the Internet. Try the recipes on yourself first as sort of a practice run. This way, you'll know how they taste and look before trying something beyond your current level of culinary expertise. Remember, you want to impress them, not distress them, and for sure, you want to avoid causing any intestinal upset after the partaking of your spread.

This is also a great way to assure Mom and Grandma that they can stop worrying that you will waste away and starve to death eating vegan. You will feel so empowered as a vegan while strutting your stuff, healthfully filling their bellies, and positively showcasing your new lifestyle, that you may even open up the lines of communication between yourself and those most opposed to or threatened by your being vegan. Many a mind has been swayed on a full stomach!

> **In a Nutshell**
>
> To help spark your vegan culinary creativity and impress your friends and family, try some of the recipes in Part 6. Vegan cookbooks and the Internet can also provide inspiration for holiday menu ideas.

Holiday Gathering Advice

Holiday gatherings can cause headaches and squabbles all on their own, but throwing veganism into the mix can add a whole new dimension. How you handle it could mean all the difference between chaos and quality time. Many holiday gatherings have either family or cultural traditions associated with them, and most have eating involved somewhere in the festivities. In America, that usually means that lots of meat and dairy foods will be involved.

In a Nutshell

Whenever we are invited to a holiday gathering, we always offer to bring something, and often bring several little things. This ensures that we will eat as well as everyone else, and we also like to tantalize others with some vegan treats. It also makes it easier for your "special diet" to not be a problem for the host, and it's a great way to open the eyes of others to the possibilities of meatless alternatives and substitutions.

The Meat in Front of You

Even though you may feel baited into it or you may just *want* to, resist the urge to condemn or negatively comment on the animal food that sits on the table before you. Remember, even though you don't want or need to eat it, someone did work very hard to prepare what they considered a good meal for their guests, and it would undoubtedly hurt their feelings to have you criticize their food during the meal. After all, you could have chosen not to take part in the meal to begin with, and you can always politely excuse yourself from the table if need be.

You can also try to situate yourself away from meat dishes and other such items, as well as from any arguments that may ensue during mealtime. Conflict is bad for relationships and everyone's digestion, and no matter how things go down, likely you will be blamed. After all, you are the vegan, and they already view you as not being "normal." Don't give them any more ammunition to use against you by ruining the meal with your comments. Instead, if you want to talk about why you choose not to eat meat, wait until the right time—preferably away from the dinner table.

A Few Holiday Dining Tips

Many holiday meal traditions revolve around a roast of some sort, but that doesn't mean you can't start some new traditions of your own. You can make hearty casseroles and entrées from all-plant-based ingredients to replace meat-based offerings. A vegan lasagna, pot pie, or stuffed squash makes a wonderful centerpiece for a winter holiday meal, instead of Tom the Turkey or Babe the Pig.

As vegans, we are often asked what we eat for Thanksgiving instead of turkey. We comment that we eat most of the normal things, such as mashed potatoes, gravy, stuffing, and so on, in addition to whatever we choose to have as our main entrée. When you really think about it, the best part of the typical Thanksgiving dinner is all the trimmings and side dishes! Yams, with their vitamins A, C, and beta-carotene; mashed potatoes and stuffing full of complex carbohydrates; and cranberries bursting with all kinds of antioxidants are all foods that give you energy. Sure, turkey has protein, but it also contains tryptophan, which tends to knock you out after the big meal instead of revving you up.

If you want to really impress your guests, hollow out a large pumpkin (the kind for eating, not carving). Make a mixture of bread stuffing, cooked grains, sautéed onions, celery, and apples, and season it to taste as you would your favorite stuffing recipe. Pack the mixture into the hollowed-out pumpkin, and bake it at 350 degrees for an hour or more or until the pumpkin is tender. Then, place it on a large platter and serve up the stuffing, as well as the pumpkin flesh, to your hungry guests. It looks impressive, tastes delicious, and will win you some rave reviews!

"May I Take Your Order?"

When it comes to dining out as a vegan, the first bit of advice we can offer you is don't be intimidated. If you're lucky, you will have a vegan, vegetarian, or *veg-friendly* establishment to frequent. Check your local paper and phone book for possible options, as well as online sources. If you have any vegan or vegetarian friends, ask them for some good restaurant recommendations, too.

Eugene, Oregon, where we live, is an example of a town that actually has several all-vegan or vegetarian restaurants, and vegans who live here feel so fortunate. Most establishments and people in the community are familiar with the terms *vegan* and *vegetarian*, which means we don't have to give a long speech every time we mention we're vegans. But living in such a progressive community is not the norm for most newbie vegans. If you

Vegan 101

If an establishment is **veg-friendly,** it has an understanding of the basics of vegan and vegetarian dietary guidelines and philosophies and provides vegan or vegetarian options.

live in a community without veg-friendly places to eat, you'll have to make full use of your vegan survival skills.

Begin by assuming that when you go to a restaurant, you will have to spend some time looking over the menu. First, check to see if the menu has a vegetarian section or selections. If it does, you're in luck, as it is usually very easy to leave off cheeses and other dairy products used as garnishes to accommodate vegan tastes. If not, check for salad and side-dish options you can use to create your own vegan meal.

Your Server: Friend and Ally

After looking over the menu, you will need to find your waiter, as you will most certainly need his assistance. Begin by being very friendly and polite, and it doesn't hurt to smile. After all, you need your server as an ally when ordering. First let him know you're a vegan, and explain that you follow a strict vegetarian diet that includes no animal products whatsoever, including meat, fish, chicken, eggs, gelatin, honey, and all dairy products and cheeses. They may or may not be familiar with veganism, so it will only benefit you in the long run to spell out your exact dietary no-no's.

Don't be afraid to ask your server for any menu suggestions. Ask how things are pre-pared and what ingredients are in a dish, especially some that may be hidden or not obvious from the menu description. If he doesn't know, ask if he could check with the chef for further clarification. A little checking ahead of time can save having to send something back that you aren't able to eat and prevent you from ingesting hidden animal products.

In a Nutshell

If you tend to dine out a lot, you may want to write out a card listing clearly which foods you eat as a vegan, which foods you avoid, along with any foods you may dis-like or be allergic to, and pass this to the chef or cook via your server when ordering. Nothing ruins a good evening faster than an unexpected bout with lactose intolerance!

"Service" Is Their Middle Name

Don't forget it's called the food *service* industry, and service is and should be their middle name. Restaurants are there to serve you, the customer, and any decent estab-lishment should have a chef or cook who is able to whip up something special with a little advance notice and instruction. And for many, this allows the chef to be creative and deviate from the standard menu items. Prior notice gives them a better chance of serving you something spectacular instead of just plain boiled or steamed veggies and white rice.

Hopefully, these tips will help make your dining experiences pleasant ones, as they should be. Be sure to let your waiter know if you were satisfied, tell him to give your compliments to the chef, and be sure to reward his efforts with a generous tip or a kudos to the manager on his behalf. Working in food service is extremely hard work and often goes underappreciated. Waiters remember who gave them a generous tip, who gave them an adequate tip, and who was a cheapskate. If you frequent a place often, you will become recognized, and if you are known as being generous, their level and quality of service will likely know no bounds.

On the Lookout for Hidden Ingredients

Being a vegan means staying on your toes, especially when you have to rely on others to eat. When cooking for yourself, you know exactly what ingredients you used and how you prepared the food. But when dining out, you don't exactly have access to a precise ingredients list or a video showing you the path your food followed on its way to your plate. As a vegan dining out at a nonvegan restaurant, you must be aware of the possibility of hidden animal ingredients in your food.

Some servers easily overlook the chicken broth used to cook the rice, the sprinkle of cheese, or the added dollop of sour cream when attesting that the offering is suitable for a vegan. So use a little common sense; if the name of the recipe includes *fromage*, *au gratin*, *Alfredo*, or *cream of this or that*, it probably contains dairy or cheese.

When in doubt, ask what exact ingredients are in the dish. Be polite and friendly, as you don't want your server to think you're difficult. He may just start telling you what he thinks you want to hear, just to appease you. If you discover there really isn't anything suitable for a vegan on the menu, you can find out if the kitchen would be able to prepare something special for you. Often, you can make an impromptu entrée by combining vegetable side dishes with grains or pasta.

> **CAUTION**
>
> **Hot Potato** _____
>
> You would think that wine, made from grapes, would be vegan, but that's not always the case. Clarifying agents, used to remove cloudiness as well as yeast and other substances from the wine, are often of animal origin. One example is *isinglass*, a gelatin made from the swimming bladder of fish. Fortunately, many manufacturers produce vegan wine. One all-vegan, sulfite-free brand of wine is Frey Vineyards. (See www.freywine.com for info.)

Dining Expectations

Of course, eating at an all-vegan restaurant is the ideal dining experience for a vegan. The first time you eat at one, you will feel incredibly spoiled at being able to peruse a menu knowing you can order anything and not worry about what may or may not be lurking in the dish. It is pure bliss. But you can't always be so lucky as to have even one completely vegan restaurant in your area.

> ### In a Nutshell
>
> Some restaurants will gladly share ingredient lists, especially where special diets are concerned. It's helpful to call ahead of your arrival, at a nonbusy time, to fully address all your specific questions and concerns.

The type of establishment you dine at can greatly influence your chances of having a satisfactory vegan meal. The level of service and experience of the kitchen staff varies greatly from restaurant to restaurant, and you can expect this to be reflected in your choice of selections, means of preparations, possibilities of substitutions, and encounters with hidden ingredients.

Fine Dining

Most people who are not independently wealthy can only afford to eat at fine dining restaurants—you know, those places that have several "stars" to their credit—on special occasions or when the boss is treating. Such restaurants usually have tons of animal-based dishes on their menus, but some are becoming more progressive and offering vegetarian, vegan, and even raw meals or "tastings," as they are currently being called.

If a fine dining restaurant is on top of its game, it will try to stay up on the latest food trends, and raw vegan is becoming the "in thing" among the health conscious and many celebrities. If the menu doesn't offer something suitable, someone in the kitchen might be able to whip up something vegan and delicious for you. Expect that your creation may take a little longer to arrive at your table, as it is being specially prepared for you.

The Average American Sit-Down Place

Eating at the average American sit-down restaurant can prove to be a bit trickier for vegans. First, check to see if it serves any vegetarian offerings that could easily have the dairy or eggs omitted. If not, check the salads and side dishes for possibilities.

Use your common sense, though, when deciding what a safe vegan option is. For instance, if they have fried fish or chicken on the menu, there's a good chance that the french fries you ordered will be fried in the same oil, in the same fryer. Or the hash browns could possibly be cooked on the grill next to some meat item. The same goes for a veggie burger, or anything fried or grilled. Some vegans request that their veggie burger be cooked in the microwave just to eliminate the possibility of coming into contact with meat.

Salads without dressing and plain baked potatoes are usually safe choices. A drizzle or two of olive oil makes a tasty vegan addition not only to your salad but to your potato as well. Margarines often contain casein, whey, or some other dairy-derived ingredient, so don't automatically consider them a dairy-free option.

> **CAUTION** **Hot Potato**
>
> In nonvegan or nonvegetarian restaurants, it's a good idea to stay away from pilafs, as they tend to be cooked in meat-based broths. Beware of mashed potatoes as well, as they are often prepared with butter, milk, and even meat-based broths.

White and brown rice are usually fine, but check for the addition of butter. Most restaurants usually don't have a problem steaming some veggies for you, so don't be afraid to ask even if it isn't listed on the menu. When in doubt about how something is prepared, ask the waiter to ask the kitchen staff. Better safe than sorry!

The Global Diner

Certain types of cuisine seem to be more veg-friendly than others. We find that many Italian, Mexican, Chinese, Japanese, Mediterranean, and Middle Eastern restaurants seem to be more accommodating of vegan diets and offer many traditional vegan or vegetarian dishes to begin with. You still may have to ask for the cheese or dairy to be left off as a garnish or sauce, and remember to inquire about whether or not an item has any other animal ingredients that are not obvious.

Vegans do need to be careful when dining on Thai or Indian food, as they like to use ghee, which is clarified butter, and fish sauce to add flavor to their dishes. You should also keep in mind that the means of preparation attributed to a certain cuisine or style of cooking may determine if you will actually be served a vegan meal or one with a few meat remnants from the meal cooked before or beside yours.

Feasting on Fast Foods

Eating on the go seems to be becoming more and more the norm for an increasing number of us, and it's often the result of trying to fit too much into our everyday lives. That's why more and more Americans are turning to fast food on a weekly, and for some, a daily basis. And no wonder; fast-food joints are everywhere you turn, and their advertising on TV and radio is relentless. Many of the more popular and heavily advertised franchises have locations across the globe, in remote places, with much the same menu as the one just down the street.

Unfortunately, these major fast-food chains have very little to offer vegans or the health-conscious. Their menu selections are made up of mostly meat and dairy-oriented foods and contain lots of simple carbohydrates; fried and heavily processed foods; and excessive amounts of fat, salt, and sugar. To say that the fruit and veggie options are limited is a massive understatement!

In a Nutshell

Most of the major fast-food franchises will supply you with their nutritional information and ingredient lists upon request, but they often do not have the information readily available at all locations. Whether you're vegan or health-conscious in general, if you're concerned about your sugar, salt, or fat consumption, fast-food joints should be on your list of places to severely limit—or better yet, avoid altogether.

The foods most major fast-food chains offer make it practically impossible to formulate a well-balanced meal with adequate protein, complex carbohydrates, and nutrients, while also being low in fat and high in fiber. Instead, most menus feature foods fried and high in protein, fat, and calories. Eat too many fast-food meals, and you could well be on the path to poor health and obesity.

There's no reason why nutritious, whole vegan foods can't be served up quickly *and* healthily to fit in with people's busy lives. In fact, several vegan and vegetarian fast-food type restaurants have already opened throughout the United States and elsewhere. Because vegan and vegetarian markets are on the increase everywhere, hopefully more of them will follow.

The Least You Need to Know

◆ Preparing your own meals—and creating a space in the kitchen for your vegan ingredients, foods, and cookware—can make it easier for a vegan to live in a meat-eating household.

◆ Bringing a tasty vegan dish or two of your own to a gathering can be a great way to ensure you will have something vegan and nutritious to eat—and might entice nonvegans to open their minds (and mouths!).

◆ Mealtime isn't a good time to argue about vegan issues, even if you're baited by others; try to save any debating for after the meal.

◆ Fully explaining your vegan dietary restrictions to a waiter or cook can make your dining experience in a nonvegan restaurant more successful and enjoyable.

Chapter 15

Supporting Your Ideals

In This Chapter

- ◆ Making a difference with organics
- ◆ Supporting merchants that reflect your values
- ◆ Examining the world of natural foods stores

Being vegan means putting your beliefs and compassion into action through the things you do, wear, say, and eat. It is a way of approaching the world around you and can certainly have a great influence on what you buy and who you buy it from. Supporting those businesses, individuals, and products that most closely embody and support your values as a vegan can be a way to make your presence known and your economic influence felt. When it comes to the way you spend your money on goods and services, your actions could end up making a world of difference to everyone involved.

Putting Your Money Where Your Heart Is

Your money, and how you choose to use it, is quite important. Informed vegan consumers who spend their dollars wisely can have a huge effect on the kinds of products manufactured, as well as the kinds of companies that become, and remain, successful. Consumers don't just greatly affect the market, they *are* the market. And if enough of them want to, they can help effect positive change for animals through the way they approach shopping.

Think of each dollar you spend as being a vote for the product you're buying and for the merchant you're buying it from. Choose to support shops and businesses that more closely reflect and support your vegan ideals first and foremost, especially the small independent companies that need you as a loyal customer to stay competitive against the big corporations.

You can also make statements with your purchases by not supporting certain businesses or large retailers that support animal cruelty and the use of resulting products, in addition to employing unfair and child labor practices. For vegans, showing compassion and opposing the abuse and suffering of others is extended to fellow human beings as well, and not just other members of the animal kingdom.

Where to Shop

Being a vegan doesn't mean you have to forego all your old haunts and shopping grounds and only shop at veg-friendly places—although you can if you want to if they exist in your area. You can also purchase many vegan food products through your local grocery. Just take a look around, and you'll be amazed at the number of foods on your supermarket shelves that are vegan and you didn't even know it. Your local market may even stock organic produce next to the conventional produce. You may have a limited number of whole-grain and organic selections in other areas, though. That's where a natural foods store can be your best bet.

Check your phone book, as most large towns and cities have at least one natural foods store somewhere in the vicinity. As you will soon learn, natural foods stores have a larger selection of products that fall within your new dietary guidelines. You'll undoubtedly discover vegan products you didn't even know existed—as well as those you couldn't have imagined in your wildest vegan fantasies. Vegan marshmallows, "nacho cheese" dip, nougat bars, doughnuts, even soy jerky are just a few of the vegan products available from coast to coast.

Many of us are fortunate enough to live in areas that have natural foods stores nearby, but for those of you who don't, fortunately you do have the Internet. By surfing the web, you can find many different ways to purchase items to stock your vegan pantry, fulfill your personal or household needs, as well as find like-minded people to connect with. You can also find the answer to just about any vegan question you might have, such as where the closest natural foods store or vegan restaurant is or where you can find a particular product or service in your area. Use your favorite search engine to get started, and see Appendix B for some great website suggestions.

You may be lucky enough to have a natural foods cooperative, or co-op, in your area. A co-op is a not-for-profit organization of members, usually families, who join together to combine their purchasing ability and share the labor of purchasing, displaying, and storing the items. The main idea is to buy in bulk and share in the costs and savings. Becoming a member of a co-op gives you access to foods and products you normally wouldn't be able to find in your area, and at a reduced rate. If you have the opportunity to join a co-op, then by all means do so!

In a Nutshell

Three of the most popular online vegan merchants are veganessentials.com, veganstore. com, and differentdaisy.com. Each has a wide assortment of vegan products, from snacks to clothing to supplements—even vegan marshmallows and marshmallow fluff, doughnuts, or the ever-elusive vegan gelatin! Surf on in to these sites whenever you can't find vegan products closer to home.

How to Shop

When shopping, whether you're in the grocery store or a natural foods store, start in the produce section. It's usually situated close to the entrance, and for a reason: to lure you in to buy attractive and colorful fruits and veggies on impulse. So go with it! This is your best place to begin for sources of good, wholesome foods in a large section of fresh and dried fruits and vegetables in all shapes, colors, and textures, from all corners of the globe. Choose organics for the most bang for your buck when it comes to health as well as environmental benefits.

Many stores also feature specials or discount sections, so use these to your advantage. Another good tip is to buy fruits and veggies when they're in season and abundant. Not only will they taste better, they'll also be more affordable. After checking out the produce section and store specials, move on to filling your dry goods and pantry needs.

Always make your freezer and refrigerated selections last. You don't want these items exposed to room temperature for any longer than they need to be, and you don't want to risk spoilage or other problems that arise from refreezing. Keep in mind your transit time, especially in warm summer months, and consider keeping a cooler in your trunk to carry frozen or refrigerated foods home in. Fewer dangers are associated with improperly refrigerated veggie-based items than with meat-based ones, but you still need to be conscious of these things, especially when it may result in the unthinkable: a half-melted carton of your favorite nondairy ice cream. On second thought, that could still be quite yummy.

> ### In a Nutshell
>
> It's best to stay focused and move systematically through the aisles of a store to efficiently make your selection. If it will help, perhaps make a shopping list ahead of time and arrange it by aisle. Wandering around aimlessly and having to retrace your steps for something on the other side of the store can greatly increase your time spent shopping and make it a much less pleasant experience.

Organics: The Natural Way

One of the best things you can do for yourself, your family, and the environment is to support organic farming practices and purchase organic and non-genetically modified products whenever possible. Better sustainability of crops and gentler use of the land is better for the farmers and for you. No pesticides or chemical fertilizers used on crops means none are passed on to you or the environment. Choose organics, and you are choosing wise, Earth-friendly agricultural practices over widespread pesticide usage and environmental harm.

> ### In a Nutshell
>
> Don't be put off by slightly higher prices for organic goods. The extra money you spend on organic food now will save you many more times that money in the future, in the form of prevented medical bills arising from conditions caused by exposure to pesticides and chemical fertilizers. Look at it as a wise investment in your future health!

What about the economics of organics? Growing organic crops is definitely good for the economy. It helps struggling farmers preserve their livelihood by nourishing their land and ensuring that they are paid a fair price for their harvests. It can especially help the smaller farms compete with the conglomerates as organics fetch a better market price than conventional produce. This gives farmers back the sense of pride they deserve as the keepers of the bounty that sustains us.

By purchasing organic products whenever possible, you can use your purchasing power to give a vote in favor of the organic approach to farming and sustaining ourselves, while voting against polluting the earth, and our bodies, with dangerous chemicals and pesticides. The major food producers will ultimately take notice and want to jump on the organics bandwagon, which they have already begun doing by buying out natural foods companies and introducing more organic items into their product lines.

Appearance Isn't Everything

Some people are under the impression that just because organic produce doesn't always look as shiny and pretty as the conventional stuff that it is somehow inferior in quality. But this couldn't be further from the truth. Not only are organics better for you, but they also actually taste better than their nonorganic counterparts because they have never come into contact with chemical fertilizers or pesticides. Eating organic is actually as close to eating fruits and veggies in their unadulterated, natural, healthy states as you're going to get—besides growing your own in your backyard or community organic garden, of course.

Fruits and vegetables are just like us; we aren't perfect, and they shouldn't be expected to look perfect either. We all have our bruises and blemishes, and we come in all shades of colors and sizes. If you feel having a perfect-looking apple is worth being exposed to residue from pesticides and chemical fertilizers, then there is certainly enough conventional produce on the market for you to choose from. Fortunately, there is a more natural alternative!

Absorbing It All

When you think about it, the extent that pesticides and other contaminants from modern industrial and agricultural practices have polluted our air, land, and water is mind-boggling. And they continue to do this at an alarming rate. But the pollutants don't end with Mother Earth. Our bodies absorb these harmful substances through what we eat, drink, apply, and wear.

Your body is like a big sponge that absorbs and holds on to contaminants it encounters. It views contaminants as invaders, and it often loses the battle against them. This is why many environmental pollutants, such as waste and fertilizer runoff, toxic chemicals, and pesticides, have been linked to many of the major health disorders plaguing the human race.

> **Hot Potato** _____
>
> Your body absorbs and holds on to the good, as well as the bad, of what you give it. Put good things into your body, and you will get good things back out of it. Put in junk, and you will get junk back, which is usually seen in the form of excess pounds, poor skin and hair, and a bad attitude. Use your head and make wise, informed, and self-supporting purchasing decisions. You will feel better about yourself and your new lifestyle.

Shopping at Natural Foods Stores

Natural foods stores, otherwise known as health food stores, are places of wonderment and havens for vegans, vegetarians, and those who have to follow special diets. Once thought of as places run by people living on the fringe of society, natural foods stores now make up a multibillion-dollar-a-year industry. The natural foods industry has really come a long way in the last 20 years in terms of selection, pricing, and availability of goods and services. Many stores started out as supplement stores and juice joints and then branched out to include produce, personal, and home-care products.

One of the best ways to judge the caliber of a natural foods store is by what it more prominently features, food items or supplements. Those stores that emphasize food first for good health and supplementation second as a backup are the true gems of the industry and our first choice for where to shop. Natural foods stores should provide people with the tools and means necessary to sustain themselves and their health. Customers come to them with the hope of enhancing or improving their health, and a good natural foods store will be able to show them all the ways to do that. As a result of a store's added effort, it will have loyal, repeat customers, not those who just come back for a refill of pills every few months.

The Whys and Hows

Shopping at natural foods stores has several advantages over shopping at your local supermarket. Among them …

   ◆ Larger selections of organic products.

   ◆ Larger and fresher all-organic or mostly organic produce sections.

- More support of local produce and products.

- Wider selection of vegan and vegetarian alternative products.

- A more expansive and inclusive bulk section.

Natural foods stores stock many meat and dairy alternative products that can assist you in preparing your meals. Check the labels for ingredients, and analyze the nutritional information when comparing brands if you have an option. Of course, seek out organic products and ingredients whenever possible.

Natural foods stores also stock prepackaged foods such as veggie pizzas; veggie meals; meat alternative products; nondairy frozen desserts and novelties; and frozen fruits, vegetables, and juices, just to name a few. All these products can make transitioning easier and come in handy when you come home hungry and too tired to cook.

Many stores also give you a discount, usually 5 or 10 percent, if you purchase a product by the case. Call in advance to ask about whether or not a store offers case discounts and check availability. It may even be able to order you a case of a product you don't see on the shelves as it has many more products available via distributors than it has shelf space for.

> **In a Nutshell**
>
> A good way to keep up on new and upcoming vegan food items is to read vegan- or veg-oriented publications. The best nationally available vegan magazine is *VegNews*, which is loaded with all kinds of product information and other useful info. See www. vegnews.com for details.

Veggie Wonderland

Most conventional grocery stores have fairly large produce sections but generally only have a small area containing organic produce. You'll find just the opposite at natural foods stores. Most carry all-organic or mostly organic produce, and many stock seasonal and specialty items you may not find anywhere else in your area. It really is like a veggie wonderland for a vegan!

Perusing the produce section can be a little like walking through an art gallery filled with vibrant colors and textures. Taking it all in,

> **Hot Potato**
>
> Most conventional supermarkets have to stock the same produce day in and day out, so their products are often rushed to market from points unknown, and the quality is often compromised. Because they're usually locked into the brands and types of produce they offer, they often aren't able to work with local suppliers or farmers for their produce needs.

visually, can fill you with wonder and excitement. It can also give you some ideas as to what you might want to eat for your next meal. Go with what looks good and is affordable, and build the rest of your meal around that.

Many natural foods stores stock locally grown produce when it's available, that is often grown within miles of the store. Buying produce from local sources means getting the freshest and best quality, as well as contributing to the livelihood of the small farmer in your own community. Foods taste their best when eaten in season and picked at their peak of ripeness and not before. Prices are usually more affordable at those times as well.

Buying in Bulk

Being able to purchase items in bulk quantities from bins is one of the best things about shopping at natural foods stores. Buying in bulk is good for you and the environment. It is good for you because you will often pay ⅓ to ½ of the price for the same product out of a bulk bin as you would in prepackaged form. Many stores offer paper or plastic bags for dry goods or encourage you to bring your own. They might also sell containers to use for bulk liquid and solid ingredients such as oils, nut butters, and syrups.

CAUTION

Hot Potato

Check the quality of bulk items, as with any ingredient you use, to ensure freshness and turnover rate. Buy in useable-size quantities to prevent spoilage and to keep from overstocking your pantry. If you have the room, and the need for it, then by all means stock up on those 10-pound bags of organic brown rice and quinoa!

Buying in bulk saves you money because it helps manufacturers reduce packaging and advertising costs, in addition to cutting down on the store's cost expended and shelf space needed for restocking. The conservation of packaging materials has a ripple effect on our environment: buying items with little or no packaging means less waste added to our landfills and less petrochemicals used in the creation of environmentally unfriendly packaging. Many organic product manufacturers prefer to use Earth-friendly packaging materials, including recycled paper and soy-based (instead of petroleum-based) inks for their labels.

The Least You Need to Know

◆ Choosing organics is best for your health and for that of the planet.

◆ Support shops and businesses that most closely reflect and support your vegan ideals.

◆ A good natural foods store has just about everything you need to sustain your vegan diet and lifestyle.

Chapter **16**

Buying Your Vegan Eats

In This Chapter

◆ Seeking out whole-grain foods

◆ Indulging good news about chocolate

◆ Understanding food labels

◆ Snacking on healthy foods

◆ Looking at vegan food products

Now that you have some ideas on where and how to shop as a vegan, it's time to learn how to be a wise vegan food shopper. Some people dread shopping for groceries, but it can actually be quite fun, with so many different vegan products available on the shelves as well as a never-ending supply of products we never even knew existed. Be an informed consumer when you go shopping. Know what you came for and what you like and dislike; buy from companies and stores you like and trust; take advantage of sales or use coupons; and don't let fancy packaging mislead you.

Be sure to read all packaging to know what you are actually getting and paying for. When purchasing prepackaged foods, start by reading the label. Some companies that market to the natural foods community clearly label if their foods are vegan, low in fat or sugar, wheat or gluten-free, nut-free, or even dairy-free. It really makes your shopping process easier and quicker when products are already labeled as vegan or in a similar manner. Let's get ready to go shopping, vegans!

Whole Grain, You're Not Refined

Vegan or otherwise, consuming and purchasing wholesome products whenever possible is a good rule of thumb to follow. Choose cereals, grain dishes, snacks, baked goods, and dessert items made with whole grains and not heavily refined ingredients. Whole-grain items contain the entire seed or kernel of the grain with all the important nutrients and fiber still intact.

Eat grains either in whole, cracked, split, or ground forms. Look for the words *whole grain*, *whole*, or *stone ground* on the label to ensure you're getting all the benefits from your grain and bread products. You can even find products, especially breads, that contain 100 percent whole-grain ingredients. Manufacturers will often also use molasses or other natural sweeteners, which are better choices for your health and your body than high-fructose corn syrup and bleached sugars.

You'll find multi-grain products—those made from a mixture of grains—on the shelves of most stores. They're a great way to increase your consumption of grains such as amaranth, buckwheat, barley, or rye, which most of us consume rarely if ever at all.

Sprouted grain products like breads, crackers, and other baked goods are also becoming more popular and readily available. Grains are soaked, rinsed, and sprouted; grinded together; and processed and baked accordingly. Sprouting increases and retains the availability of vital nutrients such as vitamins, minerals, amino acids, and digestive enzymes, which help keep your body functioning as smoothly and efficiently as it should. Sprouted grain products tend to have more protein, fiber, and complex carbohydrates than other grain products.

Ezekiel 4:9 bread by Food for Life is a commercially available organic sprouted grain bread made from a

> **CAUTION**
> **Hot Potato**
>
> Most whole-grain baked goods and breads contain no preservatives or artificial additives and are more susceptible to attracting mold, so be sure to keep such products in your refrigerator. They'll last longer.

> **Golden Apple**
>
> Take thou also unto thee wheat, and barley, and beans, and lentiles, and millet, and fitches, and put them in one vessel, and make thee bread thereof, according to the number of the days that thou shalt lie upon thy side, three hundred and ninety days shalt thou eat thereof.
> —Ezekiel 4:9 (King James Version)

mixture of sprouted whole grains and beans such as barley, millet, wheat, spelt, soybeans, lentils, and others. The bread, based on a biblical verse, is meant to sustain you, as it is full of complex carbohydrates and protein. If you are feeling a little adventurous and want to try making your own sprouted grain bread, get online. You'll find many recipes available.

Deciphering Food Labels

When buying any prepackaged product, whether it's a package of veggie burgers or a bag of chips, be sure to read the ingredient list. Items are listed by their volume as contained within the product, from largest to smallest. If you see whole-wheat flour listed first, you know there's more whole-wheat flour in the item than any other ingredient. If salt is listed last, salt is the least used ingredient by volume.

Use these tips to know what to look for—and what to avoid—on a label. Look for the word *organic* before as many ingredients as possible. Favor foods that contain whole grains, unrefined sweeteners, and other wholesome ingredients. Avoid partially hydrogenated or hydrogenated oils whenever possible, and instead look for cold-pressed or expeller-pressed oils. (We discuss proper oil choices and the reasons behind them in Chapter 18.)

Watch out for animal ingredients in the most unlikely foods. Manufacturers use gelatin; eggs; dairy products such as cheese, butter, and casein; and animal-based broths and oils in many prepackaged foods. Whey, the liquid that results from cheese making, is also a commonly used flavor enhancer. It is a cheap way for food manufacturers to give foods a creamy or cheesy flavor.

Natural flavorings is actually a catch-all term used in ingredient lists to hide secret blends of herbs and spices or other ingredients. These "natural flavorings" can be from animal or plant-based sources, and this phrase on a label can be very tricky for vegans. When you see it among the ingredients, don't buy the product unless you know the natural flavorings are vegan in origin. When in doubt, call or e-mail the manufacturer to ask whether or not its natural flavorings are suitable for vegans. In fact, when you wonder about *any* ingredient or aspect of a product, contact the manufacturer and ask them about it. Most are usually happy to clear up any confusion about its products and answer your questions, particularly if they can put your mind at ease about animal products being involved, and gain or keep a customer in the process.

Enriched foods can also contain animal-based sources of nutrients. As mentioned in Chapter 10, the supplement form of vitamin D_3 used to fortify foods is only derived from animal-based sources. So if you see vitamin D_3 listed on your box of fortified breakfast cereal, it definitely isn't vegan.

Avoid ingredients you don't recognize or can't understand, as they're usually chemical additives, artificial preservatives, or other ingredients that are far from wholesome and natural. Avoid artificial colorings and flavorings, as many are harmful or potentially derived from animal sources.

CAUTION

Hot Potato _____

Vegans, beware of foods that have been dyed red, as they may contain ground-up bugs! Carmine, also known as carminic acid and cochineal extract, is a red dye made from ground-up cochineal beetles. These beetles eat prickly pears and other cacti. They then absorb and concentrate their bright red juices in their bodies. The red dye is used to color lipsticks and other makeup, candy and confections, baked goods, maraschino cherries, spreads, juices, and other products. This takes finding a bug in your food to a whole new level!

Finally, check the sugar, fat, and sodium contents for an actual serving. Some manufacturers try to fool you into thinking their product is better for you than it actually is by considering a serving size an unrealistically small amount no one would actually limit himself to in one sitting. Be sure to multiply the fat content and other nutritional aspects by the amount of servings in the item to get the full picture of what you'll be consuming.

Helping Hands: Convenience Items

Once you go vegan, you are really going to be inspired by the foods you'll eat. And if you don't already cook for yourself, be prepared for that to change very soon, out of sheer necessity if nothing else. Unless you live in L.A., New York, or some other large veg-friendly city and can afford to dine out at veggie restaurants for all your meals, you're going to have to learn to cook. Cooking for yourself is essential to vegan survival. Don't be intimidated. Just get some cookbooks or go online for some recipes, and dive right in!

If entering your kitchen seems foreign to you or feels a little like entering a lab with all of its gadgets, metal, hard surfaces, and sharp utensils, then start small with simple dishes such as soups, salads, sandwiches, one-pot meals, or pasta. Don't be afraid of trial and error because experimenting can often be very rewarding. Even if your finished product seems to border on the inedible, remind yourself that it is vegan and that you made it yourself!

Not everyone can work quickly in the kitchen or has time for making every meal from scratch on a daily basis. With our hectic lifestyles, it's understandable and even practical to have some prepackaged foods in your pantry, refrigerator, or freezer. There's nothing wrong with using these foods in a pinch, as they can provide you with a nutritious vegan meal or snack whenever you feel the pangs of hunger. In this chapter and on into Part 5, we provide you with recommendations to help stock your pantry, refrigerator, and freezer with delicious and nutritious vegan food items.

To start you out slowly, we begin with quick-fix ideas to help you through your transition into eating as a vegan on a daily basis. Applying all your newly found vegan nutritional advice immediately to your daily diet may seem intimidating at first, but it shouldn't be. Just take it meal by meal, and day by day.

> ### In a Nutshell
>
> Veg-friendly companies with a conscience do exist! Here are some of our favorite independent companies: Eden Foods, Road's End Organics, Now&Zen, Purity Foods, Small Planet, Lumen Foods, Westbrae Naturals, Annie's Naturals, Green & Black's, Wildwood Harvest Foods, Endangered Species Chocolate Company, and Plamil. Look for them in your natural foods store.
>
> In Part 5, you learn more about how to specifically use some vegan food items that may be new to you, like dairy and meat replacements, in addition to picking up some tips that help to get you off and baking as a vegan.

Using a few helping-hand convenience items now and again can help you eat a healthy meal—not a fast-food meal—during a busy workweek or weekday schedule. Remember then, when you have more time, to prepare for yourself some homemade vegan foods and goodies from scratch.

It can also be easier to avoid "bad ingredients" if you buy all organic or mostly organic pre-packaged foods. Organic products tend to be free of unwanted additives such as man-made preservatives and artificial colors and flavors, many of which have been linked to various health problems. Look for the word *organic* in ingredient lists as much as possible.

Boxes and Mixes

So what kinds of quick-fix vegan foods can you expect to find on your store's shelves to make your life easier? Starting with breakfast, you can find boxed and bulk dry cereals full of whole grains, nuts, seeds, and dried fruits. For those who like their breakfasts hot and hearty, you can also find boxed and bulk hot cereals. You can also discover, in mix and boxed forms, vegan baked goods such as quick breads, muffins, cornbread, cookies, and cakes. Some stores even offer these types of mixes in gluten-free and sugar-free varieties as well.

For lunch and dinner, try boxed and bulk grain, rice, and pasta selections. Also available are natural meals-in-a-cup or -bowl, made with grains or pasta, veggies, beans or tofu, and a sauce, which is a great start for lunches and light meals. You can find seitan mixes, veggie burgers, and soy-based loaves and sandwich fixings in boxes and bulk. These enable you to quickly whip up your own semi-homemade creations.

Shortcuts

You can also buy precooked food items to help speed up your meal production time. Organic canned goods run the gamut from plain cooked beans, seasoned beans, and veggies, to soups, veg-based chilies, and mock meat products. These can really come in handy when you're short on time but still want to eat something healthful.

Look for bottled sauces and condiments that can turn simple vegetables and grains into exotic coconut curries, tempting teriyaki stir-fries, or new twists on comfort food. Using canned tomato products and sauces, many of which come preseasoned and in a wide variety of flavors, paired with your additions of veggies, beans, or mock meats, requires very short simmering times but can give you the same rich flavors of slow-cooked meals.

CAUTION

Hot Potato

When using precooked or prepackaged foods, be sure to read the ingredient and nutritional labels, and be conscious of sodium levels. Many prepared canned goods contain rather large amounts of sodium per serving. Drain and rinse canned beans to remove any brining liquid and its excess sodium before cooking.

Here's another tip for those who cook only for themselves or for those of you who may not be very handy with a knife or don't like to do a lot of cutting: check your produce department for precut and prewashed veggies. Prewashed organic greens and salad mixes come in all types of variety blends and make salad munching so amazingly easy. They are great to have on hand when you're in need of some quick raw goodness.

Also in the produce department or on the salad bar, if the store has one, you can often find precut vegetables or small amounts of greens you can use in your recipes. If cutting and chopping isn't your favorite thing to do and often keeps you from eating better, then by all means, pay a little extra to have someone else do it for you. Buy off the salad bar—you can often get the amount of a veggie you need at a more affordable price and with no labor involved on your part. With a quick stroll down the aisle, you can have the makings of a great stir-fry or veggie burrito in no time.

In a Nutshell

If you don't like to use canned goods, why not cook large amounts of foods, divide them into useable portions, and then freeze them? You can do this with beans, veggies, fruits, sauces, spreads, soups, stews, and casseroles. Putting a little extra aside for another time takes very little effort, and you'll thank yourself when you're in need of a quick, healthful meal and don't have the time to prepare it from scratch.

Prepared Deli and "Grab-and-Go" Items

As an ever-increasing and expanding part of the retail market, more and more grocery and natural foods stores are including in-store bakeries and delis. If your local store has these, check to see what whole-grain breads and vegan baked goods may be available. Most natural foods stores have a larger selection and more options for you and your wallet. A hearty bread can make for some great morning toast with jam, as the base of an awesome sandwich with a yummy spread and tons of veggies, or a juicy portobello mushroom sandwich or veggie burger.

For those who have little confidence in their baking skills or who may have food allergies, the bakery in your natural foods store could be an eye-opening experience. Following the current food trends, many stores are developing new products to suit vegans, special diets, and food allergies. You should be able to find cookies, cakes, pies, and other baked goods, and some even accept special orders to alter recipes to fit your specific needs. Just ask at the counter if you don't see something vegan that suits your taste.

In a Nutshell

Do a little sampling of vegan items from the natural foods store deli to try new foods or recipes. Most items are either sold by the pound or prepackaged. Be sure to read ingredient labels or ask for the ingredients if they're not posted.

Some stores have even developed their own lines of prepared grab-and-go items, which you can usually find in either the store's deli section or with the other refrigerated items. These can be anything from prepared sandwiches, salads, spreads, side dishes, and main dishes, to entire meals. It's kind of like a healthier version of fast food! Many of these items are made with all natural and organic ingredients—you can't find that in the average burger joint. For a quick meal or a healthy addition to a meal, check out what's available in a store near you.

Packaged Refrigerated and Frozen Items

After checking for fresh options in the deli area of your local grocery or natural foods store, be sure to check for vegan foods in the refrigerated and frozen foods sections. In addition to premade meal items, you can find vegan dairy substitutes, beverages, mock meats of all kinds, vegan mayonnaise substitutes, vegan puddings, and other condiments, oils, and refrigerated products.

Look in the freezer section for frozen harvested delights such as organic juices, cut fruits, vegetables, and mixed blends. Organic food companies are now even marketing such foods as french fries, onion rings, and tater tots, and many stores stock them. Freezing captures food's freshness, halts its decay, and barring any mishaps in the freezing process, helps it retain more of its nutrients. These frozen items can help you whip up a delicious smoothie, toss together a stir-fry, or round out your plate with a veggie option.

Vegan products are often stocked in specialty areas or right next to their animal-based counterparts in many conventional supermarkets. Check for frozen waffles, veggie burgers, soy sausages, veggie burritos, appetizers, and specialty dessert items near their nonvegan counterparts. You can also find many vegan meal-type foods such as noodle or grain bowls with veggies, heat-and-serve entrées, frozen vegan pizzas, and even frozen holiday alternatives like mock turkey with all the vegan fixings.

> **Vegan 101**
>
> **Sorbet** is a usually dairy-free frozen dessert made from puréed fruit, water, and a sweetener. The French traditionally use sorbet to cleanse the palate between courses of a meal.

Last, but certainly not least, you can find vegan versions of ice cream in the freezer cases of your natural foods store and even some regular grocers. Just because you go vegan doesn't mean you have to give up your sundaes and ice cream cones! Many stores carry several types of nondairy frozen desserts to choose from, including *sorbets*, soy-based and rice-based ice creams, and even a few nut-based ice creams.

In the freezer cases, you should be able to find at least one type of vegan sorbet, produced by manufacturers such as Howler, Natural Choice, Double Rainbow, and Cascadian Farms. You'll also find one or more of the following brands of nondairy ice cream: Soy Dream, Soy Cream, Soy Delicious, Rice Dream, Sweet Nothings, Whole Soy Cultured Soy Yogurt, and Tofutti. Freezees Nutcream is made with cashew milk, making it as creamy as creamy can be. You can also find all sorts of frozen vegan novelty treats as well, like frozen chocolate-covered bananas, ice cream bars of all varieties, fudgey frozen bar treats, fruit bars, ice cream sandwiches, and even ice cream cookie sandwiches.

When purchasing prepackaged refrigerated and frozen foods, be sure to read the labels before you buy. Look for wholesome and organic ingredients in the list, and check sodium, sugar, and fat contents. This will greatly assist you in making smarter choices for fueling your engine. It really does pay to put the best-quality foods into your body if you want to get positive results out of it in the form of good health and vitality.

Snacking Wisely

Most people love to munch on a little something here and there throughout the day. It's only natural. In fact, nutritionists say it's fine to snack on the right foods at the right times; some take it a step further to say we should have five to seven small meals or snacks throughout the course of the day instead of three large meals. They feel that it makes better nutritional sense for your body to receive a more steady supply of nutrients throughout the day and that it's easier for your body to digest smaller meals. Snacking could have a positive effect on any stomach or regularity issues you might be having, in addition to helping even out spikes and dips in your blood sugar levels.

Be sure to snack wisely, though. Small meals or leftovers, a piece of raw fruit or veggies, a handful of nuts, or a few whole-grain crackers are all examples of good snacks or in-between meal munchies. Chomping down on an entire bag of chips or cookies at one sitting isn't good for your waistline, skin, or physical or mental health. And you'll probably regret the indulgence later on.

You can find more healthful versions of chips and snack foods on many store shelves. As always, check the labels to discover the ingredient and nutritional information and to help you choose between brands, if necessary, to get the best deal for your money. Baked snacks tend to have less fat and calories, so buy baked varieties over fried whenever you have the choice. Remember to avoid hydrogenated and partially hydrogenated oils in your snack foods as much as possible, and omit foods cooked in lard, butter, or ghee (clarified butter). They contain tremendous amounts of saturated fats, especially harmful trans-fatty acids. Consumption of these types of fats contributes to developing heart disease and obesity.

Snacks to Avoid

When buying packaged snacks, always read the label carefully. Steer clear of animal-based flavorings and ingredients. This is more obvious with some snack foods than with others. Many product flavors—such as sour cream, honey Dijon, nacho cheese, cheddar cheese, chili and cheese, buttered, and barbecue, just to name a few—are obviously not vegan. Also, steer clear of fried pork rinds and beef jerky. Avoid products that contain the animal ingredients we've already mentioned, too, including "natural flavors," carmine, whey, and casein. Some bean dips, fried foods, and baked snack cakes could even contain lard or beef fat. Many other products have animal ingredients buried within a long list of ingredients, so put on your reading glasses and check out the whole ingredient list. Where and when these ingredients and others pop up keeps a vegan on his or her toes when shopping for food items.

> **CAUTION**
>
> **Hot Potato**
>
> Don't go shopping on an empty stomach or when you have a bad case of the munchies! It's been proven that shopping while hungry causes you to buy more of the wrong kinds of foods. It's better to go shopping after eating a healthy meal. You'll then be better able to think with your head—not with your stomach!

If you stick with wholesome organic products, you can better avoid artificial colorings and flavorings as well as animal-based ingredients. Try to also look for low-fat and baked, not fried, snacks. Choose naturally sweetened or unrefined sugar-based snacks instead of those full of high-fructose corn syrup and bleached sugar. And don't forget fiber-rich, whole-grain, or multi-grain snack foods to help kick your metabolism into high gear!

Good Snacking Ideas

Start with a nutritious breakfast or early morning meal to get started in the right direction because how you start your morning affects your nutritional and physical snacking needs later in the day. If you eat well, you might only need a handful of nuts or dried fruit to keep you going until lunch. If you eat light or hardly anything at all, then maybe reach for a granola bar, energy or protein bar, or some raw veggies and a savory dip to help satisfy your food cravings. You can repeat this pattern of eating a larger meal followed by a smaller meal or snack throughout the day to keep eating right and satisfy your caloric and nutritional needs as well as your appetite.

Of course, at times you will want to eat a little junk food–type snack instead of a piece of fruit or other healthful treat. You may be having a party or inviting friends over to watch a movie, or maybe you are just in need of a little crunchy munching. If you take a careful look at the store shelves, you can find some great-tasting snacks that are better for you than others.

Many food companies use organic ingredients in their snack foods. A few of the companies that produce healthy savory snacks include Alpsnack, Bearitos, Garden of Eatin', Geni-Soy, Guiltless Gourmet, Newman's Own, Robert's American Gourmet, Late July, Mary's Gone Crackers, Skeet & Ike's, Kettle, Terra, Boulder, Hain, Harry's, Stacy's, and many others. You can find these products in conventional or natural foods stores from coast to coast.

Satisfying Your Vegan Sweet Tooth

A few fortunate souls out there don't really favor sweets, but most Americans do have a sweet tooth they feel obliged to satisfy from time to time. Too many of us actually let our sweet tooth control us in making most of our food choices, though. Sugary sodas, chewing gums, candies, cookies, cakes, pastries, doughnuts, and other sweet treats are part of almost everyone's daily diet in one form or another. Many of these foods are loaded with empty calories, excessive amounts of sugar and fat, and all too often, preservatives and artificial ingredients.

You can find many wholesome vegan baked goods premade in natural foods stores. Some may be made in-store while others come prepackaged. A few of our favorite brands are Alternative Baking Company, Uncle Eddie's, Goodbaker, Nana's, Health Valley, Fabe's Natural Gourmet, Sun Flour Baking Company, and Newman's Own.

> **In a Nutshell**
>
> Allison's Gourmet is a wonderful online source of completely vegan baked goods, such as scrumptious cookies, brownies, fudge, and more recently, gourmet chocolates. Her goodies are made with organic ingredients and are available in different varieties each month or as samplers. She even uses eco-friendly packaging! You can visit Allison's Gourmet on the web at www. allisonsgourmet.com.

You can also sometimes find vegan baking mixes for cakes, cookies, and other baked goods. Simple Organics makes many such products; just look for them and others in the baking aisle of your local natural foods store. In Chapter 23, we give you recipes for making a few homemade vegan baked goods and desserts that will hopefully inspire you to become your own vegan baker.

If you suffer from food allergies, natural foods stores often feature baked goods to help you satisfy your sweet tooth as well. Read labels and ingredient lists carefully to avoid unwanted ingredients, and also be aware of the nutritional information for each serving.

> **Hot Potato**
>
> Keep in mind that the price often reflects the quality of ingredients used in a product. If the price of a package of cookies or cake is only $1, you can assume that even if the ingredients are free of animal products, they are made with cheap, highly refined ingredients. Whole-grain, organic, and alternatively sweetened products usually do cost more. Compare the ingredients with the serving size and nutritional information to determine if the item is worth the extra cost to you.

Vegan Chocolate

It's a common misconception that you have to give up chocolate when you go vegan. This couldn't be further from the truth because, traditionally, chocolate is made without the use of milk or other dairy products. Most fine-quality dark chocolate is still dairy-free. (Just take a look at the ingredient list to be sure.)

Many chocolates are now made with milk, although many connoisseurs would argue such products really shouldn't be considered chocolate if milk is added to the equation. U.S. manufacturers rely on heavy amounts of cream, milk, and even butter to make their chocolaty confections. However, many European and fine chocolatiers use dairy-free dark chocolate more often in their products.

Chocolate is made from chocolate liquor, which is made up of a 50-50 blend of cocoa solids and cocoa butter. The higher the percentage of cocoa solids, the finer and darker-tasting the chocolate. Dark chocolate contains up to 75 percent cocoa solids, and sometimes a sweetener such as sugar is added. (Really good dark chocolate has a slightly bitter taste as it melts on your tongue.) Additional flavorings can be added if desired, along with a stabilizer such as lecithin to help the chocolate form into a bar or mold.

If you look, you can find some really excellent vegan chocolates and chocolate products. For use in baking, you can find vegan chocolate chips in most stores. Many semisweet brands are already dairy-free, and in natural foods stores you can find brands such as Sunspire, Dagoba, Tropical Source, and Ghirardelli. You may even be able to find some of these brands in bulk as well.

> **In a Nutshell**
>
> Dark chocolate contains more flavonoids and antioxidants than white or milk chocolate, as well as up to four times the amount of polyphenols and catechins as red wine and green tea. These substances help protect your body against cancer and heart disease and lower your blood pressure and cholesterol levels.

For stocking stuffers, Valentine's Day, Easter, special occasions, or whenever you need a chocolate fix, check out any of several yummy vegan chocolate bars available. Vegan-friendly brands include Endangered Species, Dagoba, Green & Black's, Newman's Own, Tropical Source, Conscious Creations, Ecco Bella, Chocolate Decadence, Cloud Nine, Terra Nostra, and Rapunzel.

Vegan chocolate bars come in all sorts of flavors, such as almond, hazelnut, peanut butter, raspberry, truffle, espresso, orange, mint, and chili. You can chop these bars and use them to garnish desserts, top nondairy ice creams, or use in place of chocolate chips in your vegan baked goods.

> **In a Nutshell**
>
> Chimp Mints are little squares of delicious mint-flavored vegan dark chocolate. Made by Oregon-based Endangered Species Chocolate Company, it is a fair trade product made with organic ingredients. All the proceeds from these tasty bits go to the Jane Goodall Institute to help the chimps that are part of her rescue efforts. Each piece of chocolate also comes with a trading card featuring one of the chimps and his or her life story.

Vegan Candy

Most candies are nothing more than sugar, flavoring, and coloring, yet they can trigger childhood memories and bring instant giggles of delight. And you might be surprised to learn plenty of your childhood favorites are vegan. They're not necessarily good for you or free of artificial ingredients, but they *are* free of animal products.

Here is a partial list of "old school" vegan candy options for the sugar fiend, according to PETA's petakids.com website:

- Airheads Taffy
- Charms Blow Pops and Lollipops
- Chick-o-Sticks
- Cracker Jack
- Dots
- Dum-Dums
- Fireballs
- Goldberg's Peanut Chews
- Hot Tamales
- Jolly Ranchers
- Jujubees and Jujyfruits
- Lemonheads
- Mambas
- Mary Janes
- Mike and Ike
- Now and Later
- Pez
- Ring Pop Lollipops
- Smarties (U.S. brand)
- Sour Patch Kids
- Starburst
- Super Bubble
- Swedish Fish
- Sweet Tarts
- Twizzlers
- Zotz

Many natural foods stores now sell a new wave of candies flavored with fruit juices and other unrefined sweeteners instead of sugar. Let's Do Organic makes vegan Gummi Bears in several flavors. Sharkies Organic energy fruit chews are a similar gummy-style chew. St. Claire's makes mints and tarts to flavor and freshen your breath, and Organic Candy Company makes hard candies of all sorts.

For those who like chewy candy treats, check out fruit leathers, Wha Guru Chews, Panda or Tubi's licorices, and ginger candies made by several companies, including Ginger People and Reed's. You can even find sprinkles for your sundaes and desserts by Let's Do Organic in chocolate and multi-colored confetti varieties.

As you can see, sweet vegan options abound!

The Least You Need to Know

◆ Dairy-free frozen desserts such as ice creams, sorbets, and novelty products abound. Check the freezer cases of your natural foods stores and conventional grocers.

◆ Many prepared and packaged vegan food options on the shelves of your local market can make it easier for you to eat right when you don't have much time to cook.

◆ When reading product ingredient lists, be on the lookout for animal ingredients labeled as "natural flavors," cochineal extract, whey, gelatin, and others.

◆ Seek out the healthiest options when buying snack foods, but if you're in the mood for more of an indulgence, you do have many vegan options.

◆ Dark chocolate is normally made without the use of milk or other dairy products. Many fine vegan brands of chocolate are just waiting for you at your natural foods store.

Part 5

Substitution Is the Mother of Invention

If you don't eat meat and dairy, whatever will you eat? Have no fear! Many plant-based substitutes are available, with an endless array of uses.

In Part 5, you learn about the magical soybean, which you can use to replace meat, dairy products, eggs, and flours and starches, while providing protein, carbohydrates, calcium, and many other vital nutrients. Learn how to mimic with mock meats, nondairy milks, and cheese substitutes, and discover some of the available prepackaged brands. We also give you some pointers on revamping baking recipes; hints on replacing eggs, butter, and milk with ease; and tips to make things "gel" as a vegan and sweeten your treats to perfection!

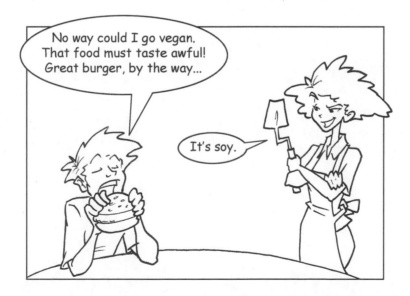

Using Protein Alternatives

In This Chapter

- ◆ Suggestions for using soy products
- ◆ Preparing beans, grains, and greens
- ◆ Understanding and serving seitan
- ◆ Using mock meats to mimic

It's our hope that by the time you reach this point in the book, you've already begun to feel secure about the issue of getting enough protein and are also familiar with which vegan foods can supply it. In this chapter, we take a look at using store-bought protein sources in your cooking, and we clear up any confusion you may still have about the products on your grocery store or natural foods store shelves. Then, in Chapters 20 through 23, we provide you with some recipes that will enable you to make some of your own homemade vegan protein powerhouses.

Cooking with Beans, Grains, and Greens

Many cultures, past and present, have sustained themselves on a diet that relies heavily on beans, grains, and greens as sources of protein, among other nutrients. Italians often eat polenta, rice, and pasta with stewed beans such as cannellini, chickpeas, Roman beans, and peas. Greens such as escarole, spinach, or Rainbow chard are enjoyed with aromatics, seasonings, fresh herbs, and olive oil. Eastern Europeans and those who live in the British Isles nourish themselves with kasha, oats, and noodles, with kale, cabbage, and other hardy greens. They also use peas, lentils, white beans, and red beans in many of their standard dishes.

In the Pacific, rice and noodles are eaten at most meals with vegetables and greens such as spinach, bok choy, and cabbage. Cooks there use soybeans in thousands of ways, and black beans and aduki beans are also used whole and to make sauces and desserts. In the Americas, a majority of foods use corn, wild rice, quinoa, and other wild-growing seeds and grain. Many native peoples developed and harvested hundreds of varieties of beans, root vegetables, and grasses. Flavorful items such as carrots, onions, herbs, dandelion, cress, and chicory are used to flavor and supplement the cooking pot.

Beans, grains, and greens are often thought of as simple and hearty "peasant foods." However, you can also use them to make gourmet fare, such as bean and roasted veggie croquettes on a bed of millet, basmati, and wild rice pilaf, with a side of chard and radicchio sautéed in chili-flavored olive oil with shallots, garlic, and sliced almonds. Sounds yummy, doesn't it? Or you can make a simple lentil and spinach soup flavored with tarragon and thyme. Stir in some small orzo pasta or brown basmati rice toward the end of the cooking time. And don't forget the traditional New Year's good luck meal of black-eyed peas and greens simmered with the "holy trinity" of Southern cooking: onions, celery, and peppers. Serve this delicious concoction with rice and cornbread—*mmm!*

Cooking a Crock o' Beans

Many people are intimidated by cooking beans, maybe because they experienced gas after eating them or maybe because they didn't season them well or fully cook them the last time. Beans do get a bad rep, but they shouldn't; they're delicious when prepared with care; nutritiously high in protein, complex carbohydrates, and B vitamins; and low in fat and calories. They're also extremely affordable in cost-per-pound comparison with nonvegan protein sources such as meat, eggs, and dairy.

You can find precooked beans in cans at most stores, and they're good to keep on hand for making quick and easy meals. However, buying dry beans in bulk or prepackaged is really the cheapest way to purchase them. Remember to sort your dry beans to remove dirt, rocks, and other debris. Some people like to do this in a colander. We like to sort beans on a large plate, in small batches, moving small amounts from one side to the other. This way we can easily and fully see any foreign material. After you've sorted through the beans, place them in a colander and rinse them under running water.

CAUTION

Hot Potato _____

A big mistake some people make while cooking beans is not cooking them in enough water or for long enough to get them fully tender. Eating undercooked beans can cause gas, abdominal pains, or both. Some people like to soak their beans first, discard the water, and then start with new water when cooking them. Soaking can reduce cooking time and potentially eliminate excess gas, but it is not a necessary step.

Here's how you can make a basic batch of beans:

1. Start with the largest and heaviest pot you have in your kitchen. Place your beans inside; cover them with at least 4 to 6 inches of filtered water; and bring the water to a boil.

2. Reduce heat, cover, and simmer for 1 to 3 hours or until the beans are tender.

3. Add additional water as the beans cook, as needed, so they remain covered with water.

The size and variety of the beans you cook determine the length of cooking time needed to fully cook the beans until tender. The best ways to tell if your beans are tender are to taste them or squish a cooked bean between your fingers. When the beans are fully soft, they're done.

You can fully cool cooked beans, portion them into small containers, and freeze them for use in quick meals later. This is a great economical alternative to using canned beans, particularly if you are using organic beans.

In a Nutshell

Some people like to add a piece of kombu, which is a sea vegetable, to the pot when cooking beans because it can help reduce gas and make beans more tender. Also, using a pressure cooker to cook beans can be a time-saver if you happen to own one.

Deeply Ingrained in Grains

Cooking grains is a lot like cooking beans as it requires a good deal of water or other liquids to soften the grains or kernels. Preparing grains is based on ratios of moisture to dry product; sometimes it's 1:1, others 1½:1 or 2:1 or a variation thereof when you're cooking large quantities of grains.

Don't be afraid to try new grain varieties you may never have eaten. Instead of buying long-grain rice every time, why not try a different variety such as basmati, jasmine, wehani, texmati, or a completely different type of grain altogether? When you're feeling a little adventurous, explore your store's bulk or prepackaged grains sections, and see what appeals to you.

In a Nutshell

Lundberg Family Farms was one of the early pioneers of organic rice growing in the United States. Since the 1960s, Lundberg has used organic and sustainable growing practices that they call "nutra-farming" in producing their rice. Today, they sell a wide variety of healthy rice varieties, including brown, wehani, basmati, black japonica, jasmine, and many others. They also offer a wide assortment of other rice products, many of which are suitable for vegans.

Most grains packages list cooking directions; when buying in bulk, check for directions near the bin. Also use cookbooks and the Internet for inspiration and ideas. Some people like to toast their grains, in a dry pan or with some oil, to bring out a nutty flavor. They then add the liquid and proceed with the cooking procedure.

You can cook your grains in filtered water, fruit or vegetable juices, vegetable stock, or coconut milk; add seasonings and herbs either prior to or after cooking. Adding some vegetables, greens, beans, or other protein can turn a simple pot of grains into a one-pot meal.

Greenery Gastronomy

Greens and all their wonderful fiber are a vegan's and dieter's dream. No matter what the variety, greens are low in fat and loaded with flavor and vitamins. Greens such as spinach and broccoli are surprisingly high in protein. Chop raw greens to make salads and slaws or add crunch to other dishes. You can even make a raw burrito by using large leaves to encase a wide assortment of your favorite raw fillings.

Some people like to stew or simmer greens in broth or water for a long time to make them so tender they fall apart. If you do this, don't discard the cooking liquid as it contains many vitamins that the cooking greens released. Drink it, sop it up with bread, or use it to add flavor to soups and stews.

Eating greens raw preserves most of their nutrients, so that's the best way to eat them. You could also sauté or stir-fry them in a little oil, alone or with other vegetables, until crisp tender or just tender. Their colors should remain bright and not turn drab and dull. Most greens are delicious when sautéed in a little olive oil with garlic and seasoned with salt, pepper, and red pepper flakes for a little kick!

Demystifying Soy Products

Soy products may be new to you, but they were developed in China centuries ago and have been used there and all over the world ever since. We have many dedicated chefs and "health nuts" to thank for taking soy to new heights in the United States. Their kitchen experiments—playing around with different cooking, cutting, and preparation techniques and trying different flavorings and seasonings with tofu—helped produce some amazing soy-based products, recipe ideas, and cookbooks. These early pioneers further inspired others to give soy a chance. They, in turn, shared the soy message and culinary ideas with other hungry souls, and the Western soy-foods phenomenon began to spread. By pushing their culinary creativity, chefs and home cooks continue to add to the popularity of soy foods and further cement them as a staple in the global diet.

Soy products confuse many people because they come in so many different forms. You can purchase soy sauce, miso or fermented soybean paste, soy flour, soy grits or flakes, tofu, or tempeh. Soy products appear as meat analogs and mock meats, soy milks, soy cheeses, soy-based dairy replacements, soy-based sauces and soups, and soy ice creams.

> **In a Nutshell**
>
> Soy is extremely versatile, easily grown throughout the world, capable of filling many of our nutritional needs, and very affordable as a food source. There's no wonder, in an effort to fight world hunger and malnourishment, more and more people across the globe are adding soy products to their daily diets and food supplies.

Gettin' Saucy: Soy Sauce

Soy sauce is a commonly used condiment and flavoring agent made from a fermented soybean mash. It comes in several varieties:

♦ **Tamari.** A rich-tasting soy sauce made from fermented miso, or from soybeans, salt, water, and koji (a beneficial mold), and usually aged for 2 years.

♦ **Shoyu.** Made the same way as tamari, but with the addition of wheat.

♦ **Nama Shoyu.** A raw version of shoyu with many live enzymes still intact.

♦ **Bragg Liquid Aminos.** Used as a substitute for traditional soy sauces, it contains all essential and many nonessential amino acids.

In general, you can freely substitute any of these soy sauces for another in recipes.

The Incredible Tofu

Tofu is one of the most amazing soy foods. A coagulant is added to creamy soy milk and then the curds and whey are separated as in traditional cheese-making. The result is silky, protein-rich tofu. This soft-textured tofu—often packaged as soft, silken, or silken-style tofu—is used to make purées and desserts (which will be discussed further in Chapter 19).

> **In a Nutshell**
>
> Tofu is often referred to as being "spongelike," for several reasons. It does have a spongelike texture; tiny holes are often visible within the soybean curd. Also, like a sponge, you can squeeze out excess moisture from tofu and soak up other liquids with it.

Other blocks of tofu are pressed to varying degrees to remove excess water to form firm and extra-firm varieties. Firm and extra-firm tofu are more suitable for use in making cubes, strips, cutlets, and substantial fillings, sandwiches, and entrées.

If you've never tried tofu or cooked with it before, don't be intimidated. Tofu is easier to work with than you might think. First squeeze out as much of the water that it was packaged with as you can. Cut the tofu into cubes, strips, big cutlet-size pieces, or whatever you desire. You can then bake it, broil it, fry it, grill it, or use a combination of these methods.

You might have heard people say tofu is bland, scary looking, and tasteless. These folks must have just had a badly prepared tofu dish or tried to eat it straight from the package. Well-prepared and flavored tofu can be heavenly, amazingly pungent and chewy, and a wonder to behold when prepared by a tofu master or talented chef!

When it comes to flavoring ideas, remember tofu's spongelike qualities. It will absorb whatever you throw at it or bathe it in, and the tofu will take on and further develop those flavors during the cooking process. You can't go wrong with using a little tamari or other form of soy sauce. Then choose an oil such as olive oil, toasted sesame oil, or a flavored oil to prevent sticking and to add flavor.

Sea salt, black pepper, turmeric, chili powder, and dried and fresh herbs such as basil, parsley, dill, and thyme all impart great flavor to your tofu. But don't stop there! Shake on a little of this, a dash of that, and you can come up with some new combinations of your own. Use barbecue sauce, tomato sauce, gravy, and other creamy toppings to make some savory flavor combinations and hearty meals when paired with some grains and veggies.

> ### In a Nutshell
>
> Nutritional yeast gives your tofu, or tempeh for that matter, a nutty, cheesy, or savory flavor. You can add it to marinades, sprinkle it on top of a dish, add it to dry breading ingredients, or use it as part of a seasoning mixture. (See Chapter 6 for more on nutritional yeast.)

Tempting with Tempeh

For someone who is new to soy products, tofu may seem a little odd upon first sight, but tempeh may appear even stranger. As you first gaze at it through the plastic packaging, you may think it has gone bad, with its colorful mold marbling and odd texture. But don't be scared. It may look like a child's science project gone awry, but it tastes absolutely wonderful. Think of it as the blue cheese of the soy world; after all, it is injected with mold spores and fermented in much the same way. The result is a highly digestible, fermented soybean cake that has an earthy flavor often described as being meaty, beefy, or mushroomy.

Tempeh is fabulous when crumbled or cubed and used in recipes commonly calling for beef. Try it in tomato sauces, chili, stroganoff, and hearty stews. Flavor and season it very much like tofu, with tamari and olive or toasted sesame oil. It can also easily handle more assertive herbs and spices such as rosemary, tarragon, cayenne, and curry powder. Large cutlets of tempeh make for delicious sandwiches, either baked or fried, and they can become great burgers, hoagies, and patty melts.

Better yet, you can make a tempeh reuben. Start by mixing soy mayonnaise, a little ketchup and relish, and some seasonings to make the creamy dressing. Then cook some tempeh cutlets that you have marinated in tamari and oil, toast some rye bread, and begin assembling your sandwich. Add your choice of toppings such as sauerkraut, tomato slices, lettuce, spinach, onions, avocado, soy cheese slices, or soy mock bacon or Canadian bacon. You can eat it after assembling or place it under a broiler for a few minutes to heat all the ingredients. Then roll up your sleeves, tuck in your napkin, and dive in to one fantastic vegan sandwich!

Playing Tricks with TVP

Textured vegetable protein, or TVP, is one of the easiest meat substitutes to use and keep on hand. You can purchase it in the bulk section of many stores in small flakes or granules or big, chunklike pellets. This type of TVP is easily stored in airtight containers for long periods of time and is easily rehydrated in liquid, making it great for traveling or camping.

CAUTION

Hot Potato

TVP can be stored for extended periods of time in its dry state, but as soon as it's rehydrated, you must refrigerate it and treat it as you would any perishable cooked food.

Recently a new prepackaged form of TVP has hit the shelves. Marketed as "ground" or "crumbles" by several companies such as Boca Burger, Morning Star, and Yves Veggie Cuisine, these come ready to use, flavored, in several varieties, and can be found refrigerated or frozen in many stores. You can easily use them as ground meat replacements, in making burgers or loaves, or stir them into sauces, stews, chilies, and entrées. The texture and flavor of these products in dishes will fool most people who will swear they're eating meat, not a soy substitute.

Mimicking with Mock Meats

If you happen to be a vegan who misses the "meaty-tasting" items in your diet, you don't have to do without. In your grocer's freezer or refrigerator cases, you can find vegan replacements for many of your childhood favorites. Craving a hot dog or hamburger? No problem, simply choose from several brands of soy-based hot dogs or burgers made with ingredients such as vegetables, grains, mushrooms, and soy products. You can also find sliced deli "meats" in bologna, ham, or turkey flavors. How about a few slices of mock Canadian bacon, pepperoni, meatballs, or sausages in spicy Italian, breakfast, or brat styles? Or maybe you're hankering for some jaw-stiffening vegan jerky? You can find that as well.

Want to have a supersize vegan hoagie or throw a tailgate party or other casual get-together? Get some vegan sliced deli meats, and go to town! Start with some hearty bread or rolls and then begin layering different varieties of slices, alternating with vegan sliced cheeses and crunchy vegetables. Sprinkle on some seasonings, and pour a great dressing over the top. You can't find anything like that in your neighborhood sub shop!

You can also take the same ingredients and turn them into a mock meat and cheese platter or an antipasto tray. Or use them to create some snazzy appetizers such as the classic pepperoni-cheese-cracker combo or a fancy version of "pigs in a blanket" using vegan ingredients. For a show-stopper, take a spear of asparagus, wrap it in Canadian bacon or a ham-style slice with a little soy cheese and a smear of Dijon mustard, and then encase the entire little package in phyllo dough and bake until crispy. This is guaranteed to wow the eyes and taste buds!

You can even host your own vegan barbecue bash. Just buy a grill of your very own (so you don't have to share with the meaty grill), and cook some grilled veggies, ears of corn, veggie burgers, and vegan hot dogs. Make a big pasta, potato, or green salad with a wide assortment of colorful raw veggies and fresh dressing. You can even have s'mores for dessert by using vegan graham crackers (try Health Valley Amaranth Graham Crackers), vegan marshmallows (which you can purchase in natural foods stores or online), and your choice of vegan chocolate. Prepare them like you did when you were a kid, and enjoy!

Seitan in Your Supper

Seitan, also known as wheat meat, is a delicious meat substitute made from the protein portion, or gluten, of wheat flour. It is nutritious, has zero cholesterol, and has little or no fat. Seitan has a firm, chewy texture that works well in recipes that call for meat.

You can find several varieties of prepared seitan, either plain, seasoned, or in sauces, made by companies such as White Wave and Lightlife Foods, in the refrigerated and freezer sections of many stores. Use them to make sandwiches, spreads, and salads. Toss in some seitan strips or chunks in your stir-frys, soups, stews, pasta or grain dishes, and entrées for a chewy and nutritious addition.

Tofurky is a widely distributed brand of seitan-based turkey alternative that manages to look and taste a lot like turkey. The manufacturer even sells a complete vegan holiday meal,

> **In a Nutshell**
>
> Make a mock chicken salad by mixing cooked seitan, diced celery, onion, and herbs with a little soy mayonnaise. Add some sliced almonds or shredded carrot for color and texture, and serve on whole-grain toast!

including gravy, stuffing, "wishstix," and dumplings. It's quite popular among vegetarians and vegans who are looking for a good turkey substitute at holiday time. Tofurky also markets an assortment of vegan deli slices, sausages, and jerky.

Now&Zen also offers a vegan UnTurkey Feast, as well as a wide range of seitan-based mock meat products such as UnChicken, UnSteak, and UnRibs. The Field Roast Grain Meat Company makes "grain meats" such as vegan sausages, deli slices, loaves, cutlets, and a stuffed celebration loaf suitable for the holiday season as well. Similar to seitan, it is made with a mixture of vital wheat gluten and other grains, vegetables, legumes, and seasonings.

You can even make homemade seitan with vital wheat gluten, available in most baking aisles or bulk bin sections. In Chapter 22, we give you a recipe to make your own Baked Seitan Roast. The Seitan Roast also makes a fabulous sandwich: thinly slice and layer the roast onto a large roll, and then serve it with the seitan cooking liquid, *au jus* style. Or go with a creamy gravy like the Groovy Onion Gravy and serve it with a side of Mouthwatering Mashed Potatoes (both recipes are in Chapter 22). Or cut the roast into cubes, strips, cutlets, make it into breaded treats, and on and on. Seitan has endless uses!

The Least You Need to Know

- ◆ Cooking with beans, grains, and greens is an easy and delicious way to add whole, natural sources of protein and other nutrients to your vegan meals.

- ◆ Prepared mock meats can provide vegan replacements for many of your meaty childhood favorites; look in your grocer's freezer or refrigerator cases to see what's available.

- ◆ Using an assortment of available soy products such as tofu, tempeh, and TVP can make it easy for you to prepare convenient and protein-rich meals.

- ◆ Using seitan in your meals, either purchased frozen or made at home, is a great way to add a "meaty" texture to your meatless dishes.

Doing Without Dairy and Cheese

In This Chapter

◆ Sampling various brands of vegan cheese

◆ Replacing and substituting dairy products

◆ Comparing butter, margarine, and oils

◆ Making your own cheesy creations

◆ Demystifying hydrogenated fats

Often, while talking with someone about what you do and don't eat as a vegan, she'll say something such as, "Oh, I could probably give up meat, but not cheese and ice cream. I would miss them too much!" By now, you know how to enlighten such people about the vegan alternatives that exist for all these products, including what's available and their health advantages over the traditional versions.

In this chapter, you learn more about how to substitute for dairy ingredients in your day-to-day eating, cooking, and baking. Some ingredients such as butter and milk are easy to replace, but others may be a bit trickier or take some getting used to. Don't expect the same end results with vegan substitutes you may have had with dairy products (like the browning or stringy characteristics of melted cheese, for instance). Some vegan items are very close, though!

Butter, Margarine, and Oils

It takes more than 2 gallons of milk to make a single pound of butter. Everything that's bad about whole milk is multiplied many times over in butter. It is a high concentration of saturated fats, and indulging in it can raise your cholesterol levels, increase your risk of cardiovascular disease (among other diseases), and lead to obesity. It's no wonder, then, that there's such a huge market for healthier alternatives to butter.

> **CAUTION**
>
> **Hot Potato**
>
> The average dairy cow produces 200,000 glasses of milk in a lifetime, which could be used to produce 12,500 pounds of butter. Aside from all the cow has to go through to produce that much milk, think of all of that artery-clogging saturated fat!

Unfortunately, most commercially available margarines aren't any better than butter and can contain just as much saturated fat, and worse. Read labels to be sure of what you're actually getting. Some margarine brands even contain whey or other dairy derivatives, so don't assume a product is vegan just because you see the word *margarine* on the label. Also, look for vegan brands such as Soy Garden that contain little or no trans-fatty acids and are nonhydrogenated. These products tend to be whipped and available in plastic tubs instead of in sticks. If you're going to use margarine at all, it should really be this variety.

The better choice over margarine and butter is the use of heart-healthy plant-based oils such as olive, safflower, flax, sesame, sunflower, and pumpkinseed. You can use these in many forms of baking and cooking, often with better results than with hardened fats such as margarine or vegetable shortening. If you were going to melt them down anyway in the preparation of your recipe, using a liquid form actually saves you time and effort. You can use margarine in cookies, pie crusts, and frostings, if you want, but oils can also work well in most cases.

Choose your oil by the recipe, the other ingredients in it, and the preparation technique you will be using. Olive oil works well in and on practically everything, so you can't go wrong keeping it well stocked in your pantry. Buy extra virgin and organic for the best flavor and the most health benefits. Store it away from light, keep the bottle tightly sealed, and don't keep it for more than a year as it will turn rancid.

What's *Hydrogenated* Mean?

Food labels contain some very confusing ingredients, particularly when it comes to fats. *Cold-pressed, expeller-pressed, partially hydrogenated, hydrogenated, nonhydrogenated*—all these terms can appear before oils and other fats on the nutritional labels of your favorite foods. *Cold-pressed* and *expeller-pressed* are both desirable terms in regard to how your oil has been processed, so seek out products with these words on the label whenever possible. But when you get to hydrogenated, read carefully because what comes before it can be very important. If the word appears at all, you want it to read *non*hydrogenated.

Hydrogenated fats, or trans fats, are the man-made "bad fats" that clog your arteries and lead to heart disease. Back when scientists were playing around with the development of margarine, they learned to use hydrogen to suspend fat molecules to make them become more saturated and hardened. Hardening was important to the nature of the product, and suspending molecules to hold or bind food together seemed all right in theory.

Unfortunately, because hydrogenated fats were something completely new in the history of the planet, the end result was quite harmful. Our bodies were and continue to be confused by hydrogenated fats. They don't recognize them as normal fats, so they don't process them accordingly for energy and fuel. Instead, these fats go directly into fat storage supplies and end up clogging arteries and adding inches to the hips and waistline. They also raise your bad cholesterol levels and decrease your good cholesterol levels. They're basically the worst kind of fat you could possibly put into your body!

> **In a Nutshell**
>
> Many vegan and vegetarian food companies are aware of the negative effects of hydrogenated fats and don't use them in their production. They often proudly draw attention to the presence of minimally processed expeller-pressed, cold-pressed, nonhydrogenated, and organic oils in their products, right on the front of their labels. This can make healthy and wise vegan shopping much easier!

The Functions of Fats

Fats function as a lubricant for your body's inner workings—similar to what they do in cooking and baking—in addition to a few other things as well. The slick characteristic of fats makes them useful in dressings, marinades, and sauces, where they provide flavor and mobility to ingredients. In baking, fats add layers between the starch or grain molecules that provide flavor and flakiness to cookies, pastries, and pie crusts.

Fats also provide a certain richness or mouth-feel to foods. But you don't need a lot of fat in your foods to achieve this sensation, which is where many cooks go wrong. Fats should flavor and not overpower or overwhelm the food. Excessively oily or greasy foods are unappealing, unappetizing, and usually bad-tasting. Start with small amounts of fat, and add more only as needed.

You could cut part of the fat called for by replacing it with other liquid ingredients such as water, juices, soy milk, or fruit purées that would complement the recipe. Cutting out additional fats in foods wherever possible is good for your waistline and your heart. It can also allow for a more guilt-free consumption of dessert if you pass up the greasy french fries or chips with your meal.

Using Nondairy Milk Substitutes

As we mentioned in Chapter 6, and as you may know from your own purchases, some truly amazing alternatives to milk, cream, yogurt, sour cream, cream cheeses, and other dairy products fill grocery store shelves. You can find products made from soy, rice, nuts, grains, and combinations thereof in most dairy cases, right next to their animal-based cousins. Availability varies from store to store and from state to state, so those living in more veg-friendly areas will have more of a selection.

Read labels and compare brands to see which ones best suit your personal tastes and needs. Some are thicker than others and come sweetened, unsweetened, plain, or flavored, so you are bound to have fun in the sampling process. These vegan versions work as fine substitutes and can help provide a thick, creamy texture to beverages, smoothies, light sauces, soups, stews, curries, and desserts.

Hot Potato

Using powdered soy beverages in recipes may yield slightly different results than when using soy, rice, or grain milks. Powdered beverages tend to be a bit watery, so you may need to increase the amount of powder used to create a thicker version suitable for your use.

Measure for Measure

You won't have to do a lot of tinkering or measurement altering when using vegan ingredients, especially when you use soy milks, rice milks, and other nondairy beverages. They usually work measure for measure as a milk substitute, and you'll find that they impart the same thick and creamy texture to your dishes. Soy-based yogurts, sour creams, and cream cheeses usually cause few problems when used measure for measure for their dairy counterparts.

If you don't think you'd be able to use an entire container of soy milk, for example, you're in luck. Soy powders and soy protein powders are available; just reconstitute and enjoy! These beverages make refreshing drinks on their own, or use them in sauces, dressings, soups, savory dishes, and desserts.

Using What, Where?

So how do you know what type of nondairy substitute to use and in what recipe to use it, particularly if your kitchen and cooking in general are new to you? Start with the liquid beverages, as they're easy to use. They add creaminess to your soups, sauces, and libations just as milk or cream would. You can thicken them with a roux or starch or thin to suit your needs and uses.

Use soy yogurt just like regular yogurt in recipes such as *raita*, curry, desserts, and smoothies, or enjoy with your morning granola and fruit. Look for soy yogurts manufactured by Whole Soy, White Wave, and Nancy's. Tofutti and several private label companies make vegan versions of sour cream and cream cheese. You can also use soy yogurt, sour cream, and cream cheese to add creaminess to sauces and dressings or in dessert recipes in place of their dairy counterparts.

> **Vegan 101**
>
> A **raita** is an Indian salad traditionally comprised of raw veggies, yogurt, and seasonings and served as a cool accompaniment to main dishes.

Whether you buy sweetened or unsweetened nondairy milks is a personal choice, but consider these thoughts: for use in soups, stews, and baked goods, it's best to stick with a plain variety or perhaps even vanilla in some cases. The other flavors, such as chocolate, carob, or nut varieties all work well in beverages, smoothies, and desserts. But feel free to experiment; cooking and baking is all based on personal preferences and tastes, so have fun and enjoy!

Prepackaged Vegan Cheeses

Americans are obsessed with cheese. They melt it on everything; nibble it up in chunks, slices, and wedges; and use it as everything from a sprinkled garnish to a heaping standalone side dish. Fortunately for vegans, quite a few nondairy cheeses exist, although availability varies from region to region. Nondairy cheeses really come in handy when you're missing the taste and feel of cheese or when you're craving a creamy addition to your meal.

Some nondairy cheese brands such as Tofutti Soy-Cheese Slices or Soymage Vegan Singles are presliced and ready to eat on a sandwich. Others come in unsliced or block form, as do Vegan Rella and Soymage Vegan, two of the most widely available brands of such vegan cheeses in the United States. Soymage Vegan also makes a vegan cream cheese, sour cream, and a Parmesan-style cheese suitable for sprinkling on pasta or pizza.

The best unsliced vegan cheese we've found so far is a brand called Vegan Gourmet Cheese Alternative, marketed by Follow Your Heart. Most vegans are in search of a cheese that melts and tastes delicious, and this one truly does both. It comes in mozzarella, cheddar, and Monterey Jack flavors. Shred fine strands onto your next pizza and then bake it until browned, bubbling, and gooey! Or sandwich thin slices of this cheese between slices of whole-grain bread for an incredible vegan grilled cheese sandwich or with other vegan goodies for a patty melt sandwich.

For those who couldn't have made it through grade school or college without macaroni and cheese, try some of Road's End Organics' several varieties of boxed macaroni and cheese. It tastes just like you remember—but better—and it's vegan! Marketed under the name Road's End Organics Chreese, you can purchase it in several flavors such as the classic elbows with vegan cheddar, shells, or even numbers for the kids at heart. Chreese also comes in some gluten-free varieties. Road's End Organics also produces some vegan gravy mixes and nacho chreese dips.

> ### In a Nutshell
>
> The average American cheese lover consumes more than 30 pounds of cheese per year. The average vegan doesn't even come close to eating that quantity of vegan cheese in a year's time, but if he did, he would only get a fraction of the saturated fat and none of the cholesterol.
>
> Some natural foods stores make their own brand of vegan cheeses or carry their own private label products, so take a look around and see what may be available!

Making Your Own Cheese Alternatives

If you don't have access to vegan cheeses in your area or you don't like the varieties available locally, you can always try making your own. It's actually pretty easy, and you can control what ingredients go into your vegan cheese.

You can usually find vegan cookbooks with recipes in your local library and bookstores. These can help you get started making vegan cheese. Joanne Stepaniak has written several great books with recipes for homemade vegan cheeses, sauces, dips, and spreads. Our favorites are *The Nutritional Yeast Cookbook* and *The Uncheese Cookbook*. You can also find many helpful vegan recipes online, including at vegsource.com and veganchef.com.

Getting Saucy

The simplest cheese substitute to make is a mock cheese sauce. In Chapter 20 we give you a basic recipe to get you started called Vegan Cheesy Sauce. It's rich and creamy and flavored with oh-so-cheesy nutritional yeast.

You can jazz it up with a little hot sauce, chili powder, wine, or additional shredded premade vegan cheese. Adding more paprika or chili powder deepens the color of the sauce; leaving them out makes it lighter. Stirring in a little Dijon or whole-grain mustard or black or white pepper gives it zip. The sauce takes on a more savory flavor with the addition of fresh herbs such as parsley, thyme, dill, and basil.

Vegan cheese sauce is excellent as a dipper for bread, like a fondue, or as a sauce over veggies, pasta, grains, mashed potatoes, or tofu. Drizzle it over sandwiches or pizza for a melted gooey treat!

Firming Things Up

Do you want your vegan cheese spreadable or sliceable? You can vary the consistency and firmness of your vegan cheese by using different coagulants. Nut butters and seed pastes, such as cashew butter and raw tahini, lend creaminess and texture to crock-style vegan cheese spreads. Starches such as *arrowroot* and cornstarch can help bind your cheese into a block, suitable for cutting into soft chunks or slices.

Agar-agar, which comes from the sea and is used as a vegan type of gelatin, is your best choice for firming your cheesy creations. It really solidifies and holds your vegan cheese together to produce nice, even slices when cutting. (We discuss the wonders of agar-agar further in Chapter 19.)

> **Vegan 101**
>
> **Arrowroot** is a starch obtained from the tubers of the tropical herb *Maranta arundinacea*. Used primarily as a thickener, arrowroot tubers are sometimes also eaten whole as a vegetable. The word is derived from the Arawak word *aru-aru*, meaning "meal of meals."

For more recipes to make crock or spreadable types of cheese, blocks, and sliceable cheeses, check out Joanne Stepaniak's books, other cookbooks, and online. You're bound to find a few cheesy creations you and your family will love!

The Least You Need to Know

♦ You can generally substitute vegan versions of dairy products measure for measure for their nondairy counterparts.

♦ When it comes to using fats, favor heart-healthy oils over those containing lots of saturated and hydrogenated fats.

♦ Quite a few vegan-friendly nondairy cheeses are suitable for vegans and can help when you're missing the taste and feel of cheese or craving a creamy addition to your meal.

♦ Make your own vegan cheesy creations, from creamy sauces to solid slices, with a little know-how and the right ingredients.

19

Vegan Baking Substitutions

In This Chapter

- ◆ Taking the dairy out of baking
- ◆ Firming up without gelatin
- ◆ Getting sweet with vegan sweeteners
- ◆ Substituting for eggs in recipes
- ◆ Using tofu in your baking

Many people believe you have to use butter, milk, and eggs to make delicious baked goods and you simply can't do without those traditional staples. Actually, vegan baking produces a variety of rich and delicious baked goods that could easily rival the best any traditional baker has to offer! Of course, how well an item turns out has a lot to do with the quality of the ingredients and the skill of the baker. Vegan baking usually begins with high-quality ingredients, so you will already be off to a good start. Now all you need to learn is a little about cooking and baking terms and some vegan baking substitutions—that's where this chapter comes in!

Vegan baking relies on a lot of seemingly magical chemical reactions with leaveners, binders, flours, fats, and fat replacements. Don't let that intimidate you; that's how all baking is, vegan or not. With a little practice and patience, you will become the wizard of your vegan kitchen. Then you can enjoy the fruits of your labor and even proudly share your creations with others to show them how delicious vegan eating can be!

> **CAUTION**
>
> **Hot Potato** _____
>
> Hey, don't be so quick to get rid of that old cookbook! Many of us learned to bake from Betty Crocker–type cookbooks, and we often have fond memories of some of those recipes. Those old favorites or sentimental dishes can be a lot of fun to try to veganize, so don't necessarily get rid of all of your vegan-unfriendly cookbooks yet. They can still give you ideas and help spark your culinary creativity!

Being Butter-Free

It's helpful to understand the role the fat, seasoning, starch, or acid is playing in a recipe, and whether it is an essential part or just a supporting component in the dish. Always start with small changes first when trying out a newly veganized recipe.

Fats are the easiest to replace. Olive oil is a great baking substitute, in most instances, for melted butter, ghee, lard, and heavily processed vegetable oils and shortening. You can also use other light oils such as sunflower, safflower, or soybean in baking. Oils work best in cakes, brownies, some drop cookies, breads, and quick breads.

Solid fats work best in pastry recipes as the chilled fat remains separated in layers from the dry ingredients and melts when baking to provide a rich flavor and flaky texture. No wonder butter is so prized by pie bakers for its rich taste, and frugal bakers rely on lard and vegetable shortening to add flake and fat to their pie crusts and biscuits at a fraction of the cost. But because these aren't suitable vegan ingredients, what should a vegan baker use? Well for one, don't use just any old margarine. Instead, use the nonhydrogenated whipped kind (see Chapter 18).

The best-tasting and most consistent measure-for-measure butter replacement is made by Smart Balance. It comes in several varieties, including Earth Balance Organic Whipped, Natucol, Soy Garden, Buttery Sticks, and Shortening. For those who can't find Smart Balance products, Spectrum Naturals makes other nonhydrogenated spreads, such as Spectrum Margarine, 100% Spectrum Spread, and Essential Omega-3 Spread.

Each of these products gives your vegan baked goods a buttery flavor with much less fat than butter and no cholesterol. Use them in place of butter in pie crusts, cookies, chilled pastry doughs, crisps, cobblers, and crumb toppings. They also whip up nicely and make vegan frostings light and creamy!

Leaving Out the Milk and Cream

In most of your baking, you can easily do without the use of cow's milk. All soy milks, rice milks, and grain- and nut-based milks can be suitable replacements in puddings, pastries, cakes, desserts, and even to prepare or thin frostings and glazes. If milk is only providing moisture in a recipe, you can also substitute other liquids such as water or juices.

Cream has a thicker consistency than milk, and the higher fat content also adds richness to recipes. You can usually easily substitute White Wave's Silk Creamer or Westsoy's Creme de la Soy in a recipe where cream is providing moisture and creaminess.

You can also use tofu to make a whipped topping replacement for whipped cream. In Chapter 23, you will find a recipe for Creamy Tofu Topping or Mousse, which is delicious and can be used on top of fruit and your favorite desserts.

> **In a Nutshell**
>
> Make a homemade vegan alternative to cream by blending ½ cup soy milk and ½ cup silken tofu or ½ cup soy milk blended with 2 to 3 tablespoons dry soy milk powder until smooth and creamy. It substitutes measure-for-measure for the cream called for in most recipes.

Some big-name nondairy whipped toppings are available at your local supermarket, but most of them still contain animal ingredients such as sodium caseinate, along with hydrogenated oils, high-fructose corn syrup, preservatives, and artificial ingredients. A more healthful and completely vegan alternative is Hip Whip made by Now&Zen. It's made from tofu and cashew butter and is sweetened with brown rice syrup and grape juice concentrate. It is available in Plain, with a hint of vanilla, or Chocolate Mousse varieties. Use it to decorate your desserts, pies, and parfaits or to provide a light and creamy sweetness to your vegan creations.

Doin' the Dozens Without Eggs

It's quite unfortunate that eggs have become a staple of many people's diets. Not only do the hens pay a heavy price for laying them, but so do those who eat them. According to the American Heart Association, the average large egg contains 213 milligrams of cholesterol, which is more than 70 percent of the daily recommendation for dietary cholesterol intake. These numbers make eggs unsuitable for heart patients as they have to keep their dietary cholesterol intake below 200 milligrams per day.

Fortunately, you can substitute for eggs in many ways. How you do it depends on the role the eggs were playing in the original recipe. Basically, the purpose of eggs in a recipe is either to act as a binder, thickener, or leavening agent or just to add moisture. For instance, in veggie burgers, sauces, or casseroles, you want a binding or thickening effect. Starches do the trick here, so try adding some arrowroot, potato starch, cornstarch, flour, oats, or breadcrumbs to reach the desired consistency. Adding a tablespoon or two of nut butter, like peanut butter, cashew butter, or raw tahini, also helps bind or hold ingredients together.

Trying to substitute for eggs in baking can be a bit trickier. If the eggs are part of the recipe simply to provide moisture, you can replace them with the same amount of water, soy milk, or juice. When you need the "binding" properties of eggs when making cookies, breads, and baked goods, you can use applesauce, puréed bananas, puréed dates, or Ener-G Egg Replacer, which is made with potato starch and tapioca flour and is widely available in natural foods stores. To achieve the "thickening" qualities of eggs in pie fillings or custards, you can use agar-agar, kudzu, arrowroot, cornstarch, or flour.

Use these basic suggestions for substituting 1 egg:

> **In a Nutshell**
>
> Here's a little tip for those who try Ener-G Egg Replacer. The directions on the box suggest you use 1½ teaspoons Ener-G Egg Replacer plus 2 tablespoons water to replace 1 egg. We have had better results by increasing the amount of Ener-G Egg Replacer to 1 tablespoon, especially when using it as a binder or thickener.

- ¼ cup silken, firm, or extra-firm tofu, puréed until smooth

- ¼ cup puréed bananas or applesauce, plus ½ teaspoon nonaluminum baking powder

- 2 tablespoons nut butter, such as peanut butter or tahini

- 1 tablespoon finely ground flax seeds, plus 3 tablespoons water, blended in a blender until frothy and allowed to rest 30 minutes to 1 hour

- 1 tablespoon Ener-G Egg Replacer whisked with 2 tablespoons water

- 1 tablespoon cornstarch or flour whisked with 1 tablespoon water

Try experimenting with some of these to see which ones work best in your recipes.

Gellin' Without Gelatin

Gelatin is a very strange food product. It turns liquids into solid or semi-solid masses, thickening a little or a lot, depending on the amount used. Some fruits and veggies such as tomatoes, beans, and peas contain natural gelling properties. (This is easily demonstrated when you look at a leftover pot of split-pea soup and see an actual layer of gel across the top.)

This type of gelatin is based on plant cellulose structure, not the collagen released from animal bones and tissues. That's right—animal-based gelatin is made of leftovers from the slaughtering process. Bones, hooves, skin, tendons, and other miscellaneous parts are boiled in water to release their natural collagen. The extracted gelatin is formed into translucent sheets, strings, or ground into a powder. It is then used in cooking to thicken sauces, jellies, desserts, candies, ice creams, marshmallows, baked goods, and many other products. Surprisingly, it also is used to clarify soups and stocks, some vinegars, juices, wines, beers, and spirits. It is used to make cosmetics, capsules for supplements, personal care products, and as an industrial stabilizer used in many everyday products. (See Chapter 26 to learn a little more about the uses of gelatin in household items.)

There's some culinary benefit to be able to bind things together or gel them, but you don't have to rely on animal by-products to do it. Vegans and vegetarians have several alternatives to use. A few companies, such as Emes and Hain, even make boxed plain and flavored vegan gelatin; look for them in grocery and natural foods stores. You can also experiment with other gelling agents such as flax seeds, agar-agar, starches, and other all-natural plant ingredients. You'll be amazed by the solidifying results!

Flax Seeds: Fiber and Form

A mixture of flax seeds and water was once a popular hair-setting solution. After making the standard flax-seed gel recipe of 1 tablespoon flax seeds and 3 tablespoons water, either boiled or blended together, and then letting it sit for a while, you'll see why. It turns into a very gummy, gel-like substance. Strain out the flax seeds through a cheesecloth before using it to set your hair in rollers or with spikes; you don't have to do this in cooking and baking.

Flax seeds have a slightly nutty flavor, which they impart to your baked goods. As a result, they are especially good paired with recipes that contain nuts and seeds. The gelling properties of the flax seeds and water can work as a binder or egg replacement

Hot Potato _____

Always store your flax seeds in the refrigerator or freezer, and use them up within 6 months or less. Like most seeds, their high fat content can easily lead to rancidity, so help them keep their cool!

in your baking recipes, so they'll work well in your vegan quick breads, pie fillings, and cookies.

Grind flax seeds in a coffee grinder, blender, or food processor to a fine powder for ease of use. Do this ahead of time, in small batches, keep the mixture in an air-tight container in the refrigerator, and use it as needed.

Flax seeds are very nutritious, high in beneficial omega-3 fatty acids, vitamins, minerals, and protein. They are also a high-fiber and protein-rich food source good for your skin, brain, immunity, and weight control. These tiny seeds are also rich in lignans, which provide so many health benefits and safety nets. They have anticancer, antitumor, antiviral, antibacterial, and antifungal properties as well.

You can purchase flax seeds in brown and golden varieties, either whole, ground, or as an oil. See your friendly neighborhood natural foods store to find out what's available.

Agar-Agar (Not an '80s Band)

Duran Duran, Mister Mister, Oingo Boingo, and Agar-Agar? The first three may be popular bands from the 1980s, but the last one certainly isn't! It's actually a widely used seaweed derivative that's odorless, tasteless, nearly colorless, and has amazing gelling properties. It's available in sticks, flakes, or as a powder, and the amount you use varies with each variety and depends on the amount of gelling required.

You can find agar-agar in many Asian specialty markets, grocery stores, and natural foods stores. Use it to thicken your own fruit juices to make jiggly treats, like kanten! Kanten is a dish that suspends fruits, beans, nuts, and seeds in a gelled agar-agar mixture and is very much like the gelatin desserts most of us grew up with at family functions and as part of our school lunches. Also add agar-agar to thicken sauces, frostings, puddings, fillings, and other custardlike desserts.

Stiffening with Starch

You can also use many starches to help your sauce or pie filling gel. Try a little Ener-G Egg Replacer, arrowroot, cornstarch, potato starch, _kudzu_, tapioca flour, or other flour diluted in a little water or other liquid to give substance to your creation. Cook the starch-liquid mixture to begin the thickening process and to remove any starchy taste.

Vegan 101

Kudzu, or *kuzu*, is a starch-based thickening product made from the tuber of the kudzu plant. People in Japan and throughout much of Asia eat the leafy foliage cooked like other greens; they also use the large tubers as a thickening agent. This quick-growing vine was brought from Japan to the southern United States, where it is referred to as "the vine that ate the South" because it now covers nearly 7 million acres of land!

Arrowroot and tapioca give your finished sauce or filling a glossy shine; cornstarch and flour often leave things dull, cloudy, or creamy-looking. Arrowroot also works better with acidic ingredients, which sometimes inhibit cornstarch. In general, it takes 1 tablespoon starch diluted in 2 tablespoons liquid to thicken 1 cup of a mixture such as a sauce, stock, or juice.

Acceptin' Pectin

Many fruits and vegetables contain a natural dietary fiber known as pectin. Pectin can help keep your digestive system running properly and regulate your blood cholesterol and sugar levels, thus helping you fight off chronic degenerative diseases, heart disease, and diabetes. In addition to its health benefits, you can also use pectin as a thickening agent.

These are examples of pectin-rich foods:

- Apples
- Avocados
- Bananas
- Blueberries
- Carob
- Cherries
- Currants
- Grapes
- Oranges and other citrus fruits
- Peaches
- Pineapples
- Raisins
- Raspberries
- Sunflower seeds
- Tomatoes

The pectin contained in these foods acts as a gelling agent, binder, thickener, and stabilizer, especially after its fiber is broken down and mixed with water. The thickening process starts immediately, so you can use them to thicken raw foods or cook them to release more of their thickening properties. Use them to make jellies, jams, sauces, puddings, and other delicious desserts. Fruit pectin is also commercially available in powdered and liquid forms.

The Endless Uses of Tofu

Tofu may be the most versatile of all vegan ingredients, so you should definitely make every effort to become friends with it. Keep it regularly stocked in your kitchen, in both regular and silken-style varieties. Regular tofu requires constant refrigeration or freezing, while silken-style tofu packaged in aseptic containers usually requires refrigeration only after opening, making it perfect for traveling or camping.

Use tofu to quickly whip up a hearty breakfast meal, savory sandwich, tasty treat, or delicious dessert. As mentioned earlier in the egg section, use a little puréed tofu to replace eggs when revamping your favorite recipes to fit your vegan diet. Also use a little puréed tofu to replace some of the fat called for in a recipe—sometimes up to one third the amount—without altering the end result a bit. As a binder or thickener, puréed tofu works well in cakes, quick breads, cookies, and other baked goods.

You can use puréed tofu, thinned with a little water or soy milk, and a little lemon juice, apple cider vinegar, or other acid, to make vegan yogurt, sour cream, or cream cheese substitutes to use in baking. Puréeing tofu turns a simple block into a light and creamy base with endless possibilities. Sweeten and flavor it with some sugar, maple or brown rice syrup, agave nectar, and fruit juices and purées to make toppings, puddings, fillings, frostings, and cheesecakes. Or blend in a little cocoa or carob powder—or better yet, some melted vegan chocolate or carob chips—and you can turn puréed tofu into a vegan chocolate mousse!

Baking and chilling will thicken your tofu purée mixture, so we recommend this step when making cream pies and cheesecakes. You can also use puréed tofu to make creamy sauces or to thicken your sauces. Homemade vegan ice creams and sherbets come out thicker and creamier with the addition of a little puréed tofu. Use crumbled or lightly puréed tofu to replace cottage cheese or ricotta cheese in pastries, blintzes, and even Italian favorites like lasagna or stuffed shells.

Being Fruitful with Fruit

Fruit purées that contain high concentrations of natural pectin thicken beautifully to make delicious fruit toppings and pie fillings. In Chapter 20, you'll find a recipe for Breakfast Fruit Parfaits with a creamy raw banana topping you can also use on fruits or desserts—or enjoy all by itself for a fat-free treat. Frozen bananas puréed with a little cocoa or carob powder make a quick frozen dessert similar to ice cream. Thinned with soy milk or other liquid, it makes a delicious smoothie. Chapter 20 also contains a smoothie recipe that might provide you with some inspiration for blending up some fruity refreshments of your own.

In Chapter 23 is a raw pie recipe called Raw Mixed Berry and Mango Pie that illustrates the wonderful binding properties of fruit and their natural sweetening capabilities. Fruits contain concentrated natural sugars and provide tastes that range from the lightest and most delicate to the most dramatically sweet, bitter, and pungent. You can use fruit purées and juices to sweeten your desserts or as part of the liquid ingredients called for in your recipe.

Fruit purées add moisture and can also be used to replace part of the fat called for in a recipe, from one quarter to one third of the amount. This often results in a more cakelike texture (rather than chewy) in your baked goods.

Pureed bananas can serve many functions in your baked goods. Use them to replace part of the fat or oil called for in a recipe, as well as an egg or two because they provide a lot of moisture. This often results in moist-textured, rather than dry, baked goods. Try them in cakes, cookies, and quick breads. Other fruit purées, such as applesauce or puréed dates or prunes, also work as fat and egg replacements while providing moisture enhancement.

> **In a Nutshell**
>
> Once thawed, fruit juice concentrates, which are found in the freezer section of most stores, can be used measure-for-measure as replacements for other liquid sweeteners in your favorite recipes. Be sure to use organic brands or ones that are made of 100 percent fruit juice, instead of those that contain high-fructose corn syrup and artificial colorings or flavorings.

When puréeing bananas or other fruits, be sure to do it for at least 2 minutes to whip in a lot of air. The air stays suspended in the purée and gives height to your baked goods. Adding a little nonaluminum baking powder also gives extra rise to your baked treats.

Chapter 23 contains a recipe for Chewy Walnut Brownies, a fabulous egg- and butter-free vegan brownie that beautifully illustrates the use of the puréed banana and baking powder combination. Make them for your friends and family, and they'll find it hard to believe the treats are dairy- and egg-free.

Sweeteners to Use and Avoid

Many of us love to eat sweet-tasting foods more than salty, sour, or even spicy foods. Sugars do provide energy, but consuming too much sugar, especially in heavily refined foods, can be detrimental instead of beneficial to your health. White sugar, in particular, is the enemy of the health-conscious and the vegan alike. Most of the major sugar companies in the United States bleach their sugar to make it white. Not only do manufacturers strip away beneficial nutrients in the process, but the bleaching process itself is usually not even vegan.

Cane Sugar and Beyond

In particular, sugar produced from sugar cane, also known as cane sugar, is bleached using a special filtration process that cleanses away its nutty brown color and leaves a polished ivory-colored mass. It is often filtered through activated charcoal that can come from animal as well as plant sources. Often, the process uses a special charcoal made from animal bones, which is commonly referred to as bone char or boneblack. Using bone char in the bleaching process is only done with cane sugar, not beet sugar. In Europe, the production of almost all bleached cane sugar is done without the use of bone char and, therefore, is suitable for vegans. The opposite is true for most of the big U.S. producers, though.

Powdered and brown cane sugar are often processed using bone char as well, particularly those produced by manufacturers that normally use bone char in their bleaching process. For them, brown sugar is simply bleached cane sugar with some molasses added back in, and powdered or confectioners' sugar is bleached cane sugar that's been finely processed

> **CAUTION**
>
> **Hot Potato**
>
> Three of the largest U.S. sugar manufacturers—Domino, California & Hawaiian Sugar Company (C&H), and Savannah Foods—use bone char in their cane sugar bleaching processes. Their sugar is sold as various supermarket and generic brands as well. Sucanat and Florida Crystals are two widely available brands of sugar that do not involve the use of bone char and are therefore suitable for vegans.

with cornstarch to prevent caking. Brown or powdered sugar based on beet sugar rather than cane sugar is suitable for vegans as are those sugars produced by companies that do not use bone char. Florida Crystals makes a great vegan powdered sugar as well as several varieties of brown sugar, based on evaporated cane juice. Also try Muscovado sugar, a vegan moist brown sugar available at natural foods stores.

To know for sure you're getting a truly vegan sugar, you can contact the company directly and ask them for information. You can also avoid problems by looking for products labeled as *evaporated cane juice, organic unbleached sugar, raw sugar, turbinado sugar, demerara sugar,* or *beet sugar.* These are all vegan. You can also substitute maple sugar (made from dehydrated maple syrup) and date sugar (made from pulverized dried dates) in place of cane or beet sugar. Maple sugar and date sugar are especially delicious in cookies that contain nuts or seeds.

Syrupy Sweetness

Some vegans prefer to stay away from granular sugar altogether and stick with using liquid sweeteners such as molasses, maple syrup, barley malt syrup, brown rice syrup, concentrated fruit juice syrups, agave nectar, and sorghum. These sweeteners tend to keep your blood sugar at more even levels, with fewer spikes and dips than those caused by refined cane sugar.

To ensure that your maple syrup is pure, buy only certified organic. Also, avoid "maple flavored syrup," which is usually made from sugar or corn syrup mixed with artificial colorings and flavorings and maybe a tiny percentage of actual maple syrup. There's really no comparison between the two products, and they are only interchangeable on pancakes and waffles, not in cooking or baking.

> **CAUTION**
>
> **Hot Potato**
>
> You might have heard one of the many rumors floating around that maple syrup isn't vegan because it is often clarified. Fortunately, most commercially available brands of maple syrup in the United States no longer use lard in the foaming process and instead use oil. When in doubt, contact the manufacturer.

Stevia is known as the "sweet herb" to the people of Paraguay and Brazil, where it originates. People of these regions have chewed on the leaves and twigs of the plant for centuries. They also add it to their foods and beverages, like mate tea concoctions. Stevia has been growing in popularity in the United States since the 1990s, and you can find it in liquid and powdered forms in most grocery and natural foods stores. It is a highly concentrated sweetener, and only very little is needed to replace a cup of sugar or other sweetener. So far there are no known side effects to its usage.

Honey, You're Not So Sweet

Honey is another sweetener vegans avoid. What's wrong with honey? Simply put, honey is the regurgitation of the food bees eat, and as a result, is not vegan by any stretch of the imagination. Honey was also listed as one of the foods vegans abstain from in the original aims of the Vegan Society.

> **In a Nutshell**
>
> Surprising as it may be, honey also sometimes contains botulism, which is the reason why it's widely recommended that honey never be fed to children under the age of 1. Between 70 and 90 cases of infant botulism are reported in the United States annually, and Sudden Infant Death Syndrome has been linked, in part, to infant botulism.

Vegans consider it cruel to take the honey away from the bees, as the bees created it for themselves to meet their own dietary needs. Honey is food bees make from the nectar of flowers and flowering trees to feed the hive and sustain the young. The honey production of a single bee, over the course of a lifetime, is only around $\frac{1}{12}$ teaspoon. That's a lot of work to produce very little honey! Each tablespoon of honey represents the life's work of 36 bees.

Also, to obtain honey on a commercial level, the bees have to be smoked out of their hives, which isn't pleasant. Who likes to get smoke in their eyes and respiratory system? Often, bees are also killed in the process of obtaining honey, the comb, and beeswax.

Flour Power

The importance of purchasing whole-grain flours is really apparent in vegan baked goods, as they bind, thicken, coat, and encapsulate so many foods and food items. The nutty, almost sweet flavors of whole-grain flours give more depth to the flavors of your baked goods, in addition to a deep golden brown color after baking. Also, all the vital bran, germ, and other nutritional benefits of the whole grains are all still contained within your baked goods instead of having been stripped away. Because whole grains contain fiber, which is good for your digestion and colon, they can make for some pretty tasty good-for-you desserts.

Try experimenting with using new flours such as whole-wheat flour, whole-wheat pastry flour, barley flour, and oat flour, alone or in combinations, to replace bleached white flour in recipes. To try your hand at gluten-free baking, stock up on some gluten-free flours such as quinoa, amaranth, brown rice, and tapioca flours, which work most successfully in combinations, to replace wheat. Using a ratio of two parts brown rice flour to one part of either quinoa, amaranth, or tapioca flour, or a combination of two or more of them, works in most pastries, cookies, cakes, and other baked goods.

Buy flours in bulk for the best price, and rotate your stock often to ensure the freshest quality.

Hot Potato _____

Flours can go stale and rancid, as well as attract bugs, so always keep your flours stored in airtight containers.

Experimenting and Accepting

It may take you a while to get used to using some of your new vegan ingredients, but be patient and keep trying, especially if baking and cooking are new to you. Accept the fact that you won't be able to duplicate everything with vegan ingredients. For instance, foods that are made entirely of eggs, such as meringues and soufflés—forget about it. They can't be done vegan because there are too many eggs holding the mix together. You can make other vegan goodies instead of meringues, or use tofu whipped toppings to "kinda sorta" replace the meringue on a pie. You can also have some tofu scramble instead of a soufflé for brunch or breakfast or a tofu cheesecake to replace a dairy version.

There will be times when you want to duplicate or imitate a once-favorite food item and others when you will be inspired to strike out in a different direction with the same ingredients to create a new vegan gastronomical nirvana. Different can be better! Tinker and experiment in your kitchen to accommodate your own tastes or lack or abundance of ingredients. If you stumble upon something really great-tasting, be sure to write it down so you'll be able to duplicate the recipe another time. Also, don't forget to share your vegan goodies with others; they can be a great way to spread the vegan message and turn others on to this great way of eating and living!

The Least You Need to Know

- Nonhydrogenated vegan whipped margarines work extremely well as a replacement for butter in your baked goods, and nondairy milks can substitute for cow's milk with ease.

- Agar-agar is a vegan alternative to gelatin that you can use to thicken your sauces, frostings, puddings, fillings, and other custardlike desserts. Several brands of vegan gelatin are also available commercially.

◆ Tofu is a versatile ingredient that you can use in a variety of ways to replace fat, eggs, and cream in your vegan baked goods.

◆ Bananas and other pectin-rich fruits can act as binders and fat replacers in a recipe. They also add height and moisture to the finished product.

◆ In the United States, most bleached cane sugar is processed using bone char, a special charcoal made from animal bones. This is not the case with beet sugar or other vegan sugars.

◆ Choose whole-grain flours whenever possible, as they will yield the best results for your baked vegan creations while supplying nutritional benefits.

Part 6

Vegan Food for the Soul

Now that you know how to shop wisely, it's time to stock up on your vegan cooking and baking supplies. Pull out the pots, pans, bowls, colanders, and cutting boards; sharpen your knives; gather your utensils; and get ready to create some delicious vegan goodies!

No matter what your level of kitchen skills, we offer you vegan recipes to suit all your wants, needs, and cravings. From the quick and easy, to the basics needed to create meals at holiday time or as a special treat for someone you love, you'll find it all in Part 6. From breakfast to dessert, we give you lots of options and ideas for fueling yourself with good vegan foods!

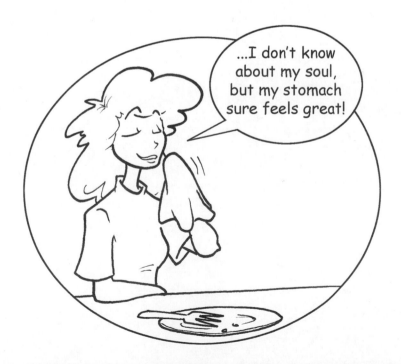

20

Breakfast Ideas

In This Chapter

♦ Cool and healthy fruity beginnings

♦ Veganizing old breakfast favorites

♦ Hearty and hot vegan breakfast ideas

Going vegan doesn't mean you have to miss out on delicious breakfasts like the ones many of us fondly remember our mothers and grandmothers making for us when we were growing up. You can easily make vegan versions of dishes such as French toast, scrambled eggs, sausages, and other hearty fare with a little bit of know-how and culinary creativity!

In this chapter, you will find a dozen recipes for creating some awesome and filling vegan breakfasts, and most of them will help you start your day on an even better foot than Mom's versions ever did. Hers may have been loaded with cholesterol and featured limited amounts of veggies, with servings of fruit often being limited to only a small glass of juice or half a grapefruit. Most vegan breakfasts contain great sources of complex carbohydrates, protein, and calcium, in addition to several servings each of fruits and vegetables. What better way to jump-start your day!

Many of us have hectic morning schedules or just don't move so quickly in the morning. As a result, we have to eat breakfast "on the go" more often than we like. That's why, in this chapter, you will find recipes for quick fruit-based breakfasts such as fruit salads, smoothies, and even a breakfast parfait. Then we offer a few hearty choices like tofu scramble, potato and veggie home fries, tempeh sausages, and two traditional breakfast breads—biscuits and cornbread. We even have a few recipes to impress the vegan skeptics out there.

You can make many of the heartier recipes in large batches ahead of time and reheat them in smaller batches as needed to satisfy your morning grumblings with a nutritious breakfast even when you're hard-pressed for time.

Tropical Teaser Smoothie

1 large banana, peeled and cut into 2-inch pieces

1½ cups mixed frozen berries, such as strawberries or blue-berries

1 cup mango, peeled, pitted, and diced

1 cup pineapple chunks

1 cup fresh or bottled orange juice

1 cup soy milk, rice milk, or other nondairy milk of choice

1 TB. ginger, peeled, and grated

Yield: 4 servings
Prep time: 5 minutes

1. Place banana, frozen berries, mango, pineapple chunks, orange juice, soy milk, and ginger in a blender, and blend until smooth.

2. Serve immediately in tall glasses with straws, if desired. Store any extra in the refrigerator for up to 1 or 2 days, and blend again before serving.

Variation: Feel free to substitute other fresh and frozen fruits to suit your own personal tastes. You can also use other fruit juices or omit them completely and use all soy milk or even water to help purée the fruit and achieve a creamy consistency.

CAUTION

Hot Potato

Drinking smoothies is a great way to get two to three servings of fruit all in one glass, but be sure to drink them slowly and chew the contents slightly. This will allow your saliva to mix with the contents, which will help your body access and utilize more of the beneficial antioxidants, vitamins, and minerals.

Soy Buttermilk Biscuits

Yield: 12 biscuits
Prep time: 15 minutes
Cook time: 10 to 15 minutes

In a Nutshell

You can also add 2 tablespoons unbleached sugar to the dough for extra sweetness when preparing the biscuits. Then, mix together some fresh-cut fruits such as berries, peaches, and plums; sprinkle them with a little additional sugar; and leave them to macerate for a while. Then use the biscuits and macerated fruit to make vegan shortcake!

¾ cup soy milk, rice milk, or other nondairy milk of choice

2 TB. fresh or bottled lemon juice

2¼ cups whole-wheat pastry flour

½ cup soy flour

2 TB. nonaluminum baking powder

¾ tsp. sea salt

⅓ cup olive oil

2 TB. pure maple syrup

1. Preheat the oven to 400°F. Whisk together soy milk and lemon juice in a small bowl or measuring cup, and set aside to thicken for 10 minutes. In another bowl, add whole-wheat pastry flour, soy flour, nonaluminum baking powder, and sea salt, and stir well. Drizzle olive oil over dry ingredients. Using a pastry blender, two knives, or your fingertips, cut in olive oil until mixture resembles coarse crumbs. Add thickened soy milk and pure maple syrup, and stir well to form a ball of dough.

2. Place dough on a floured surface, and knead for 1 minute. Roll or pat dough to a ½-inch thickness. Using a 3-inch biscuit cutter or glass, cut out 12 biscuits. Carefully transfer them to a nonstick cookie sheet.

3. Bake for 10 to 12 minutes or until golden brown on the bottom. Serve biscuits hot, either plain, with jam, or split and topped with gravy.

Variation: For a change of pace, add chopped fresh herbs such as dill, thyme, parsley, or chives, or even a little shredded vegan soy cheese to the dough before cutting out biscuits.

Vegan Cornbread

2½ cups yellow cornmeal

2 cups whole-wheat pastry flour

3 TB. nonaluminum baking powder

½ tsp. sea salt

1⅓ cups soy milk, rice milk, or other nondairy milk of choice

1⅓ cups filtered water

½ cup pure maple syrup

½ cup olive oil

1 tsp. pure vanilla extract

Yield: 1 (9×13-inch) pan or 12 squares
Prep time: 5 to 10 minutes
Cook time: 20 to 25 minutes

1. Preheat the oven to 375°F. Using a little olive oil, lightly oil a 9×13-inch pan and set aside. In a large bowl, sift together yellow cornmeal, whole-wheat pastry flour, nonaluminum baking powder, and sea salt. In a medium bowl, add soy milk, water, maple syrup, olive oil, and vanilla extract, and stir well.

2. Add soy milk mixture to dry ingredients, and stir until just combined. Pour mixture into the prepared pan. Bake for 20 to 25 minutes or until a toothpick inserted in the center comes out clean. Allow to cool slightly before cutting into squares.

Variations: This is a basic cornbread recipe you can jazz up with a few additions, such as the following:

◆ **Green onion:** Add ½ cup sliced green onions, 1 tablespoon nutritional yeast flakes, and 1 tablespoon chili powder.

◆ **Jalapeño:** Add 2 jalapeños, seeds and ribs removed, and finely chopped.

◆ **Green chilies:** Add 1 (4-ounce) can diced green chilies, drained.

◆ **Cheezy:** Add ½ cup shredded vegan soy cheese, 2 tablespoons nutritional yeast flakes, and 1 teaspoon paprika.

◆ **Corn and chive:** Add ½ cup cut corn and 3 tablespoons chopped chives.

◆ **Corn muffins:** Pour prepared cornbread batter into oiled or paper-lined muffin tins, filling them ⅔ full, and bake at 425°F for 15 to 20 minutes or until lightly browned around the edges.

Hot Potato

Store your cornmeal in an airtight container in the refrigerator or freezer to prevent it from going rancid or attracting bugs. It can last for several months this way. Also, use organic, non-GM (non-genetically modified) cornmeal because there have been problems in recent years with corn supplies being tainted with modified "Starlink" corn, which is not approved for human consumption.

Almond Spice French Toast

In a Nutshell

Nuts make for a great pick-me-up snack. Most are nutritional power-houses, and almonds especially are high in fiber and low in fat. They also contain all 9 essential amino acids, calcium, iron, magnesium, copper, zinc, phosphorus, vita-mins B and E, and of course tons of protein. Store your almonds and other nuts in the refrigerator or freezer to keep them fresh and prevent rancidity.

¾ cup sliced almonds

1¼ cups filtered water

¼ cup brown rice syrup or pure maple syrup

1 tsp. unbleached sugar

1 tsp. pure almond extract

1 tsp. pure vanilla extract

1 tsp. ground cinnamon

½ tsp. ground nutmeg

½ tsp. sea salt

8 slices whole-grain bread or other bread of choice

1. Place almonds in a food processor, and process for 30 seconds to roughly chop. Add ½ cup filtered water and brown rice syrup, and process for 1 minute or until smooth. Add remaining water, unbleached sugar, pure almond extract, pure vanilla extract, ground cinnamon, ground nutmeg, and sea salt; process mixture an additional 2 minutes or until very smooth and creamy.

2. Transfer almond mixture to a 9×13-inch baking pan. Place 4 bread slices in almond mixture, flip them over to coat other side, and allow bread slices to soak in mixture for 2 minutes. Using olive oil, lightly oil a large, nonstick skillet (or griddle), and set it over medium heat. Using a fork, carefully remove soaked bread slices from almond mixture, and add them to the hot skillet.

3. Cook slices over medium heat for 1 to 2 minutes or until golden brown. Carefully flip them over with a slotted spatula and cook an additional 1 to 2 minutes or until golden brown on the other side. While cooking the first batch, repeat the soaking procedure for remaining 4 bread slices. Transfer French toast to a large plate. Lightly oil the skillet again, and repeat the cooking procedure for remaining bread slices. Keep slices warm in a 250°F oven while preparing second batch. Serve French toast with your choice of jams, preserves, syrups, or fresh fruit.

Mixed Melon, Berry, and Pineapple Salad with Mint

3 cups cantaloupe, cut in 1-inch cubes

3 cups honeydew, cut in 1-inch cubes

3 cups seedless watermelon, cut in 1-inch cubes

3 cups pineapple, cut in 1-inch cubes

2 cups strawberries, hulled and quartered

2 cups blueberries

½ cup fresh orange juice

⅓ cup chopped fresh mint

Yield: 14 cups
Prep time: 10 minutes

1. Combine cantaloupe, honeydew, watermelon, pineapple, strawberries, and blueberries in a large glass bowl, and toss gently.

2. Sprinkle orange juice and mint over top of fruit, and toss gently again. Cover and chill in the refrigerator or serve immediately.

Variation: Substitute other fresh fruits to suit your taste and seasonal availability. You can also sprinkle chopped or sliced nuts such as almonds or seeds or shredded unsweetened coconut over the fresh fruit to add a little extra crunch and texture.

In a Nutshell

Fruit salads that are left over for more than a day or two often lose their eye appeal but are still quite edible and tasty. Throw leftover fruit salads in the blender and purée until smooth for a great impromptu smoothie!

Breakfast Fruit Parfaits

Yield: **4 servings**
Prep time: 5 minutes

In a Nutshell

These breakfast parfaits are made of layers of fruit, fruit purée, and granola in a similar fashion to an ice-cream sundae. Who says you can't have dessert for breakfast?

1 cup blueberries

1 cup blackberries, cut in half lengthwise

1 cup strawberries, hulled and sliced

1 mango, peeled, pitted, and diced

1 kiwi fruit, peeled and diced

¼ cup fresh or bottled apple juice

5 large bananas, peeled and cut into 2-inch pieces

2 tsp. fresh or bottled lemon juice

1 cup shredded unsweetened coconut

4 cups store-bought or homemade granola

1. Combine blueberries, blackberries, strawberries, mango, kiwi, and apple juice in a medium bowl. Toss gently to combine, and set aside.

2. In a food processor, process bananas and lemon juice for 1 minute or until smooth. Scrape down the sides of the container. Add shredded coconut, and process an additional 2 to 3 minutes or until extremely light and creamy. Transfer mixture to a glass bowl.

3. To assemble parfaits: in the bottom of 4 large glasses or dessert dishes, add ½ cup mixed fruit mixture, ½ cup granola, and follow with ½ cup banana–coconut cream mixture. Repeat layers, ending with banana–coconut cream mixture. Serve immediately.

Variation: Use nondairy plain or flavored soy yogurt as a substitute for the banana–coconut cream mixture.

Breakfast Potato and Pepper Home Fries

6 cups red-skinned potatoes, scrubbed and diced

2 cups onions, diced

1½ cups green bell pepper, seeds and ribs removed, and diced

1½ cups red bell pepper, seeds and ribs removed, and diced

2 TB. olive oil

1½ TB. garlic, minced

¼ cup chopped fresh parsley

2 TB. chopped fresh thyme, or 2 tsp. dry thyme

½ tsp. paprika

½ tsp. sea salt

¼ tsp. freshly ground black pepper

Yield: 6 to 8 servings
Prep time: 10 minutes
Cook time: 15 minutes

In a Nutshell

You can make home fries or fried potatoes and veggies with any kind of potatoes you have on hand. Try using Yukon Gold, fingerlings, Russian Blue, or even a garnet yam in your morning veggie sauté for a delicious change of pace.

1. Sauté red-skinned potatoes, onions, green bell pepper, red bell pepper, and olive oil in a large nonstick skillet over medium-high heat, stirring occasionally, for 7 to 10 minutes.

2. When potatoes are tender and lightly browned, add garlic and sauté an additional 2 minutes. Add parsley, thyme, paprika, sea salt, and black pepper; sauté an additional 2 minutes. Serve immediately as a side dish.

Sammy's Spicy Tempeh Sausages

Yield: 10 sausage patties

Prep time: 5 minutes, but 1 hour chilling time required

Cook time: 10 to 15 minutes

In a Nutshell

These tempeh sausage patties can be prepared in larger batches, precooked, and frozen in an airtight container for later use. Then, simply reheat in the oven or in a nonstick skillet until heated through.

2 (8-oz.) pkg. tempeh

½ cup whole-wheat flour

1½ TB. tamari, nama shoyu, or Bragg Liquid Aminos

1½ TB. balsamic vinegar

1 TB. olive oil

1 tsp. dried basil

1 tsp. dried oregano

1 tsp. dried thyme

1 tsp. garlic powder

1 tsp. onion powder

1 tsp. ground fennel

½ tsp. crushed red pepper flakes

¼ tsp. freshly ground black pepper

1. Using your fingers, crumble tempeh into a medium bowl. Add the remaining ingredients and stir well to combine. Line a cookie sheet with parchment paper, and set aside. Using a ¼-cup measuring cup, portion tempeh sausage patties by gently packing tempeh mixture into the cup with the back of a spoon. Flip the measuring cup over onto the prepared cookie sheet, and tap it to release patty. Repeat portioning procedure, yielding 10 patties. Cover with plastic wrap, and refrigerate for 1 hour or more.

2. Using olive oil, lightly oil a large nonstick skillet. In batches, cook tempeh sausage patties over medium heat for 5 to 7 minutes or until well browned. Carefully flip over patties with a spatula and cook an additional 5 minutes, or until golden brown and crisp around the edges. Transfer cooked patties to a large plate. Add additional olive oil to the skillet, as needed, to prevent patties from sticking and between batches.

3. Serve as a side dish, sandwich filling, pizza topping (crumbled); or use to add to sauces, pasta or grain-based salads, or main dishes.

Variation: To make Tempeh Maple Sausage, a great breakfast version of this recipe, omit all the dried herbs and crushed red pepper flakes, and replace them with 2 teaspoons Herbes de Provence. Add ½ cup apple, peeled and finely chopped. Also, replace tamari and balsamic vinegar with ¼ cup pure maple syrup and 2 tablespoons apple juice. Then, prepare tempeh sausage patties in the same manner as described here.

Tempeh Sausage and Golden Bean Gravy on Biscuits

½ batch Soy Buttermilk Biscuits (recipe earlier in this chapter)

½ batch Sammy's Spicy Tempeh Sausages (recipe earlier in this chapter)

1 (15-oz.) can baby butter beans or other white beans, drained and rinsed

¾ cup vegetable stock

½ cup onions, finely diced

¼ cup nutritional yeast flakes

1 TB. garlic, minced

½ tsp. sea salt

¼ tsp. freshly ground black pepper

¼ tsp. rubbed (dried) sage

> *Yield: 3 cups gravy or 6 servings*
>
> **Prep time:** 15 minutes
> **Cook time:** 30 to 35 minutes

In a Nutshell

Golden Bean Gravy is also excellent served over mashed potatoes, grains, or vegetables. Or add it to soups or stews to give them richness in flavor and texture.

1. Prepare Soy Buttermilk Biscuits and Sammy's Spicy Tempeh Sausages according to recipe instructions, and allow to cool slightly. Using your fingers, crumble sausage patties into a bowl, and set aside.

2. In a blender or food processor, add baby butter beans, vegetable stock, onions, nutritional yeast flakes, garlic, sea salt, black pepper, and sage. Blend for 1 to 2 minutes or until smooth and creamy.

3. Transfer bean mixture to a small saucepan, and stir in crumbled sausage. Set the saucepan over low heat, and cook until heated through, stirring often.

4. Split biscuits in half, and place each individual serving on a plate, and top with desired amount of tempeh and bean gravy. Serve immediately.

Tofu Scramble, Western Style

Yield: *4 servings*
Prep time: 5 minutes
Cook time: 10 minutes

1 lb. firm tofu, patted dry

1 tsp. onion powder

1 tsp. garlic powder

¼ tsp. turmeric

½ cup onions, diced

⅓ cup green bell pepper, seeds and ribs removed, and diced

⅓ cup red bell pepper, seeds and ribs removed, and diced

1 TB. olive oil

2 TB. nutritional yeast flakes

2 TB. chopped fresh basil, or 2 tsp. dried basil

2 TB. chopped fresh parsley

½ tsp. sea salt

¼ tsp. freshly ground black pepper

1. Using your fingers, crumble tofu into a small bowl. Sprinkle onion powder, garlic powder, and turmeric over the top. Toss well to evenly coat tofu, and set aside.

2. Place onions, green bell pepper, red bell pepper, and olive oil in a large nonstick skillet. Sauté over medium-high heat for 3 minutes, stirring occasionally, or until vegetables are soft. Add reserved tofu and nutritional yeast flakes, and stir well. Sauté an additional 5 minutes, while stirring often, until tofu is dry and slightly browned. Add basil, parsley, sea salt, and black pepper; stir well to combine. Serve immediately as a side dish, main dish, or enjoy rolled in a tortilla with salsa as part of a breakfast burrito.

Variations: You can make many different tofu scrambles to suit your taste and to accommodate what you have on hand:

- **Savory:** Replace onions and peppers with ½ cup sliced green onions, and replace chopped basil with an additional 2 tablespoons chopped fresh parsley.

- **Florentine:** Substitute 2 cups roughly chopped fresh spinach, ½ cup sliced mushrooms, ½ cup sliced green onions, and ½ cup diced sun-dried tomatoes.

- **Spanish:** Omit turmeric and substitute chili powder, add ⅓ cup sliced olives to sautéed vegetables, and add ¼ cup chopped fresh cilantro.

In a Nutshell

With the same ingredients, you can make a vegan frittata. Simply sauté the vegetables in olive oil and place in an oiled 10-inch springform pan. In a food processor, combine tofu, seasonings, nutritional yeast, salt, pepper, and add ½ cup soy milk, 2 tablespoons arrowroot, and 1½ teaspoons agar-agar flakes. Process for 1 to 2 minutes or until very smooth. Pour tofu mixture over sautéed vegetables. Bake at 375°F for 35 to 45 minutes or until firm and golden brown around the edges.

Vegan Cheezy Sauce

½ cup nutritional yeast flakes

3 TB. whole-wheat or spelt flour

4 tsp. arrowroot

½ tsp. sea salt

½ tsp. dry mustard

½ tsp. garlic powder

¼ tsp. paprika

1½ cups soy milk, rice milk, or other nondairy milk of choice

1 TB. olive oil

Yield: 1½ cups	
Prep time: 5 minutes	
Cook time: 5 minutes	

In a Nutshell

This vegan version of cheese sauce has an endless array of uses, from a sauce over vegetables, pasta, or grain dishes, to an addition to soups or stews, or as an accompaniment to main dishes. You can even use it to make a yummy vegan macaroni and cheese by mixing it with cooked elbow macaroni!

1. In a saucepan, whisk together nutritional yeast flakes, whole-wheat flour, arrowroot, sea salt, dry mustard, garlic powder, and paprika.

2. Add soy milk and olive oil, and whisk until very smooth. Cook over low heat, whisking constantly to avoid lumps, for 3 to 5 minutes or until sauce thickness. Serve hot as a sauce, or allow to cool for use as a dip or spread. Store covered in the refrigerator for up to 5 days. Reheat in a saucepan as desired.

Vegan Eggs Benedict

In a Nutshell

You can also make a vegan version of that popular fast-food muffin breakfast sandwich by skipping the Vegan Cheezy Sauce and tomato, and instead layering the Yves Canadian Veggie Bacon and Tofu Scramble between a split Soy Buttermilk Biscuit or English muffin.

2 English muffins

4 slices Yves Canadian Veggie Bacon

½ batch Tofu Scramble, Western Style, made using the Savory variation (recipe earlier in this chapter)

½ batch Vegan Cheezy Sauce (recipe earlier in this chapter)

4 thick tomato slices

Chopped fresh dill, for garnish

Chopped fresh parsley, for garnish

1. Split English muffins and toast them until golden brown. Set aside.

2. Prepare Yves Canadian Veggie Bacon according to package instructions. Also prepare Tofu Scramble, Western Style, using the Savory variation and Vegan Cheezy Sauce recipe according to recipe instructions.

3. To assemble each serving: in the center of a large plate, place ½ toasted English muffin. Top with a slice of Yves Canadian Veggie Bacon, ¼ prepared savory Tofu Scramble, and 1 slice of tomato. Drizzle with ¼ prepared Vegan Cheezy Sauce over the top, and garnish with a sprinkle of freshly chopped dill and parsley.

Chapter 21

Lunch and Lighter Fare

In This Chapter

- ◆ Packing homemade vegan lunches
- ◆ Creating delicious and nutritious sandwiches
- ◆ Tossing up some light and fresh salads

It isn't smart to start your day off on an empty stomach, but due to time constraints and daily routines, many people go without a morning meal. For those who skip breakfast, lunch is the first meal of the day, so it really needs to count and provide enough fuel to give them energy and keep them running at full capacity throughout the rest of the day.

What you eat and *if* you eat breakfast should definitely influence your lunch choices. If you had a hearty breakfast, you may still feel quite full and want to eat a lunch on the lighter side, having only a soup or salad or a combination of the two. If you traded 10 extra minutes of sleep for your usual morning bowl of oatmeal and fruit, then you should have something more substantial. Good choices could include a big bowl of soup or salad, a hearty sandwich or burger, or maybe a combination of all of the above if your appetite is up for it.

Those who attend school or work outside the home have to enjoy their lunches away from the comforts of their vegan kitchen. But you don't have to buy your lunch every day; you can pack lunches for yourself and your loved ones and have lunch on the go! Making your own vegan meals and taking them to work or school is much more economical, environmentally friendly, and of course nutritious than buying lunch. What you would save in a week by not tipping alone would pay for a treat like a quart of nondairy ice cream and cookies or a night at the movies. And by making your own meals, you know exactly what is in each dish and that it is truly up to your vegan standards. In this chapter, you will find recipes suitable for eating at home, but more important, most of them can travel well as part of your packed lunch.

In a Nutshell

For those who want to get lots of veggies, want to drop a few pounds, or simply love to nibble, we suggest the Garden Patch Gazpacho with One Heck of a Chef's Salad, and a generous serving of Lemon-Garlic Hummus with an assortment of fresh vegetable crudités for an afternoon snack. If you want to make your co-workers or friends jealous, you could pack one of the hearty burgers or sandwiches in this chapter. They won't believe they're vegan!

You can pack your own healthy snacks to round out your lunch—maybe a few raw veggies or a piece of fruit, or whole-grain crackers or some pretzels, depending on what is already in your lunch basket. You can also pack nuts, fruit leathers, or dried fruits such as raisins or figs for an afternoon snack. Leftovers from the night before often make for some of the best and easiest lunchtime options. Chopped leftover veggies, grains, and pasta dishes become impromptu salads with little effort. Lunching and munching well as a vegan can be fabulously easy and delicious at the same time!

Garden Patch Gazpacho

2 cups tomato-vegetable juice, store-bought or home-made

1 cup tomatoes, diced

1 cup cucumber, diced

⅓ cup orange bell pepper, seeds and ribs removed, and diced

⅓ cup red bell pepper, seeds and ribs removed, and diced

⅓ cup red onions, and diced

⅓ cup celery, diced

¼ cup radishes, halved and thinly sliced

¼ cup green onions, thinly sliced

¼ cup chopped fresh cilantro

¼ cup chopped fresh parsley

1 jalapeño pepper, seeds and ribs removed, and finely diced

2 TB. fresh lime juice or apple cider vinegar

1 TB. olive oil

1 TB. garlic, minced

1 tsp. chili powder

½ tsp. ground cumin

½ tsp. sea salt

¼ tsp. freshly ground black pepper

¼ tsp. hot red pepper sauce

Yield: 4 to 6 servings

Prep time: 15 to 20 minutes, with 1 to 2 hours chilling time

Vegan 101

Gazpacho is believed to have originated in the Andalusia region of southern Spain. It's derived from the Latin *caspa,* which means "fragments" or "little pieces," a reference to the small pieces of bread found in the Andalusian version. Field hands took their rations of bread, oil, and water, along with some fresh summer vegetables, and pounded them all together with a mortar and pestle to make a nourishing meal.

1. Combine tomato-vegetable juice, tomatoes, cucumber, orange bell pepper, red bell pepper, red onions, celery, radishes, green onions, cilantro, parsley, jalapeño pepper, lime juice, olive oil, garlic, chili powder, cumin, sea salt, black pepper, and hot red pepper sauce in a large bowl, preferably glass. Stir well.

2. Cover and chill in the refrigerator for 1 to 2 hours to allow flavors to blend. Taste and adjust seasonings as needed.

3. Serve in chilled bowls. Store covered in the refrigerator for up to 3 days.

Variation: Substitute other fresh vegetables to take advantage of seasonal availability. You can also purée gazpacho in a blender, in batches, to make a tomato-vegetable juice suitable for drinking or for use as a base of a soup or stew.

Quick-and-Easy Veggie and Bean Chili

In a Nutshell

This chili is so versatile: serve as a side dish, as a filling for sandwiches, mixed with grain dishes for a hearty entrée, or as a chunky dip for tortilla chips or crackers. Garnish with sliced green onions, shredded soy cheese, diced avocado, or tofu sour cream. Or substitute other vegetables or beans to suit your taste. Make it milder by cutting back on the chili powder—or if you like it hot, add more!

4 cups sweet potatoes, peeled and diced

1½ TB. olive oil

1½ cups onions (or red onions), diced

1 cup celery, diced

2 cups zucchini, diced

1 cup cut corn (fresh or frozen)

1 cup green bell pepper, seeds and ribs removed, and diced

1 cup red bell pepper, seeds and ribs removed, and diced

¼ cup jalapeño pepper, seeds and ribs removed, and finely diced

½ cup green onions, thinly sliced

2 TB. garlic, minced

2 (28-oz.) cans crushed tomatoes

2 (15-oz.) cans black beans, drained and rinsed

2 (15-oz.) cans red beans, drained and rinsed

1 (16-oz.) can tomato sauce

2 TB. chili powder

1 TB. ground cumin

1 TB. dried oregano

1 tsp. sea salt

½ tsp. freshly ground black pepper

¼ cup fresh cilantro, chopped

¼ cup fresh parsley, chopped

1. Sauté sweet potatoes in olive oil in a large pot, over medium heat for 5 minutes, stirring occasionally. Add onions and celery, and sauté an additional 5 minutes, stirring often. Add zucchini, corn, green bell pepper, red bell pepper, and jalapeño pepper, and continue to sauté for 5 additional minutes. Add green onions and garlic, and sauté an additional 3 to 5 minutes or until vegetables are tender.

2. Add crushed tomatoes, black beans, red beans, tomato sauce, chili powder, ground cumin, oregano, sea salt, and black pepper to the pot, and cook an additional 10 minutes over low heat to allow flavors to blend. Stir in cilantro and parsley, taste, and adjust seasonings as needed.

Radical Rootin' Tootin' Root Salad

2 cups red beets, finely julienned

2 cups carrots, finely julienned

2 cups golden beets, peeled and finely julienned

2 cups watermelon daikon, peeled and finely julienned

½ cup green onions, thinly sliced

¼ cup chopped fresh parsley

2 TB. apple cider vinegar

2 TB. filtered water

1 TB. olive oil or raw sesame oil

1 TB. ginger, peeled and grated

1 tsp. ground cinnamon

½ tsp. sea salt

¼ tsp. freshly ground black pepper

Yield: 8 cups or 6 to 8 servings	
Prep time: 10 to 15 minutes, with 30 minutes chilling time	

In a Nutshell

This salad is perfect for raw foodists, and it's chock-full of antioxidants, folic acid, and vitamins A and C. Check the produce section of your favorite natural foods or grocery store for watermelon daikon and many more varieties to tempt your taste buds. You're probably used to eating root vegetables cooked, but they are surprisingly sweet in their raw state.

1. Place red beets in a small bowl. Cover and refrigerate until serving.

2. Combine carrots, golden beets, watermelon daikon, green onions, and parsley in a large bowl, and toss gently. In a small bowl, whisk together apple cider vinegar, water, olive oil, ginger, ground cinnamon, sea salt, and black pepper. Pour dressing over top of vegetables, and toss gently to thoroughly coat.

3. Cover and refrigerate for 30 minutes to allow flavors to blend. Just before serving, add red beets and toss the mixture only enough to incorporate them. Serve this as a salad or side dish, as part of a veggie sandwich, or on a bed of greens or grains, if desired.

Variation: You can omit or substitute other roots such as yams in the vegetable combination. Also, adding fruit such as orange segments or julienned apples to the salad makes it sweeter.

One Heck of a Chef's Salad

Yield: 6 to 8 servings

Prep time: 15 to 20 minutes

5 cups spinach, triple rinsed, patted dry, stemmed, and torn into bite-size pieces

3 cups red-tipped loose-leaf lettuce, rinsed, patted dry, and torn into bite-size pieces

3 cups Romaine lettuce or other green lettuce, rinsed, patted dry, and torn into bite-size pieces

2 cups red cabbage, shredded

2 cups mung bean sprouts, rinsed

1 (15-oz.) can kidney beans or other beans of choice, drained and rinsed

1 cup red beets, finely julienned

1 cup carrots, finely julienned

1 cup cucumber, seeds removed, quartered lengthwise, and sliced

1 cup radishes, halved and thinly sliced

1 cup cheddar-style soy cheese, shredded

⅓ cup sunflower seeds

Salad dressing of choice

1. In a large bowl, add spinach, red-tipped loose-leaf lettuce, Romaine lettuce, and red cabbage; toss gently to combine. Transfer mixed greens to a large platter.

2. In rows over top of mixed greens, arrange the following in order: mung bean sprouts, kidney beans, beets, carrots, cucumbers, and radishes. Sprinkle shredded soy cheese and sunflower seeds over the top.

3. Top individual servings with salad dressing of choice. Herbal vinaigrettes, sweet and sour, Thousand Island, and French dressings are some of the most commonly offered dressings with a classic chef's salad.

In a Nutshell

Make your own delicious salad dressings from scratch in minutes! Simply mix 1 part oil to 1 to 2 parts vinegar (your choice for both), or replace up to half the oil with filtered water for a lighter dressing. Then add some Dijon mustard, sugar or maple syrup for sweetness, fresh or dried herbs (your choice), spices, sea salt, and freshly ground black pepper for endless flavor combinations. Use more vinegar than oil for an extra zing, or replace part of the oil with filtered water to cut down on the fat.

Vegan Soy-licious Mayonnaise

1 lb. firm tofu

¾ cup filtered water

¾ cup olive oil

2 TB. Dijon mustard

2 TB. apple cider vinegar

1 TB. maple syrup

2 tsp. onion powder

2 tsp. garlic powder

½ tsp. sea salt

Yield: *4 cups*
Prep time: 5 minutes

1. Using your fingers, crumble tofu into a blender or food processor. Add water, olive oil, Dijon mustard, apple cider vinegar, maple syrup, onion powder, garlic powder, and sea salt. Process for 1 to 2 minutes or until very smooth and creamy. Scrape down the sides of the container, and process an additional 30 seconds.

2. Use immediately or cover and refrigerate. Mayonnaise will thicken tremendously after being chilled. Store in an airtight container in the refrigerator for 7 to 10 days.

In a Nutshell

Most natural foods stores and many grocery stores carry vegan soy-based mayonnaise, in both refrigerated and non-refrigerated varieties, but it's so easy to make your own. You can use this vegan mayonnaise recipe measure-for-measure in place of regular mayonnaise in your favorite recipes, as a spread for sandwiches, and as the base for dressings or sauces. Add chopped herbs for an herb mayonnaise or extra Dijon mustard and maple syrup to make a tangy Dijon dressing.

Truly Eggless Egg Salad

<table>
<tr><td>

Yield: 3 cups

Prep time: 10 minutes, with 70 minutes of chilling time

</td></tr>
</table>

In a Nutshell

You can omit the relish and add a little chopped red pepper, shredded carrots, or other vegetables for added color and crunch in the Truly Eggless Egg Salad. Or omit the turmeric and substitute the same amount of powdered kelp (available at natural foods stores) to make a mock tuna salad.

1 lb. firm tofu

1½ tsp. fresh or bottled lemon juice

½ tsp. sea salt

¼ tsp. onion powder

¼ tsp. turmeric

¼ tsp. celery seed

⅛ tsp. freshly ground black pepper

⅓ cup celery, finely diced

¼ cup green onions, thinly sliced

¼ cup chopped fresh parsley

2 TB. prepared pickle relish

½ cup Vegan Soy-licious Mayonnaise (recipe earlier in this chapter)

1. Holding block of tofu over the sink, squeeze it to remove as much water as possible. Using your fingers, crumble tofu into small pieces into a medium bowl. Add lemon juice, sea salt, onion powder, turmeric, celery seed, and black pepper; toss well to thoroughly coat tofu with seasonings. Cover and refrigerate for 10 minutes.

2. Add celery, green onions, parsley, and pickle relish to tofu mixture, and toss to combine. Add Vegan Soy-licious Mayonnaise, and stir well to thoroughly combine all ingredients.

3. Cover and chill for 1 hour to allow flavors to blend. The color will also turn more yellow as it chills. Enjoy as a salad on a bed of greens, use as a filling for sandwiches or hollowed out vegetables, or pipe on slices of squash or tomatoes and serve as a side dish or appetizer. You can also enjoy it with crackers, tortilla chips, toasted pitas, or other flat breads as a snack or appetizer.

Lemon-Garlic Hummus

2 (15-oz.) cans chickpeas, drained and rinsed

⅓ cup fresh or bottled lemon juice

6 to 8 large cloves garlic

3 TB. filtered water

2 TB. raw tahini

2 TB. olive oil

1 tsp. ground cumin

½ tsp. sea salt

¼ tsp. freshly ground black pepper

¼ cup chopped fresh parsley

Yield: 4 cups	
Prep time: 5 minutes, with 30 minutes chilling time	

1. In a food processor, combine chickpeas, lemon juice, garlic, water, tahini, olive oil, ground cumin, sea salt, and pepper. Process 1 to 2 minutes until smooth and creamy. Scrape down the sides of the container, add parsley, and process an additional 30 seconds. Taste and add more seasonings or lemon juice to desired taste.

2. Store in an airtight container in the refrigerator for 5 to 7 days. Serve with pita bread or assorted raw vegetables for a snack or appetizer, or use as a filling for sandwiches, wraps, or hollowed-out or sliced vegetables.

Variations: You can vary hummus tremendously by adding additional ingredients and changing the spices and oil. Experiment all you like, or try some of these suggestions:

♦ Add 1 to 2 tablespoons puréed sun-dried tomatoes or 1 to 2 roasted red peppers to make a vivid red variation.

♦ Add a small amount of finely chopped vegetables such as spinach, carrots, peppers, black olives, or green onions.

♦ Add 1 to 2 tablespoons additional herbs such as dill, cilantro, or basil.

♦ Use roasted garlic instead of fresh, or toasted sesame oil instead of olive oil, to give your hummus a smoky flavor.

♦ Add 1 to 2 teaspoons chili powder or curry powder to change the color and give it some spice.

Vegan 101

The word *hummus* comes from the Arabic word for chickpea, known also as the ceci or garbanzo bean. Many cultures in these regions have incorporated the chickpea into their meals. What most of us know as hummus is really called *hummus bi tahina*, made by puréeing or mashing chickpeas with tahini, olive oil, lemon juice, garlic, herbs, and seasonings.

Cornucopia Veggie Wraps

Yield: 4 wraps

Prep time: 10 to 15 minutes

In a Nutshell

Wraps are popular lunch and dinner options, but more breakfast-style wraps are emerging, too, such as the breakfast burrito. Make a vegan breakfast burrito with the Tofu Scramble, Western Style, and crumbled Sammy's Spicy Tempeh Sausages (recipes in Chapter 20), veggies, a little salsa, and diced avocado or shredded soy cheese. Just wrap all the ingredients up in a tortilla and go!

---

4 (8-inch) white, whole-wheat, or flavored flour tortillas

Spread of choice (see variation)

4 leaves loose-leaf lettuce or lettuce of choice, rinsed and patted dry

½ cup yam, peeled and shredded

½ cup zucchini, shredded

½ cup yellow summer squash, shredded

½ cup carrot, shredded

3 Roma tomatoes, thinly sliced

1 cucumber, thinly sliced

1. To assemble each wrap: place 1 tortilla flat on a cutting board, and spread desired amount of spread of choice over the top ½ of tortilla, leaving a 1-inch border around edges. Place 1 lettuce leaf in center of tortilla so a little of it hangs over the top edge. Top with 2 tablespoons shredded yam, 2 tablespoons shredded zucchini, 2 tablespoons shredded summer squash, 2 tablespoons shredded carrot, 3 Roma tomato slices, and 6 cucumber slices in 2 rows. Fold bottom of tortilla up to the center, then fold in each side, one overlapping the other to enclose vegetables, and secure wrap with a toothpick.

2. Repeat assembly procedure for remaining tortillas and ingredients. Serve immediately, or wrap veggie wraps in plastic wrap or parchment paper or put in an airtight container, and refrigerate for up to 3 days.

Variation: Substitute any of your favorite vegetables, such as shredded beets, spinach, sliced radishes, chopped veggies, sprouts, and so on. Try some spreads from this chapter, such as Lemon-Garlic Hummus, Truly Eggless Egg Salad, and Vegan Soy-licious Mayonnaise, or perhaps some plain Dijon mustard. You can also add slices of vegan cheese, marinated and baked tofu, or tempeh.

Ray's Special Submarine Sandwiches

6 Italian rolls or other rolls of choice

6 Romaine lettuce leaves or other lettuce of choice, rinsed and patted dry

1½ cups red onions, thinly sliced

2 cups green bell pepper, seeds and ribs removed, and julienned

2 cups cucumber, thinly sliced

Olive oil

Red wine vinegar

Dried oregano

Freshly ground black pepper

6 slices vegan mozzarella-style cheese or other vegan cheese of choice

Yield: 6 servings
Prep time: 5 to 10 minutes

In a Nutshell

Versions of these types of sandwiches are often called grinders, hoagies, subs, or panini on restaurant menus.

1. Split Italian rolls in half, open them, and place them on a large cutting board.

2. Divide Romaine lettuce leaves, red onions, green bell pepper, and cucumber evenly, and place them in order on bottom half of rolls. Drizzle a little olive oil and red wine vinegar over vegetables and then season them generously with oregano and black pepper. Place 1 slice vegan cheese on top of each, and replace top half of roll. Slice each sub sandwich in half and serve.

Variation: Add additional vegetables and seasonings as you like. Sub sandwiches are also good with a little mustard and crushed red pepper flakes for a spicy twist.

Try the Rustic Roasted Vegetables or Glorious Grilled Garden Vegetables (recipes in Chapter 22) in place of the fresh vegetables called for in the recipe, and serve it either hot or cold.

Real Roman Bean Burgers

Yield: 8 burgers

Prep time: 15 minutes plus 30 minutes chilling time

Cook time: 15 to 20 minutes

In a Nutshell

These burgers are great topped with lettuce, onion and tomato slices, nondairy cheese, pickles, and condiments such as ketchup, Dijon mustard, or Vegan Soy-licious Mayonnaise (recipe earlier in this chapter).

1 cup onions, finely diced

1 TB. olive oil

½ cup carrot, finely diced

½ cup red bell pepper, seeds and ribs removed, and finely diced

½ cup zucchini, finely diced

2 TB. garlic, minced

1½ tsp. dried basil

1 tsp. dried oregano

¼ tsp. rubbed (dried) sage

2 (15-oz.) cans Roman or cranberry beans, drained and rinsed

3 TB. tamari or shoyu

3 TB. ketchup

2 TB. Dijon mustard

½ tsp. sea salt

¼ tsp. freshly ground black pepper

1½ cups rolled oats

8 whole-grain hamburger buns or rolls, split

1. Sauté onions in olive oil in a large skillet over medium heat for 1 minute. Add carrot, red bell pepper, and zucchini, and sauté an additional 3 minutes. Add garlic, basil, oregano, and sage; sauté an additional 2 to 3 minutes or until vegetables are lightly browned. Remove the skillet from heat and set aside.

2. Place Roman beans in a large bowl, and roughly mash beans using a potato masher. Add tamari, ketchup, Dijon mustard, sea salt, and black pepper; stir well to combine. Add sautéed vegetables, and fold them into bean mixture. Add rolled oats, and stir thoroughly to combine. Wipe out the skillet with a clean, lint-free towel, and reuse for cooking burgers.

3. Line a large cookie sheet with parchment paper. Using a plastic ½-cup measuring cup, portion out 8 burgers onto the parchment paper, and press to flatten them slightly. Chill for 30 minutes.

4. Using a little olive oil, lightly oil the skillet (or spray with a light mist of oil). In batches, cook burgers until well browned on each side, about 3 to 5 minutes per side. Add more oil to the pan, if needed, to prevent burgers from sticking. Serve on buns with your choice of toppings and condiments.

Portobello Mushroom Burgers with Sun-Dried Tomato Aioli

6 sun-dried tomatoes

¼ cup hot filtered water

⅔ cup chopped fresh basil

2 TB. minced garlic

1 cup Vegan Soy-licious Mayonnaise (recipe earlier in this chapter)

3 TB. olive oil

2 TB. balsamic vinegar

2 TB. tamari, shoyu, or Bragg Liquid Aminos

6 portobello mushrooms, stemmed and wiped with a damp, lint-free towel

6 whole-grain hamburger buns or rolls, split

Lettuce, onion slices, tomato slices, soy cheese, or other toppings of choice (optional)

Yield: 6 servings
Prep time: 15 to 20 minutes
Cook time: 10 to 15 minutes

In a Nutshell

If you don't have an outdoor grill, cook these mushroom burgers on a grill pan on the stove-top or under a broiler until golden brown and slightly crispy around the edges. Then assemble according to the recipe instructions. Slice or chop leftover mushroom burgers, and add to pasta, grain dishes, or side dishes to give them a smoky and earthy flavor.

1. Preheat the grill. In a small bowl, add sun-dried tomatoes, pour hot water over them, and set aside for 15 minutes to rehydrate. In a food processor, combine rehydrated sun-dried tomatoes and their water, ⅓ cup chopped basil, 1 tablespoon garlic, and Vegan Soy-licious Mayonnaise, and process for 1 minute. Transfer mixture to a small bowl, and set aside.

2. In a small bowl, whisk together remaining chopped basil and garlic, olive oil, balsamic vinegar, and tamari; set aside. Dip each mushroom in marinade, and place on the hot grill stem side down. Grill mushrooms for 5 minutes, carefully flip them over with tongs, and grill an additional 4 to 5 minutes or until tender.

3. Lightly toast buns on the grill, if desired. Serve grilled mushrooms on buns with lettuce, onion slices, tomato slices, soy cheese, or your choice of toppings and a few spoonfuls of sun-dried tomato aioli or other condiments of choice.

Italian Tempeh "Meatball" Sandwiches

Yield: 6 sandwiches

Prep time: 20 to 25 minutes

Cook time: 30 to 40 minutes

In a Nutshell

You can also forego the buns and use the tomato sauce and Sammy's Spicy Tempeh Sausage Meatballs to make a delicious vegan version of spaghetti and "meatballs." Simply cook some spaghetti or linguine; top individual servings with a little sauce and "meatballs"; and then sprinkle with a little shredded soy mozzarella-style cheese, vegan Parmesan cheese, or nutritional yeast flakes.

½ cup onions, diced

1 TB. olive oil

1 TB. garlic, minced

1 tsp. dried basil

1 tsp. dried oregano

1 tsp. sea salt

¼ tsp. freshly ground black pepper

1 (28-oz.) can crushed tomatoes

1 batch Sammy's Spicy Tempeh Sausages (recipe in Chapter 20)

Olive oil

6 (6-inch) submarine rolls, other soft rolls, or hot dog buns

Shredded vegan soy mozzarella-style cheese or other vegan cheese of choice (optional)

1. Preheat oven to 400°F. Sauté onions in olive oil in a medium saucepan for 3 minutes to soften. Add garlic and sauté an additional minute, stirring constantly, until fragrant but not browned. Add basil, oregano, sea salt, and black pepper; sauté an additional 30 seconds. Add crushed tomatoes, stir well to combine, reduce heat to low, and simmer mixture for 10 minutes to blend flavors.

2. Prepare Sammy's Spicy Tempeh Sausages mixture according to the recipe instructions. Using olive oil, lightly oil a cookie sheet, and set aside. Using your hands or a small scoop, shape tempeh sausage mixture into 1¼-inch balls, and place them on the prepared cookie sheet. Using your fingers, rub a little olive oil over the top of each "meatball."

3. Bake for 25 to 30 minutes or until "meatballs" are dry to the touch and lightly browned on the outside.

4. To assemble each sandwich: split open submarine roll, spoon a little of prepared sauce on bottom half, add 4 baked "meatballs," top with some additional sauce, and sprinkle a little shredded vegan soy mozzarella-style cheese over the top (if using). Serve immediately.

22

Main and Side Dishes

In This Chapter

- ◆ Creating the center of your vegan meal
- ◆ Making vegan "meat and potatoes"
- ◆ Wowing your dinner guests with colorful and delicious veggie side-dishes

If you don't have complete confidence in your own vegan cooking abilities yet, fear not. Just keep practicing. Start with the side dishes. In this chapter, we lay out the basics of roasting and grilling vegetables, as these methods have endless uses and provide many meal possibilities. You can use roasted veggies to make hearty sandwiches when layered between slices of bread or in tortillas as wraps. Or dice them and add them to grains or cooked pasta, with a little vinaigrette, to make a filling meal. Grilled veggies are delicious eaten alone or with some stewed beans or baked tofu for a satisfying supper.

You also will find marvelous mashed potatoes and gravy recipes with several variation ideas. You can transform mashed potatoes in many ways by using different potato varieties, adding additional ingredients such as roasted garlic or sun-dried tomatoes, and seasoning with fresh herbs such as dill or rosemary. You also can use potatoes to thicken soups or stews or to make quesadillas. And knowing how to make a good gravy is just as important as your mashed potato know-how, especially for vegans. Through these pages, we give you several suggestions for using vegan onion gravy, and you are sure to come up with several others on your own.

In a Nutshell

Have leftover mashed potatoes but are stumped as to what to use them for? Make potato quesadillas! Spoon a generous serving of mashed potatoes on one half of a flour tortilla, sprinkle on a little nutritional yeast flakes or shredded soy cheese, and fold over tortilla to enclose the filling. Bake at 400°F for 15 minutes or until golden brown and crisp for a low-fat version. Or cook in olive oil in a skillet until browned on both sides and heated through. Then serve with your choice of salsa and tofu sour cream.

Beans are stars in these recipes, too. Beans mixed with grains, greens, and other veggies showcase foods from Thailand with a black bean and rice dish to the American South with a greens and beans stew. Or try the Mexican-influenced veggie, black bean, and corn cakes that are cooked much like a pancake and served with accoutrements.

You learned how to make quite a few vegan mock meats or protein alternative recipes in Chapters 20 and 21, and this chapter gives you a few more to extend your repertoire. Seitan, tofu, and tempeh provide the most filling and varied options when you want to make something to share with friends or family. Your diners may even find it hard to believe they're eating a vegan meal!

By the end of this chapter, you will have enough recipes—and we hope an equal amount of inspiration—to create many fabulous vegan meals. Feel free to showcase your new vegan culinary talents by inviting friends or family over for a meal. Positive example is the best teacher. By serving them a delicious and nutritious vegan meal, you can put their minds at ease and also satisfy their curiosity as to what exactly you eat as a vegan.

Rustic Roasted Vegetables

4 cups eggplant, cut into 2-inch cubes

4 cups zucchini, quartered lengthwise and sliced 1 inch thick

4 cups yellow summer squash, quartered lengthwise and sliced 1 inch thick

3 cups onions, cut from end to end into ½-inch-thick half-moons

2 cups green bell pepper, seeds and ribs removed, and cut into 1-inch dice

2 cups red or orange bell pepper, seeds and ribs removed, and cut into 1-inch dice

2 TB. garlic, minced

2 TB. olive oil

2 TB. chopped fresh rosemary or 2 tsp. dried rosemary

2 TB. chopped fresh thyme or 2 tsp. dried thyme

2 tsp. dried basil

2 tsp. dried oregano

1 tsp. sea salt

½ tsp. freshly ground black pepper

Yield: 6 to 8 servings
Prep time: 15 minutes
Cook time: 30 to 40 minutes

In a Nutshell

Roasting brings out the delicate sweetness of vegetables. The carmelization of the natural sugars on the skins and cut surfaces adds a rich, earthy flavor to dishes. Winter squashes and root vegetables are especially delicious when roasted. Use other herbs and spices to vary and intensify flavors even more.

1. Preheat the oven to 425°F. In a large bowl, combine eggplant, zucchini, summer squash, onions, green bell pepper, red bell pepper, garlic, olive oil, rosemary, thyme, basil, oregano, sea salt, and black pepper. Toss well to thoroughly coat vegetables. Lightly oil a large roasting pan or cookie sheet with olive oil. Transfer vegetable mixture to the pan, and spread into a single layer.

2. Bake for 20 minutes. Stir vegetables and spread into a single layer again. Roast an additional 10 to 15 minutes or until vegetables are just tender and slightly browned in places.

3. Transfer vegetables to a bowl or platter for serving. Taste and adjust seasonings as needed. Enjoy these vegetables as a side dish, part of a main dish, or diced and added to pasta, rice, or grain dishes. They're also great served as a sandwich, on rolls or bread, with a creamy or tahini-based sauce, or with a little additional olive oil and red wine vinegar.

Variation: Get creative by throwing in an assortment of your own favorite veggies.

Glorious Grilled Garden Vegetables

¼ cup olive oil

¼ cup vegetable stock or filtered water

2 TB. garlic, minced

2 zucchini, diagonally sliced ½ inch thick

2 yellow summer squash, diagonally sliced ½ inch thick

2 orange or yellow bell peppers, seeds and ribs removed, and cut into 1-inch strips

2 red bell peppers, seeds and ribs removed, and cut into 1-inch strips

2 red onions, thickly sliced

6 Roma tomatoes, sliced in half lengthwise

Sea salt

Freshly ground black pepper

1. Preheat a gas grill. In a small bowl, combine olive oil, vegetable stock, and garlic.

2. Spread out zucchini, summer squash, orange bell peppers, red bell peppers, red onions, and Roma tomatoes on a cookie sheet. Add olive oil mixture, and toss well to combine. Then season vegetables to taste with sea salt and pepper.

3. Place vegetables on the hot grill, and cook for 3 to 5 minutes or until brown grill marks appear on vegetables' surface. Carefully turn over with tongs, and grill on the other side until grill marked and lightly browned, about 3 to 5 minutes more.

4. Transfer veggies to a platter for serving. Enjoy as a side dish; part of a main dish; or diced and added to pasta, rice, or grain dishes. These veggies are also great served on rolls or bread as a sandwich with a creamy sauce and herbs or with a little additional olive oil and red wine vinegar.

Variation: Feel free to substitute other fresh vegetables to take advantage of what's currently in season in your area. Asparagus, green beans, green onions, carrots, bitter greens, mushrooms, and eggplant are also delicious grilled. Place vegetables at a 45-degree angle to the grill grate to make those must-have grill marks. This placement will also help prevent the veggies from falling through the grate and into the grill.

Mouthwatering Mashed Potatoes

3 lb. Yukon Gold potatoes, peeled and cut into cubes

Filtered water

¾ to 1 cup soy milk, rice milk, or other nondairy milk of choice

2 TB. nonhydrogenated margarine or olive oil

1 tsp. sea salt

½ tsp. freshly ground black pepper or white pepper

Yield: 4 to 6 servings
Prep time: 10 to 15 minutes
Cook time: 20 to 25 minutes

1. Place potato cubes in a large pot, cover with water, and bring to a boil. Reduce heat to low, and simmer for 20 minutes or until potatoes are tender. Drain, reserving cooking liquid (for making soup or for use in another dish), and return cooked potatoes to the pot.

2. Add soy milk and, using a potato masher, mash potatoes, making the mixture as smooth or chunky as desired. Add margarine, sea salt, and pepper; stir well to combine. Taste and add additional seasoning or margarine if desired.

Variations: Here are a few mouthwatering suggestions for alternative mashed potato dishes:

- **Roasted garlic:** Roast ½ to 1 cup unpeeled garlic cloves in a 350°F oven for 15 to 20 minutes or until golden brown. Peel cloves and add to potatoes during mashing.

- **Roasted onion or shallot:** Roast pieces of 1 peeled onion or 2 whole shallots in a 400°F oven for 15 to 20 minutes or until golden brown, roughly chop, and then add to potatoes during mashing.

- **Country style:** Use unpeeled Yukon Gold or red-skinned potatoes; sauté a small amount of onion, shallots, green onions, and/or garlic; and roughly mash everything together. Leave some chunks for character.

- **Cheezy:** Stir in a little nutritional yeast flakes, Vegan Cheezy Sauce (recipe in Chapter 20), or shredded vegan soy cheese to the finished mashed potatoes.

- **Sun-dried tomato:** Sauté a little chopped garlic and rosemary in olive oil and add to potatoes along with ½ cup rehydrated and chopped sun-dried tomatoes and some chopped fresh parsley.

In a Nutshell

If you prefer your mashed potatoes chunky or with a few lumps, use an old-fashioned hand potato masher. If you prefer very creamy mashed potatoes, use a mixer (not a food processor) on low speed to whip the potatoes to your desired consistency. You can make mashed potatoes ahead of time and keep them warm in a covered casserole in a 250°F oven or in a slow cooker on low.

Groovy Onion Gravy

In a Nutshell

If you like your gravy smooth, purée the finished gravy or strain it through a sieve to remove the onion pieces. You can also make this gravy in large batches, portion it into servings, and freeze it. Then just simply thaw and reheat before using.

⅔ cup whole-wheat flour

1 cup onions, diced

1 TB. olive oil

1 TB. garlic, minced

4 cups vegetable stock or filtered water

½ cup nutritional yeast flakes

2 TB. tamari, nama shoyu, or Bragg Liquid Aminos

1½ tsp. rubbed (dried) sage

1½ tsp. sea salt

¼ tsp. freshly ground black pepper

1. In a medium saucepan, cook flour over low heat, stirring constantly, until lightly browned and fragrant, about 2 to 3 minutes. Transfer browned flour to a medium bowl and set aside.

2. In the same saucepan, sauté onions in olive oil over low heat for 3 to 5 minutes or until soft. Add garlic and sauté an additional 2 minutes.

3. Add vegetable stock, nutritional yeast flakes, tamari, sage, sea salt, and black pepper to browned flour, and whisk well to combine. Add wet ingredients to sautéed onion mixture. Whisk well to combine, and continue to cook mixture, whisking constantly, until thickened. Taste and adjust seasonings as desired. Serve this gravy on top of your favorite vegetables, mashed potatoes, biscuits, or main dishes. Use it to make sauces for casseroles or add it to soups or stews.

Variations: Reducing the amount of onions and adding additional ingredients results in different gravies, such as …

◆ **Roasted garlic:** Roast ½ to 1 cup garlic cloves in a 350°F oven for 15 to 20 minutes or until golden brown. Use in place of or in addition to the sautéed onion mixture.

◆ **Roasted onion or shallot:** Roast pieces of an onion or 2 whole shallots in a 400°F oven for 15 to 25 minutes or until golden brown. Roughly chop and use in place of the sautéed onion mixture.

◆ **Mushroom:** Sauté 1 cup chopped mushrooms along with the onion mixture and add an additional 1 tablespoon tamari for a richer flavor.

◆ **Creamy:** Whisk in a little soy milk and 1 to 2 tablespoons additional nutritional yeast flakes to lighten the gravy's color and flavor.

Bangkok Coconut Rice and Black Beans

4 cups filtered water

2 cups brown basmati or jasmine rice

2 TB. ginger, peeled, and grated

1 TB. garlic, minced

1 tsp. sea salt

½ tsp. freshly ground black pepper

½ cup canned coconut milk

Juice of 1 orange

Juice of 2 limes

1 TB. toasted sesame oil

1 (15-oz.) can black beans, drained and rinsed

½ cup red bell pepper, seeds and ribs removed, and diced

½ cup orange bell pepper, seeds and ribs removed, and diced

½ cup green onions, thinly sliced

½ cup chopped fresh cilantro

⅓ cup sliced almonds

Yield: 4 to 6 servings
Prep time: 10 to 15 minutes
Cook time: 30 minutes

In a Nutshell

This rice-and-black-bean combo also makes a great filling for lettuce rolls. Simply add a spoonful of the chilled rice mixture in the center of a crisp lettuce leaf and roll up like a burrito. Or use it as a filling for a burrito or wrap, either hot or cold.

1. In a large saucepan, combine water, basmati rice, ginger, garlic, sea salt, and black pepper. Bring to a boil, cover, reduce heat to low, and simmer for 20 minutes or until all water is absorbed and tiny holes appear on top of rice. Remove from heat, leave covered, and set aside for 10 minutes to allow rice to steam.

2. Transfer rice to a large bowl, and fluff with a fork to loosen grains. Add coconut milk, orange juice, lime juice, and toasted sesame oil; toss gently to combine. Add black beans, red bell pepper, orange bell pepper, green onions, cilantro, and almonds; gently fold to combine. Serve plain or on a bed of chopped greens.

Variation: Chill rice mixture in the refrigerator for 1 hour or more and eat as a cold salad on a bed of chopped mixed greens.

Mean Greens and Beans

In a Nutshell

Greens and beans are excellent served over rice or quinoa. Cook rice or quinoa in a ratio of 2 parts water to 1 part rice: simply bring 2 parts water to a boil, add quinoa or rice, cover, reduce to low, and simmer for 15 minutes. Remove pan from heat, and leave covered for 10 minutes. Remove cover, fluff with a fork, and serve!

2 cups onions, diced

2 TB. olive oil

3 cups red bell pepper, seeds and ribs removed, and diced

2 TB. garlic, minced

2 cups vegetable stock or filtered water

2 bunches collard greens, washed, stemmed, and roughly chopped

2 bunches kale, washed and roughly chopped

2 bunches Rainbow Swiss chard, washed and roughly chopped

2 (15-oz.) cans butter beans or other bean of choice, drained and rinsed

3 TB. nutritional yeast flakes

1 TB. dried thyme

1 tsp. crushed red pepper flakes

1 tsp. sea salt

½ tsp. freshly ground black pepper

¼ tsp. cayenne

Hot red pepper sauce for garnish (optional)

1. Sauté onions in olive oil in a large stock pot over medium heat for 5 to 7 minutes or until soft and lightly browned. Add red bell pepper and garlic, and sauté an additional 2 minutes. Add vegetable stock, and bring mixture to a boil. Add collard greens, kale, and Rainbow Swiss chard to the pot in batches, covering pot between batches to help greens wilt.

2. Add butter beans, nutritional yeast flakes, thyme, crushed red pepper flakes, sea salt, black pepper, and cayenne; stir well to combine. Cover, reduce heat to low, and simmer for 15 to 20 minutes or until greens are tender. Taste and adjust seasonings if needed. Serve with hot pepper sauce for topping (if desired).

Variation: Substitute other greens such as spinach, turnip greens, mustard greens, and beet greens, as well as other beans, like black-eyed peas or red beans as you like. In the South, it's customary to enjoy your greens and beans with a little something to sop up the juices, such as biscuits and cornbread. Find vegan recipes for both of these in Chapter 20.

Confetti Corn Cakes

1 cup yellow cornmeal

1 cup soy milk, rice milk, or other nondairy milk of choice

1 TB. nonaluminum baking powder

1 TB. light miso

1 tsp. chili powder

1 tsp. olive oil

½ cup cooked black beans, drained and rinsed

⅓ cup frozen cut corn, thawed

¼ cup green bell pepper, seeds and ribs removed, and diced

¼ cup red bell pepper, seeds and ribs removed, and diced

¼ cup green onions, thinly sliced

¼ cup chopped fresh cilantro

Salsa and/or tofu sour cream for garnish

Yield: 4 to 6 servings
Prep time: 10 minutes
Cook time: 12 to 20 minutes

1. In a bowl, combine yellow cornmeal, soy milk, baking powder, light miso, chili powder, and olive oil, stirring until just blended. Gently fold in black beans, corn, green bell pepper, red bell pepper, green onions, and cilantro. Let batter sit for 5 minutes to activate baking powder.

2. Heat an electric griddle or skillet over medium heat. Using olive oil, lightly oil the pan. Working in batches, drop batter by ¼ cupfuls onto the hot pan, spaced 1 inch apart.

3. Cook corn cakes until lightly browned, about 3 to 5 minutes per side. Gently turn over with a spatula, and cook until lightly browned on the other side, about 3 to 5 additional minutes. Transfer to a large, ovenproof dish, and keep warm in a 250°F oven while repeating cooking procedure for remaining batter. Serve with choice of salsa and/or tofu sour cream as desired.

In a Nutshell

Most Latin foods are great served with a little avocado accompaniment such as guacamole. For quick guac, mash together 2 avocados, a little lime or lemon juice, some minced fresh garlic or garlic powder, sea salt, and black pepper. Leave it chunky, or mash it with a fork until it's smooth and creamy. Or add a little diced jalapeño, green onions, tomato, red bell pepper, or cilantro.

Baked Seitan Roast

In a Nutshell

Dice or cut leftover
seitan roast into strips
and add to soups,
stews, casseroles,
salads, pasta, rice, and
grain dishes. Or use it
as a filling for sand-
wiches or wraps.

1 cup onions, finely diced

2 TB. olive oil

3 TB. garlic, minced

2 TB. ginger, peeled and
grated

4 cups vegetable stock or filtered water

½ cup nutritional yeast flakes

⅓ cup tamari or nama shoyu

2 TB. toasted sesame oil

1 TB. onion powder

1 TB. garlic powder

1 tsp. dried thyme

1 tsp. rubbed (dried) sage

¾ tsp. sea salt

¾ tsp. black pepper

4½ cups vital wheat gluten

¾ cup whole-wheat flour

1. Preheat oven to 350°F. Sauté onions in olive oil in a skillet
   over low heat for 7 minutes or until lightly browned. Add
   garlic and ginger, and sauté an additional 2 minutes. Remove
   the skillet from heat, and allow to cool slightly.

2. Transfer sautéed onion mixture to a blender or food processor. Add vegetable stock, nutritional yeast flakes, tamari,
   toasted sesame oil, onion powder, garlic powder, thyme, sage,
   sea salt, and black pepper; process for 2 minutes or until
   smooth. Divide wet ingredients, transferring ½ to a small
   bowl, and set aside; use other ½ to mix seitan.

3. In a large bowl, add vital wheat gluten and whole-wheat flour,
   and stir well to combine. Add a little of wet ingredients to dry
   ingredients, and stir well to combine. Continue to add additional liquid, as needed, to form a firm dough. Using your
   hands, knead dough in the bowl for 2 minutes.

4. Using olive oil, lightly oil a 9×5×3-inch loaf pan. Stretch
   dough slightly and then press it in the pan. Pour ½ of
   reserved wet ingredients over top of seitan roast.

5. Bake for 45 minutes. Remove pan from oven, and pour
   remaining reserved wet ingredients over roast. Reduce oven
   temperature to 325°F, bake roast an additional 20 to 25 minutes or until all liquid is absorbed and roast is very firm to the
   touch. Allow to cool 10 minutes in the pan.

6. Remove roast from pan. Use a sharp knife to cut roast into
   slices, and transfer the slices to a large platter for serving.

Ginger-Teriyaki Tofu

2 lb. firm tofu

½ cup tamari, nama shoyu, or Bragg Liquid Aminos

¼ cup brown rice vinegar

3 TB. toasted sesame oil

3 TB. pure maple syrup

2 TB. garlic, minced

2 TB. ginger, peeled and grated

2 tsp. dry mustard

½ tsp. crushed red pepper flakes

Yield: 6 to 8 servings
Prep time: 15 minutes, plus 30 minutes to press tofu
Cook time: 40 to 50 minutes

1. Set 2 blocks tofu between 2 large plates, place them in the sink, and weight them down with several large cans or other heavy objects to press out excess moisture. Leave tofu to press and drain for 30 minutes.

2. Preheat oven to 350°F. Cut each block of tofu in half lengthwise, turn each half cut side down on the board, cut through the outer edge of the block 3 times to yield 4 tofu cutlets from each half. (So each block of tofu yields 8 tofu cutlets.)

3. Add tofu cutlets in a single layer to a large casserole dish. In a small bowl, whisk together tamari, brown rice vinegar, toasted sesame oil, maple syrup, garlic, ginger, dry mustard, and crushed red pepper flakes. Pour this mixture over tofu in dish.

4. Bake for 20 minutes. Turn tofu cutlets with a spatula, and cook an additional 20 to 30 minutes or until most of glaze is absorbed.

5. Serve 2 or 3 tofu cutlets per person as a main dish, side dish, or filling for a sandwich with fresh veggies. Or cube tofu and add to soups, stir-fries, salads, pasta, rice, or grain dishes.

Variation: You can cut tofu into small cubes, mix with marinade, and bake according to the recipe instructions. You can also substitute large tempeh cubes.

In a Nutshell

Tofu and tempeh are delicious when tossed with tamari, olive oil, a little nutritional yeast flakes, and seasonings of choice, and baked until golden brown and crispy around the edges.

Baked Breaded Tofu Cutlets

2 lb. firm tofu

1¼ cups soy milk, rice milk, or other nondairy milk of choice

2 TB. fresh or bottled lemon juice

1½ cups whole-wheat flour

1 cup yellow cornmeal

½ cup nutritional yeast flakes

1 TB. onion powder

1 TB. garlic powder

1 TB. dried parsley

2 tsp. dried basil

2 tsp. dried oregano

1 tsp. paprika

1 tsp. sea salt

½ tsp. freshly ground black pepper

1. Set 2 blocks tofu between 2 large plates, place them in the sink, and weight them down with several large cans or other heavy objects to press out excess moisture. Leave tofu to press and drain for 30 minutes.

2. Preheat oven to 400°F. Cut each block of tofu in half lengthwise, turn each half cut side down on the board, and cut through the outer edge of the block 3 times to yield 4 tofu cutlets from each half. (So each block of tofu yields 8 tofu cutlets.) Using olive oil, lightly oil a cookie sheet, and set aside.

3. In a small bowl, whisk together soy milk and lemon juice, and set aside for 10 minutes to thicken. Place whole-wheat flour on a large plate, and dust tofu with flour to thoroughly coat. Remove tofu from flour and set aside. Add yellow cornmeal, nutritional yeast flakes, onion powder, garlic powder, parsley, basil, oregano, paprika, sea salt, and black pepper to flour. Stir well to combine, and set aside.

4. Dip floured tofu into soymilk mixture; then add tofu to seasoned flour mixture, press down slightly, flip over, and repeat to thoroughly coat tofu cutlets on all sides. Place breaded tofu cutlets on the prepared cookie sheet, spaced so they aren't touching.

5. Bake cutlets for 10 to 15 minutes or until lightly browned. Turn over tofu cutlets with a spatula, and bake an additional 10 to 15 minutes or until lightly browned.

6. Serve 2 or 3 tofu cutlets per person as a main dish, side dish, or filling for a sandwich with fresh veggies on a bun, roll, or in a tortilla with a creamy sauce or some Vegan Soy-licious Mayonnaise (recipe in Chapter 21). Or cube them and add to soups, stews, salads, pasta, rice, or grain dishes.

Variations: Breading tofu or vegetables, similar to how you'd make chicken or fish, can result in endless possibilities:

◆ **Tofu nuggets:** Cut tofu into small cubes, bread, and bake according to the recipe instructions. Serve with a mixture of maple syrup and mustard, ketchup, or other dipping sauce of choice.

◆ **"Filet-o-Tofu" version:** Replace dried basil and oregano in breading mixture with 2 tablespoons powdered kelp for added nutrition and flavor.

◆ **Spicy version:** Replace dried basil and oregano in breading mixture with 2 teaspoons chili powder, ½ teaspoon ground cumin, and ⅛ teaspoon cayenne. Serve with barbecue sauce.

◆ **Breaded tempeh:** Substitute large cut pieces or cubes of tempeh for tofu. Bread and bake them in the same manner.

◆ **Breaded veggies:** Add slices or whole veggies such as eggplant, mushrooms, squash, cauliflower, or broccoli through the breading procedure, and bake them according to the recipe instructions. Eat as an appetizer or snack with a creamy dipping sauce, or use as a filling for a sandwich with fresh veggies, on a bun or roll, with a creamy sauce or some Vegan Soy-licious Mayonnaise (recipe in Chapter 21), similar to a New Orleans "Poor Boy" sandwich.

Hot Potato

Watch out for unnecessary fat! You can fry the breaded tofu in a little olive oil for a crispier crust, but be sure to drain them well and blot off any excess oil before eating.

Crunchy Sesame Vegetables over Soba Noodles

Yield: 6 servings

Prep time: 5 to 10 minutes

Cook time: 10 to 15 minutes

In a Nutshell

You can find many varieties of Asian-style noodles, including those made from brown rice, mung beans, mugwort, yams, buckwheat, wheat, and in combination with chilies, green tea, and added spices.

1 (12-oz.) pkg. soba noodles	3 cups spinach, triple rinsed, stems removed, and roughly chopped
⅓ cup fresh or bottled lime juice	2 cups red cabbage, shredded
¼ cup tamari, nama shoyu, or Bragg Liquid Aminos	1½ cups carrots, shredded
¼ cup toasted sesame oil	1½ cups red bell pepper, seeds and ribs removed, and diced
¼ cup unbleached sugar or Sucanat	
1 jalapeño pepper, seeds and ribs removed, and finely diced	1½ cups cucumber, peeled and diced
1 TB. ginger, peeled, and grated	1 cup green onions, thinly sliced
1 TB. garlic, minced	½ cup chopped fresh cilantro
	⅓ cup sesame seeds (raw or toasted)

1. Bring a large pot of salted water to a boil. Add soba noodles, and cook according to package instructions or until al dente. Drain well and transfer noodles to a large bowl.

2. In a blender or food processor, combine lime juice, tamari, toasted sesame oil, unbleached sugar, jalapeño pepper, ginger, and garlic; process for 1 minute. Pour dressing over cooked soba noodles, and toss well to thoroughly coat.

3. Add spinach, red cabbage, carrots, red bell pepper, cucumber, green onions, cilantro, and sesame seeds; toss well to combine. Serve immediately as a main dish, or chill in the refrigerator and serve as a salad.

Variations: Use other types of noodles to make many nutritious, delicious, and varied flavor combinations, and substitute other vegetables to suit your tastes. Add cashews or peanuts for additional crunch and protein, or add cubes of tofu marinated and baked like the Ginger-Teriyaki Tofu (recipe earlier in this chapter).

Creamy Lemon-Herb Farfalle

2½ cups vegetable stock

¼ cup nutritional yeast flakes

3 TB. white wine

3 TB. lemon juice

1½ TB. onion powder

1 TB. garlic, minced

1 tsp. sea salt

½ tsp. freshly ground black pepper

⅓ cup whole-wheat flour

3½ TB. plus 1 tsp. olive oil

2 TB. chopped fresh dill or 2 tsp. dried

2 TB. chopped fresh parsley

1 (12-oz.) pkg. whole-wheat or vegetable *farfalle* pasta

½ cup carrots, julienned

½ cup zucchini, julienned

½ cup green bell pepper, seeds and ribs removed, and diced

½ cup red bell pepper, seeds and ribs removed, and diced

½ cup red onions, diced

½ cup Roma tomatoes, seeds removed, and diced

½ cup frozen peas, thawed

Additional chopped fresh parsley and vegan soy Parmesan-style cheese or additional nutritional yeast flakes as garnish (optional)

Yield: 6 servings
Prep time: 10 to 15 minutes
Cook time: 10 to 15 minutes

Vegan 101

Farfalle (the Italian word for "butterflies") pasta is made from rectangular strips of pasta with zigzag or pinked edges and crimped in the center—they look like bow ties. Farfalle comes in a range of sizes, from small farfallini to large farfallone, and is ideal in soups, salads, or main dishes. Cook farfalle until just al dente, and handle gently to avoid breaking.

1. In a medium saucepan, combine vegetable stock, yeast flakes, white wine, lemon juice, onion powder, garlic, sea salt, and black pepper. Whisk well and simmer over low heat.

2. In a small bowl, whisk together whole-wheat flour and 2 tablespoons plus 1 teaspoon olive oil to form a smooth paste. Whisk flour-oil mixture, a little at a time, into simmering stock. Continue to cook over low heat, whisking constantly, until sauce is thickened. Whisk in dill and parsley. Set aside.

3. Bring a large pot of salted water to a boil over high heat. Add farfalle pasta, and cook according to the package instructions. Drain well and set aside.

4. In the same pot used to cook pasta, sauté carrots, zucchini, green bell pepper, red bell pepper, and red onions in remaining 1½ tablespoon olive oil over medium heat for 3 minutes. Add Roma tomatoes and peas, and sauté an additional 2 minutes. Add cooked farfalle and reserved sauce, and stir well to combine. Transfer to a large platter, and garnish with parsley and soy Parmesan-style cheese or nutritional yeast flakes.

Curried Vegetable and Chickpea Stew with Lemon Couscous

Yield: 6 to 8 servings

Prep time: 15 minutes

Cook time: 35 to 40 minutes

Vegan 101

Curry powder is an Indian spice blend typically made of turmeric, coriander, chilies, cumin, mustard, ginger, fenugreek, garlic, cloves, salt, and any number of other spices, all ground together. It comes in various colors, from bright yellow to deep red, and different levels of heat, from mild to extra hot. It also contains many powerful antioxidants and anti-inflammatory compounds.

2 cups onion, diced

1 cup green bell pepper, seeds and ribs removed, and diced

1 cup red bell pepper, seeds and ribs removed, and diced

1 TB. olive oil

2 TB. garlic, minced

2 tsp. *curry powder*

2 tsp. ground cumin

1 tsp. ground coriander

½ tsp. ground cinnamon

3 tsp. sea salt

1 tsp. freshly ground black pepper

3 cups sweet potato, diced

2 cups zucchini, quartered lengthwise and sliced

1 (15-oz.) can chickpeas, drained and rinsed

1 (14.5-oz.) can diced tomatoes

5 cups vegetable stock or filtered water

6 TB. fresh or bottled lemon juice

3 cups whole-wheat couscous

1. Sauté onion, green bell pepper, and red bell pepper in olive oil in a large pot over medium heat for 5 to 7 minutes or until softened. Add garlic, curry powder, cumin, coriander, cinnamon, 1½ teaspoon sea salt, and ½ teaspoon black pepper; sauté an additional 2 minutes. Add sweet potato, and sauté an additional 5 minutes.

2. Add zucchini, chickpeas, diced tomatoes, ½ cup vegetable stock, and 2 tablespoons lemon juice; stir well to combine. Cover, reduce heat to low, and simmer 15 to 20 minutes or until vegetables are tender.

3. While vegetables are simmering, combine remaining 4½ cups vegetable stock and 4 tablespoons lemon juice in a medium saucepan, and bring to a boil over high heat. Add couscous, remaining 1½ teaspoon sea salt, and remaining ½ black pepper, and stir to combine. Cover, remove the saucepan from heat, and set aside for 5 minutes to allow couscous to absorb liquid. Remove the lid and fluff couscous with a fork to loosen grains. Serve individual servings of stew over couscous.

Chapter 23

Baked Goods and Desserts

In This Chapter

- Getting hints for successful vegan baking
- Baking scrumptious cakes, cookies, and pies
- Satisfying your sweet tooth with raw, fruity snacks and a sweet raw pie

Being a great cook or chef takes skill and requires more than a little practice. But when it comes to cooking, the process can be more forgiving when you're altering a recipe or making it up as you go along; adding an extra dash here or handful there won't necessarily have a dramatic impact on the end result. But that's not the case with baking. Baking is more of a precise science, like chemistry in the kitchen. Leaveners' chemical reactions can cause great heights or end in bitter-tasting disappointment.

Vegan baking can be a bit trickier than the heavily egg- and dairy-laden baked goods and desserts most people are familiar with. Egg alternatives provide the height and texture to cakes, breads, and cookies. Exact measurements of leaveners and their triggering ingredients are necessary to ensure the proper end result.

The ratio between dry and wet ingredients determines if you will have a dry- or moist-tasting product. You can swap ingredients in certain instances, but keep the ratio in mind when playing around with substitutions. Additional add-on ingredients such as chocolate chips, dried fruits, or nuts will usually have less impact, and you can vary the amounts to suit your tastes.

You can find some vegan baked goods in grocery and natural foods stores, but they may not meet all your quality standards. If you want to survive as a vegan and satisfy your sweet tooth on your own terms, you're going to have to learn to be a vegan baker. However, there's nothing to be intimidated by! Just follow along with us; roll up your sleeves, open your pantry, and get baking!

In this chapter, you will find a baker's dozen of recipes, which seems only fitting in a chapter on vegan baked goods and desserts! Vegan baked goods may be indulgences, but in general, they are lower in fat, sugar, and calories than their egg and dairy counterparts. Also, these vegan recipes use more wholesome ingredients and provide you with a little something extra, instead of just filling you with empty calories and fat.

> **In a Nutshell**
>
> Having a well-stocked pantry helps you bake when the urge hits you. Buy commonly used baking items in bulk to save money and eliminate excess packaging. Be sure to store your dry goods in airtight containers to keep them fresh and free of pests, and label them appropriately to avoid any confusion later on.

We have included two naturally sweetened raw treats for the raw food devotee, the curious, or those trying to avoid refined sugars and sweeteners. Dried fruit and nut-rolled combinations are great for snacking and providing quick energy, and a raw fruit pie makes for a light, healthy, and delicious dessert, just perfect for the warm summer months when fruits are widely available.

You'll also find a few cookies, bars, and brownies. Bake several batches of these tasty treats and share them with your friends and co-workers. They won't believe you made them and they're all vegan! These treats are also suitable for taking to school bake sales and other such functions. You may even want to send a vegan treat along with your child when he or she is invited to birthday parties. This way he won't have to miss out on cake, just the one meant for the guest of honor.

Rounding out this chapter are some show-stopping vegan desserts, most of which also include variation suggestions to help you create even more decadent desserts. Humble pastry transforms into sweet berry hand pies. Tofu is pulverized to bits but manages to find its way into a creamy, mousselike topping, a vegan version of cheesecake, and even cake and frosting. Three recipes help fill that void in your recipe file and provide you with ideas for your next birthday or special occasion.

Flavorful Fruit Snacks

¾ **cup raisins**

¾ **cup raw walnuts**

¾ **cup medjool dates, pitted**

¾ **cup dried apricots**

¾ **cup shredded unsweetened coconut, plus more for rolling**

2 TB. fresh orange juice

Zest of 1 orange

Yield: 14 to 16 pieces
Prep time: 10 minutes

 Hot Potato

Many dried fruits are preserved with sulfites, so be sure to buy organic and unsulfured dried fruit. Also, always wash citrus fruits before zesting them, and be sure to use organic fruits for zesting to avoid getting a little pesticide residue along with your zest.

1. In a food processor, combine raisins, walnuts, medjool dates, and dried apricots. Pulse several times to roughly chop and then process for 1 to 2 minutes to finely chop. Add coconut, orange juice, and orange zest; process an additional 1 to 2 minutes or until mixture comes together to form a ball.

2. Place some shredded coconut on a plate and set aside. Dampen your hands with water, roll fruit mixture into 1-inch balls, and roll fruit balls in coconut. Place in an airtight container, and store in the refrigerator or freezer.

Variations: You can make other dried fruit snacks by substituting or omitting ingredients. Here are a few sweet and chewy combinations:

◆ **Cherry-walnut:** Replace raisins, dried apricots, coconut, orange juice, and orange zest with 1½ cups raw walnuts, 1½ cups pitted medjool dates, and 1½ cups dried cherries. Process and shape as described here. Roll in finely chopped walnuts instead of coconut.

◆ **Cranberry-pecan:** Replace dried apricots, coconut, and orange juice with 1½ cups raw walnuts, 1½ cups pitted medjool dates, 1½ cups dried cranberries, and zest of 1 orange. Process and shape as described here, but do not roll in coconut.

◆ **Blueberry-cashew:** Replace raisins, dried apricots, coconut, orange juice, and orange zest with 1½ cups raw cashews, 1½ cups pitted medjool dates, and 1½ cups dried blueberries. Process and shape as described here, but do not roll in coconut.

◆ **Fig and nut:** Replace raisins, dried apricots, coconut, and orange juice with 1 cup raw walnuts, 1 cup pitted medjool dates, 1 cup dried figs, 1 cup raw cashews or other nuts, and zest of 1 orange. Process as described here, except shape "dough" into 2-inch logs and then roll in shredded coconut.

Raw Mixed Berry and Mango Pie

1¼ cups raw sliced almonds

1 cup raw sunflower seeds

2 cups medjool dates, pitted

½ cup unsweetened banana chips

1 tsp. ground cinnamon

1 tsp. ground cardamom

2 cups blueberries

2 mangoes, peeled, pitted, and diced

¾ cup rinsed, hulled, and sliced strawberries

1 TB. ginger, peeled and grated

Sliced strawberries, blueberries, diced mango, raw sliced almonds, and/or other fruit of choice for garnish

1. In a food processor, combine almonds and sunflower seeds, and process for 1 to 2 minutes to finely chop. Add medjool dates, banana chips, ½ teaspoon cinnamon, and ½ teaspoon cardamom; process for 2 to 4 additional minutes or until ingredients are finely ground and mixture comes together.

2. Transfer mixture to a 9-inch pie pan. Using your hands, press mixture evenly over the bottom and up the sides of the pie pan. Place pie crust in the refrigerator, and chill for 20 to 30 minutes or until firm.

3. Wipe out the food processor with a clean, lint-free towel. Combine blueberries, mangoes, strawberries, remaining ½ teaspoon cinnamon, remaining ½ teaspoon cardamom, and ginger; process for 1 to 2 minutes. Scrape down the sides of the container, and process an additional minute to form a smooth purée.

4. Remove chilled pie crust from refrigerator, and pour in filling. Place pie back in the refrigerator, and chill for 30 to 45 minutes or until filling is set and slightly firm. Score top of pie into 8 pieces, and decorate each piece with a few fresh strawberries, blueberries, diced mango, and sliced almonds.

Health Nut Hermits

1 cup Sucanat or brown sugar from sugar beets

1 cup unsweetened apple-sauce

½ cup cold brewed coffee

1 tsp. pure vanilla extract

¼ tsp. pure almond extract

3 cups whole-wheat pastry flour

¾ cup soy flour

¾ cup wheat germ

2 TB. arrowroot

1 tsp. baking soda

1 tsp. ground cinnamon

½ tsp. ground ginger

½ tsp. ground nutmeg

¼ tsp. sea salt

⅓ cup raisins

⅓ cup roughly chopped walnuts

⅓ cup raw sunflower seeds

⅓ cup dried currants

⅓ cup dried cherries

⅓ cup dried cranberries

Yield: 4 dozen
Prep time: 5 to 10 minutes
Cook time: 15 to 20 minutes

In a Nutshell

Hermit cookies are a long-time New England favorite. The cookies are believed to be the result of the abundance of new spices from the spice trade. Rumor has it a version of these cookies—packed with dried fruits, nuts, coffee, and spices—was placed in canisters or tins and taken out to sea with sailors who voyaged all over the world.

1. Preheat the oven to 375°F. In a large bowl, combine Sucanat, applesauce, coffee, vanilla extract, and almond extract; stir well to combine. In a medium bowl, combine whole-wheat pastry flour, soy flour, wheat germ, arrowroot, baking soda, cinnamon, ginger, nutmeg, and sea salt. Add dry ingredients to wet ingredients, and stir well to combine. Add raisins, walnuts, sunflower seeds, dried currants, dried cherries, and dried cranberries; gently fold them into cookie dough.

2. Using olive oil, lightly oil 2 cookie sheets. Working in batches, drop cookie dough by tablespoonfuls onto the oiled cookie sheets, spacing them 2 inches apart.

3. Bake for 8 to 10 minutes or until lightly browned on bottom. Allow cookies to cool on cookie sheets for 2 minutes before transferring them to a rack with a spatula to cool completely. Repeat portioning and baking procedure for remaining cookie dough. Place cookies in an airtight container for storage.

Variation: Feel free to substitute other dried fruits and nuts to suit your tastes. You can also spread hermit cookie dough into 2 oiled (9-inch) square pans. Bake for 25 to 30 minutes or until firm to the touch and slightly browned around the edges. Allow to cool before cutting into squares.

Orange Chocolate Chunk and Cashew Cookies

Yield: 3 dozen

Prep time: 5 to 10 minutes

Cook time: 15 to 30 minutes

In a Nutshell

The cashew is a seed from a special tree apple in Brazil. The cashew apple is a delicacy there, and the cashew nut is an added bonus. A ¼-cup serving of cashews provides 22 percent of your daily requirement of magnesium, which helps with your body's absorption of calcium, as well as 38 percent of your copper needs.

2 cups barley flour

2 cups oat flour

Zest of 2 oranges

1 tsp. ground cinnamon

1 tsp. nonaluminum baking powder

1 tsp. baking soda

1 tsp. sea salt

⅔ cup pure maple syrup

⅔ cup brown rice syrup

⅔ cup olive oil or safflower oil

1 TB. pure vanilla extract

1 cup roughly chopped raw cashews

2 (2.8-oz.) pkg. vegan orange-flavored dark chocolate bars, cut into bite-size chunks

1. Preheat the oven to 350°F. In a large bowl, combine barley flour, oat flour, orange zest, cinnamon, nonaluminum baking powder, baking soda, and sea salt; stir well to combine. Add maple syrup, brown rice syrup, olive oil, and vanilla extract; stir well to form a soft dough. Add cashews and chopped chocolate, and fold gently to combine.

2. Using olive oil, lightly oil 2 cookie sheets. Working in batches, drop cookie dough by tablespoonfuls onto the oiled cookie sheets, spacing them 2 inches apart.

3. Bake for 12 to 15 minutes or until lightly browned on bottom. Allow cookies to cool on cookie sheets for 2 minutes before transferring them to a rack with a spatula to cool completely. Repeat portioning and baking procedure for remaining cookie dough. Place cookies in an airtight container for storage.

Variation: You can substitute other chocolate or carob chips, dried fruits, seeds, and nuts to suit your tastes. You can also spread cookie dough into 2 oiled (9-inch) square pans. Bake for 25 to 30 minutes or until firm to the touch and slightly browned around the edges. Allow to cool before cutting into squares.

Almond-Chocolate Chip Blondies

⅓ cup filtered water

3 TB. Ener-G Egg Replacer

1½ cup Sucanat

⅓ cup safflower oil or almond oil

2 tsp. pure vanilla extract

1 tsp. pure almond extract

1½ cups whole-wheat pastry flour

1½ tsp. nonaluminum baking powder

½ tsp. sea salt

⅔ cup vegan chocolate chips

⅓ cup sliced almonds

Yield: 1 (9×13-inch) pan or 12 squares
Prep time: 5 to 10 minutes
Cook time: 25 to 30 minutes

1. Preheat the oven to 350°F. In a bowl, combine water and Ener-G Egg Replacer; whisk for 1 minute or until very frothy. Add Sucanat, safflower oil, vanilla extract, and almond extract; whisk well to combine.

2. In another bowl, place whole-wheat pastry flour, nonaluminum baking powder, and sea salt; stir to combine. Add dry ingredients to wet ingredients, and stir well to combine. Gently fold vegan chocolate chips and almonds into batter.

3. Using safflower oil, lightly oil a 9×13-inch pan. Pour batter into pan, and bake for 25 to 30 minutes or until a toothpick inserted in the center comes out clean. Be careful not to over-bake; top and edges will appear dry and brown and the center will remain a little soft. Cut into 12 squares while still warm. Allow to cool completely before storing in an airtight container.

Variation: Substitute other nuts, raisins, or other dried fruit for almonds and chocolate chips. Or bake these plain with an additional 1 teaspoon almond extract to make butterscotch-tasting blondies.

In a Nutshell

For those allergic to chocolate, carob substitutes quite well in baking and making other sweet treats. Carob is a long brown pod, sometimes called locust bean or St. John's bread, from an evergreen tree. The pods are ground raw or after roasting to make carob powder. Carob chips are especially good for use in baking and can be substituted in most recipes.

Chewy Walnut Brownies

1 (12-oz.) pkg. vegan chocolate chips

¼ cup nonhydrogenated margarine

⅔ cup walnuts

3 medium bananas, peeled and cut into 2-inch pieces

1 tsp. pure vanilla extract

1½ cups whole-wheat pastry flour

1 cup unbleached sugar

½ tsp. nonaluminum baking powder

½ tsp. sea salt

1. Preheat the oven to 350°F. In the top of a double-boiler, combine vegan chocolate chips and margarine, and heat until thoroughly melted. In a food processor, place walnuts and pulse several times to finely chop. Transfer chopped walnuts to a small bowl and set aside. Place bananas and vanilla extract in the food processor, process for 2 minutes, scrape down the sides of the container, and process an additional minute to form a light and creamy purée. Set aside.

2. In a large bowl, stir together whole-wheat pastry flour, unbleached sugar, nonaluminum baking powder, and sea salt. Add banana purée to dry ingredients, and stir well to combine. Add melted chocolate-chip mixture, and stir well to thoroughly combine.

3. Using olive oil, lightly oil the bottom only of a 9×13-inch pan. Pour batter into the pan, sprinkle reserved chopped walnuts over top, and press them in gently with your hands.

4. Bake for 30 to 40 minutes or until center is set. Allow to cool completely, at least 1 hour, before cutting into 12 squares.

Whole-Wheat Pastry Dough

3 cups whole-wheat pastry flour

¼ cup unbleached sugar

1 tsp. sea salt

⅔ cup nonhydrogenated margarine

¼ to ⅓ cup cold filtered water

Yield: enough for 2 (9-inch) crusts
Prep time: 5 minutes, with 30 minutes of chilling time required

1. In a large bowl, combine whole-wheat pastry flour, unbleached sugar, and sea salt; stir to combine. Using a pastry blender, two knives, or your fingertips, cut in margarine until mixture resembles coarse crumbs. Drizzle in cold water, a little at a time, mixing lightly. Add additional water as needed until dough just starts to hold together. Form dough into a ball, cover with plastic wrap, and chill in the refrigerator for 30 minutes.

2. Place chilled dough between 2 pieces of parchment paper to help rolling out and transferring to pans. Bake as directed in your recipe. Use as pastry for both sweet and savory pies, turnovers, and tarts.

Variation: Substitute whole-grain spelt flour for whole-wheat pastry flour.

In a Nutshell
Chill your pastry dough to make it easier to roll out. When cooled, the fats in the dough harden and form layers throughout the dough, giving a pleasant flavor when baked. It also allows the gluten in the dough to relax and not get overworked, which could result in a heavy crust instead of a crisp and flaky one. You can also roll out the pastry dough on a floured work surface; then simply brush off excess flour before placing in or on a baking pan. Rolling the dough out between pieces of parchment paper makes rolling much easier and prevents sticking.

"Basketful of Berries" Hand Pies

<table>
<tr><td colspan="2" align="center">*Yield: 8 hand pies*</td></tr>
<tr><td colspan="2">**Prep time:** 15 minutes, with 30 minutes of chilling time

Cook time: 15 to 20 minutes</td></tr>
</table>

½ batch Whole-Wheat Pastry Dough (recipe earlier in this chapter)

½ cup strawberries, hulled and sliced

½ cup blackberries

⅓ cup blueberries

⅓ cup red raspberries

⅓ cup plus 1 tsp. unbleached sugar

1 TB. whole-wheat pastry flour

1 TB. fresh or bottled lemon juice

⅛ tsp. ground cardamom

1. Prepare Whole-Wheat Pastry Dough according to the recipe instructions and chill. Line a cookie sheet with a piece of parchment paper and set aside.

2. In a small bowl, add strawberries, blackberries, blueberries, red raspberries, ⅓ cup unbleached sugar, whole-wheat pastry flour, lemon juice, and ground cardamom. Toss gently to combine, and set aside.

3. Preheat the oven to 375°F. Transfer chilled dough to a floured work surface. Working with one half at a time, roll out dough to ⅛ inch thickness, and cut it into 5-inch circles. Using a spatula, carefully transfer circles to the prepared cookie sheet. Add trimmings to remaining pastry dough, and repeat rolling, cutting, and traying to yield 8 circles.

4. Evenly divide berry filling among dough circles, placing it in the center of each circle. Carefully fold over one side of pastry dough, press down around edges to seal, and then crimp edges with a fork. Sprinkle tops of hand pies with remaining 1 teaspoon unbleached sugar.

5. Bake for 15 to 20 minutes or until lightly browned. Serve either hot or cold. Allow to completely cool before individually wrapping to preserve freshness. Store in an airtight container if freezing.

Variation: Substitute other fruits and flavorings for mixed berries, alone or in a combination, such as strawberries, assorted raspberries, peaches, plums, apples, or cherries, blended with vanilla, almond, maple, or mint as flavoring enhancers.

In a Nutshell

To adapt this recipe to make a fruit pie: roll out dough and place it in a 9-inch pie pan. Cut off any excess, and flute the edges, if desired. Double the amount of filling called for in the recipe, but use the same combination of fruits. Bake it plain or with a crumb topping, or make the full Whole-Wheat Pastry Dough recipe, cover with another crust, and cut slits or decorate in a lattice pattern before baking at 375°F for 40 to 50 minutes or until crust is golden brown around the edges. Cool before cutting.

Creamy Tofu Topping or Mousse

2 (12.3-oz.) pkg. Mori-Nu
silken-style tofu, extra firm

⅔ cup pure maple syrup or
brown rice syrup

1 TB. pure vanilla extract

Yield: 3 cups
Prep time: 5 minutes, with 1 hour chilling time

1. In a food processor, combine silken tofu, maple syrup, and vanilla extract; process for 1 minute. Scrape down the sides of the container, and process an additional 1 to 2 minutes or until very smooth and creamy.

2. Transfer tofu topping to an airtight container, and chill in the refrigerator for 1 hour. Serve as a topping for fruit, granola, pies, cakes, and desserts—or enjoy all on its own.

Variations: Change the flavor and texture of tofu topping and mousse by adding additional ingredients in dreamy combinations:

◆ **Zest-kissed:** Add 2 to 3 teaspoons orange, lemon, lime, tangerine, or other citrus fruit zest to the food processor, and blend with other ingredients.

◆ **Lightly flavored fruit topping:** Add ½ cup fruit juice, such as raspberry, blueberry, or strawberry, to the food processor, and blend with other ingredients.

◆ **Fruit-flavored mousse:** Add 2 to 3 cups fresh or frozen fruit to the food processor, and blend with other ingredients.

◆ **Chocolate or carob:** Add 2 cups melted chocolate or carob chips to the food processor. Reduce maple syrup to ⅓ cup, and blend ingredients together.

In a Nutshell

Use this creamy tofu mousse and any of its variations to make a tofu cream pie. For a cool and creamy pie, fill a prebaked pie crust or graham cracker crust with mousse mixture, and chill in the refrigerator for several hours before cutting. Or bake the pie at 350°F for 30 to 35 minutes and allow to cool completely before cutting. Garnish pies with fresh fruit, additional dollops of tofu topping, chopped nuts, shredded unsweetened coconut, or chopped chocolate.

Vegan New York–Style Tofu Cheesecake

Yield: 1 (9-inch) cheese-cake or 12 pieces

Prep time: 10 minutes

Cook time: 35 to 40 minutes

1 (7-oz.) pkg. Health Valley Amaranth Graham Crackers

1 tsp. ground cinnamon

¼ cup nonhydrogenated margarine

2 lb. extra-firm tofu

½ cup plus 2 TB. unbleached sugar

½ cup pure maple syrup

3 TB. pure vanilla extract

3 TB. fresh lemon juice

Zest of 2 lemons

⅓ cup tofu sour cream

Hot Potato

Most pre-packaged graham crackers labeled "honey grahams" are not suitable for vegans. Health Valley Amaranth Graham Crackers are vegan and contain 70 percent organic ingredients. If you can't find these where you live, try looking for a vegan animal cracker or vanilla-, lemon-, spice-, or chocolate-flavored plain cookie you can crush to make crumbs for the crust.

1. Preheat the oven to 350°F. In a food processor, combine graham crackers and cinnamon, and process for 1 minute to crush to fine crumbs. Add margarine and process an additional minute. Using olive oil, lightly oil a 9-inch springform pan, and transfer crust mixture to the pan. Using your hands, firmly press mixture into bottom of the pan. Set aside.

2. Wipe out food processor with a clean, lint-free towel. Cut tofu blocks in half, and using your hands, squeeze as much of the excess water as possible out of each block. Then break blocks into smaller chunks and place them in the food processor. Add ½ cup unbleached sugar, maple syrup, vanilla extract, lemon juice, and lemon zest; process mixture for 3 minutes. Scrape down the sides of the container, and process an additional 2 minutes or until smooth and creamy.

3. Pour filling over crust, and smooth with a spatula. Bake for 30 minutes.

4. Meanwhile, in a small bowl, stir together tofu sour cream and remaining 2 tablespoons unbleached sugar, and set aside. After cheesecake has baked for 30 minutes, remove it from oven. Spread topping over top of cheesecake, leaving a 1-inch border around the edges. Return cheesecake to oven, and bake an additional 7 minutes or until topping's sheen changes from shiny to slightly dull. Do not allow to brown.

5. Remove cheesecake from oven and allow to cool for 20 minutes. Place springform pan on a large plate, and then place in refrigerator to chill several hours, preferably overnight. Loosen sides of cheesecake with a thin metal spatula or knife, and then remove the ring from the springform pan. Dip a knife in warm water for ease in cutting.

Lemon-Vanilla Cake with Creamy Vegan Butter-Cream Frosting

3 cups whole-wheat pastry flour

1½ cups unbleached sugar

1 TB. baking soda

½ tsp. sea salt

¾ cup filtered water

¾ cup plus 1 TB. fresh or bottled lemon juice

¼ cup safflower oil

4 TB. pure vanilla extract

2 TB. apple cider vinegar

½ cup nonhydrogenated margarine

3 cups powdered sugar

2 TB. soy milk, rice milk, or other nondairy milk of choice

> **Yield:** 1 (9×13-inch) cake or 12 pieces
>
> **Prep time:** 15 to 20 minutes
>
> **Cook time:** 20 to 25 minutes

1. Preheat the oven to 350°F. Using safflower oil, lightly oil a 9×13-inch pan and set aside. In a large bowl, combine whole-wheat pastry flour, unbleached sugar, baking soda, and sea salt. In another bowl, whisk together water ¾ cup lemon juice, 3 tablespoons vanilla extract, and apple cider vinegar. Add wet ingredients to dry ingredients, and whisk well to combine.

2. Pour batter into the prepared pan. Bake for 20 to 25 minutes or until a toothpick inserted in the center comes out clean. Remove cake from oven, and allow cake to cool completely before frosting.

3. For frosting, using an electric mixer or in a large bowl with a handheld mixer, beat margarine for 1 minute on medium speed. Add powdered sugar, soy milk, remaining 1 tablespoon lemon juice, and remaining 1 tablespoon vanilla extract; beat 2 to 3 minutes or until very light and creamy. Using a knife or small spatula, decoratively apply frosting to top of cake.

Variation: Do not frost the cake; instead, stir 2 tablespoons poppy seeds into batter before baking. Or serve cake with fresh fruit and just a dusting of powdered sugar instead of butter-cream frosting.

Hot Potato

Lemons at room temperature (or warmer) will release more of their juice more easily than ones straight from the refrigerator. Rolling or pounding a lemon on a hard surface before juicing can also help free up those juices. An average-size lemon will typically yield 1 to 2 teaspoons grated zest and 2 to 3 tablespoons juice.

Polynesian Pineapple-Coconut Cake with Tofu Frosting

> *Yield: 1 (9-inch) cake or 12 pieces*
>
> **Prep time:** 30 to 35 minutes
>
> **Cook time:** 15 to 20 minutes
>
> **Bake time:** 25 to 30 minutes

¾ cup shredded unsweetened coconut

¾ cup macadamia nuts

¾ cup medjool dates, pitted

⅔ cup plus 1 TB. filtered water

1½ cups frozen pineapple juice concentrate, thawed

2 TB. safflower oil

½ tsp. plus ⅛ tsp. coconut extract

¼ tsp. pure almond extract

¾ tsp. rum extract

2 cups whole-wheat pastry flour

2 TB. arrowroot

2 tsp. nonaluminum baking powder

2 tsp. baking soda

⅓ cup crushed pineapple

2 TB. pure maple syrup

½ tsp. apple cider vinegar

1 (12.3-oz.) pkg. Mori-Nu silken style tofu, extra firm

1. Preheat the oven to 325°F. Place shredded coconut and macadamia nuts on separate cookie sheets. Bake for 3 to 7 minutes or until lightly toasted and fragrant. Allow macadamia nuts to cool and then roughly chop them. Transfer 3 tablespoons each of chopped macadamias and shredded coconut to a small bowl, and set aside for garnishing frosted cake. Place remaining chopped macadamias and shredded coconut in another small bowl, and set aside.

2. Increase oven temperature to 350°F. Using safflower oil, lightly oil a 9-inch springform pan and set aside. In a small saucepan, place dates and ⅓ cup water, and cook over medium heat for 8 minutes or until dates have softened and most of liquid has been absorbed. Remove saucepan from heat, and set aside to cool for 2 minutes.

3. Transfer slightly cooled dates and any remaining cooking liquid to a food processor. Add 1 cup pineapple juice concentrate, ⅓ cup water, safflower oil, ½ teaspoon coconut extract, almond extract, and ¼ teaspoon rum extract; purée for 2 minutes or until smooth.

4. Sift together whole-wheat pastry flour, 1 tablespoon arrow-root, nonaluminum baking powder, and baking soda in a large bowl. Add wet ingredients to dry ingredients, and whisk until smooth. Add reserved macadamia nut–coconut mixture (larger amount) and crushed pineapple, and gently fold into batter.

5. Pour batter into the prepared springform pan. Bake for 25 to 30 minutes or until golden brown and a toothpick inserted in the center comes out clean. Allow cake to cool for 15 minutes and then remove ring from springform pan. Allow cake to cool completely before frosting.

6. For frosting, in a small saucepan, combine ½ cup pineapple juice concentrate, maple syrup, and cider vinegar. Bring to a boil, reduce heat to low, and simmer for 5 minutes. In a small bowl, whisk together remaining 1 tablespoon arrowroot and 1 tablespoon water. Whisk mixture into simmering juice mixture, and continue to cook, whisking constantly, until mixture thickens.

7. In a food processor, place silken tofu, thickened juice mixture, remaining ½ teaspoon rum extract, and ½ teaspoon coconut extract, and purée for 1 to 2 minutes or until very smooth and creamy. Spread tofu frosting over top only of cooled cake and then sprinkle remaining reserved macadamia nut–coconut mixture over frosting. Dip a knife in warm water for ease in cutting.

In a Nutshell

Macadamia originate from Australia and were only introduced to Hawaii in the late 1800s, but most of us identify them with Hawaii, which is the world's leading producer and exporter. Like most nuts, macadamias are high in fat, but they are high in monounsaturated fatty acids, which help reduce blood cholesterol levels. They also contain many antioxidants such as vitamins A and E, thiamine, riboflavin, niacin, iron, omega-3 fatty acids, and flavenoids, which help protect your body against cancer, heart disease, and high blood pressure.

Mexican Chocolate Almond Cake

Yield: 1 (8-inch) cake or 8 pieces

Prep time: 5 to 10 minutes

Cook time: 45 to 50 minutes

In a Nutshell

The Mayan culture was the first to develop chocolate into foods and beverages and flavor it. Mexican culinary traditions sweeten it with sugar and grind the roasted cocoa beans with nuts and spices—most commonly almonds and cinnamon. Then it's formed into bars and discs. This traditional blend of chocolate, sugar, almonds, and cinnamon also forms the basis of many Mexican desserts and confections.

⅓ cup safflower oil

1 cup soy milk, rice milk, or other nondairy milk of choice

¾ cup pure maple syrup

4 oz. Mori-Nu silken-style tofu, extra firm

2 tsp. pure almond extract

2 tsp. pure vanilla extract

1 tsp. apple cider vinegar

1½ cups whole-wheat pastry flour

½ cup cocoa powder

1 tsp. nonaluminum baking powder

¾ tsp. baking soda

½ tsp. ground cinnamon

⅛ tsp. sea salt

⅔ cup sliced almonds

1. Preheat the oven to 350°F. Using safflower oil, lightly oil bottom and sides of an 8-inch springform pan, and set aside. In a food processor, combine ⅓ cup safflower oil, soy milk, maple syrup, silken tofu, almond extract, vanilla extract, and vinegar; process for 1 to 2 minutes or until smooth and creamy.

2. In a medium bowl, combine whole-wheat pastry flour, cocoa powder, nonaluminum baking powder, baking soda, cinnamon, and sea salt. Add wet ingredients to dry ingredients, and whisk until smooth. Reserve 2 tablespoons sliced almonds for top of cake, add remaining almonds to batter, and fold in gently to combine.

3. Pour batter into the prepared pan and sprinkle reserved almonds over top. Bake for 45 to 50 minutes or until a toothpick inserted in the center comes out clean. Allow cake to cool for 15 minutes, remove ring from springform pan, and allow cake to cool completely before cutting.

Variation: If you're allergic to chocolate, replace cocoa powder with carob powder. You can also make a mint chocolate-chip cake with a few substitutions and changes: replace almond extract with 1 teaspoon peppermint extract, and omit cinnamon and sliced almonds. Replace vegan chocolate chips for sliced almonds, placing most of them in batter and scattering a few on top of cake before baking. Bake according to the recipe instructions and then cool and dust with a light sprinkle of powdered sugar.

Part 7

Vegan Lifestyle Choices

Being a vegan is about much more than not eating animals; it encompasses multiple aspects of your life choices. Veganism is a lifestyle. The more experienced and aware you become as a vegan, the more you'll discover new and hidden animal-based items in your life.

In the final chapters of this book, we provide a few bits of advice on buying vegan beauty and household products, finding cruelty-free clothing, taking photos, and caring for companion animals. We also give you some travel tips to help make you a wise—and well-fed—vegan traveler!

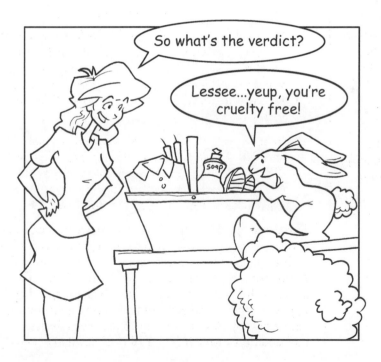

Chapter 24

Body Care and Personal Items

In This Chapter

- ◆ Choosing body care products
- ◆ Looking at vegan cosmetics
- ◆ Avoiding animal testing
- ◆ Brushing up on vegan brushes and sponges
- ◆ Checking out sources of body care items

The products that go onto your body, used for personal care in a variety of ways, are just as important to vegans as those products that go into it. As you might imagine, now that you're trying to live your life as cruelty-free as possible, you'll have to consider some issues when it comes to buying, using, and applying things such as shampoo, makeup, soap, and even dental floss.

In this chapter, we take a look at some of the issues surrounding these and other personal care items, ranging from the presence of animal ingredients to the practice of testing products on animals, and to those items that pose a risk to humans as well as other animals.

Animal Testing Issues

Being a cruelty-free vegan consumer as much as possible means being informed and making wise purchasing decisions. When it comes to stocking things such as the contents of your makeup case or your hair and skin care products, the most serious issue to be aware of is animal testing, also known as vivisection.

Many new products are routinely tested on living, unanesthetized animals in laboratory environments. These tests are carried out in the name of consumer safety by cosmetics, personal care, pharmaceutical, and household goods manufacturers.

Animal testing is a heavily debated issue, but it shouldn't be. There really isn't any logical argument for animal testing in any instance. Why? Because the rabbits, mice, rats, cats, frogs, and guinea pigs used in these tests don't share enough in common with humans, in terms of genetic makeup, to provide accurate enough data as to how humans would react to the same substance. What applies to a rat or a cat doesn't necessarily apply to humans when viewed from a physiological perspective.

> **Golden Apple**
>
> Animal studies are done for legal reasons and not for scientific reasons. The predictive value of such studies for man is meaningless.
>
> —Dr. James D. Gallagher, director of medical research, Lederle Laboratories, *Journal of the American Medical Association*, March 14, 1964

Even the chimpanzee, which is a 99 percent match for human DNA, doesn't work for accurately testing human responses to medications, cosmetics, and cleaners. Their systems would react differently, based on the simple fact that despite how closely related we are, we are still two completely different species. Knowing how a chimp, rabbit, or cat reacts to the exposure to any given substance does not guarantee that a human's system will react in the same way.

> **Hot Potato**
>
> The Draize eye test involves dropping substances, often cosmetics, into the eyes of restrained albino rabbits. In use for more than 40 years, the Draize test has a poor track record in accurately predicting the effects those substances have on human eyes. In a recent comparison of Draize test results with the actual experiences of humans using the products in question, the Draize tests only correctly predicted the human responses less than half the time.

Purchase products that say the company does not conduct animal testing, and look for the cruelty-free bunny logo. Many companies that are aware of their customers' sensitivities to these issues go out of their way to include such labeling on the product packaging. They know these consumers can be very loyal and will spread the word to others, thus increasing their sales and customer base. To be sure you don't accidentally buy a product tested on animals, you can go online and find lists of companies that test on animals. See www.stopanimaltests.com for lots of helpful information.

Most companies are aware of the facts surrounding animal research and testing. Because it isn't mandatory in most cases and due to growing public outcry over these practices, some are shying away from animal testing altogether. Instead, they are using actual human cells and tissues, artificial skin and eyes, and now computers to carry out the same scenarios in testing product safety.

The only reason the practice continues is because of a company's fear of being sued due to personal injury as a result of its product. Rather than use animal testing to prove its products are safe for human use, perhaps such companies should start with better, more natural ingredients that don't cause harm in the first place.

Natural vs. Synthetic Ingredients

The wisdom of using safe, natural ingredients over dangerous and artificial ingredients seems so apparent that you'd think every company and corporation would do it. Unfortunately, the bottom line is that companies make as much profit as possible, and often the quality and safety of ingredients takes a backseat to profitability.

In the early days, most body care and personal items did have more naturally based ingredients, made from herbal and botanical extracts and oils, often in water and alcohol bases. The preservatives, if used, were mostly natural, as things weren't really supposed to stick around on the shelf for long periods of time anyway.

Harmful and often toxic substances thought safe at the time were also used and later banned. This still happens quite a bit today.

> **CAUTION**
>
> **Hot Potato**
>
> Many preservatives, dyes, and scents can cause skin irritation, respiratory problems, and toxicity concerns. More and more people are finding themselves with chemical and environmental sensitivities resulting from the use and interaction of synthetic ingredients, chemicals, and contaminants in the products they use. This is called multiple chemical sensitivity or environmental illness.

Even with all the testing products undergo, many of them that end up causing harm to humans still make it onto store shelves.

The best way to protect yourself is to read labels and seek out more natural, organically based products. Such products really are the best for you and your loved ones. Exposing yourself to unnecessary chemicals and contaminants when you don't have to makes no sense. Become an educated consumer, read ingredient labels to know want you're buying and using, and use safer, more natural alternatives whenever possible.

Reading product labels, with their long words and strange-sounding names, can often be a little confusing. The fact that some ingredients can come from multiple sources, both plant and animal-based, or from artificially created imitations doesn't make it any easier. When in doubt about the ingredients in a product, go online and do some searching, either for the ingredients in question or for the specific product.

You can also write to the manufacturer with your concerns, usually quickly and easily via their website. Optimistically, if enough people write or call, a manufacturer might rethink its sources, especially if you supply information for a better vegan alternative.

Don't Mess Up Your Makeup

As the sayings go, beauty is in the eye of the beholder, and beauty is only skin deep. These may be clichés, but everyone really is beautiful in his or her own way. Some choose to let their natural beauty shine through with just a simple cleansing and maybe some moisturizer, while others like to give their natural beauty a little assistance with lotions, toners, masks, cosmetics, and other concoctions.

When it comes to applying something to your skin and your face in particular, it's important to pay attention to ingredients. Many hidden animal ingredients are used in the making of cosmetics and other beauty products.

Bet you didn't know that fish scales are sometimes used to give lipsticks, nail polishes, and hair products an iridescent sparkle. Or that crushed beetles are used to tint blushes, lip liners, and lipsticks, and crushed silkworm cocoons are included to give your face powder a smooth finish. Sounds like the makings of a potion made by the wicked witch, not something for a cover girl!

> **In a Nutshell**
>
> Avoiding all the animal ingredients that may be lurking in your beauty products can be tough, so educate yourself. You can find lists of commonly used animal ingredients on the Internet. PETA has a very informative list at www.caringconsumer.com/ingredientslist.html.

You don't have to pay a lot of money to help yourself look more beautiful or appealing, vegan style. Creative vegans have been using simple kitchen ingredients for centuries to make homemade beauty products. Use oils for lotions, hair treatments, and conditioners or to add gloss to lips. Use oatmeal scrubs to loosen dry skin and avocados to moisturize it. If you want to learn more about how to make your own natural beauty products, check out your local library, bookstore, or the Internet for some great books and ideas.

If you want to purchase vegan cosmetics, you can find products in all price ranges and in many retailers, drug stores, natural foods stores, through the Internet, and direct from the company. Be aware, though, as with all products that contain better-quality and cruelty-free ingredients, you get what you pay for, and some of the better products do cost a bit more.

These are some companies that make cosmetics and beauty care products suitable for vegans:

- Aveda
- Beauty Without Cruelty
- Ecco Bella
- Hemp Organics
- Herbs of Grace
- Kiss My Face
- Merry Hempsters
- No Miss
- Zia
- Zuzu Luxe

Personal Care Items

Store shelves are flooded with so many personal care products—toothpastes, mouthwashes, lotions, moisturizers, shaving creams, shampoos, conditioners, soaps, body washes, perfumes, body sprays, powders, and scrubs. Stores house rows and rows of products of all kinds, with so many to choose from and more of them appearing on shelves every day. Be sure to read the packaging and labels of these products before buying them as they, too, can contain many obvious and not-so-obvious animal-based ingredients.

Many of the top perfume manufacturers use animal musk in their perfumes. Scent glands of civets, relatives of the mongoose, produce the musk, and these glands are painfully squeezed and drained every week or two to collect the

> **In a Nutshell**
>
> Once you discover the products you truly love, use the most, and can't do without, you can search out alternative ways to purchase them to save money. Try to take advantage of specials and sales, buy company-direct, or purchase in large quantities or bulk.

musk. Musk deer are also used in the collection of animal musk, and they have been hunted to near extinction for their scent glands. Be sure to avoid any products that contain natural or even synthetic musk, as much painful animal testing and musk collection went into the development of the synthetic form of musk.

Vegans try to avoid animal ingredients, but they also try to avoid ingredients that cause harm to themselves, others, and the environment. Besides animal ingredients, many personal care products also contain substances that can be harmful to your health. For instance, many deodorants contain aluminum in their creamy white bases, which may have links to Alzheimer's. Toothpastes may contain fluoride, which is toxic and responsible for thousands of accidental poisoning cases each year. As you become an educated consumer, feel free to share the information with others who may be unaware, and you may even save a life in the process.

Taking Care of Your Smile

You brush, floss, rinse, and go to the dentist regularly and are pretty much doing everything you can to take good care of your teeth. But are you really? Now that you've gone vegan, at least you know drinking lots of cow's milk isn't the way to get a winning smile. You know tofu and leafy greens can do a lot more to strengthen your teeth and bones, and the fiber present in these foods requires you to properly and fully chew it, which is good for your molars and jaw muscles. But are you buying the right vegan products to keep your teeth strong and healthy and your breath fresh?

Do you buy a natural, chalk-based toothpaste that hasn't been tested on animals? Chalks mixed with natural salts, herbs, and botanicals help scrub away food particles, plaque, and film. You can find natural toothpastes in most retailers and natural foods stores in tubes and powdered form. You can also make your own cruelty-free tooth-polishing powder by mixing baking soda, a little hydrogen peroxide, and sea salt. This mixture also whitens your teeth over time and improves the health of your gums.

What about fluoride? Is it friend or foe? The practice of adding fluoride to consumer products, using it in dentistry practices, and adding it to our drinking water are highly controversial and often-debated topics. Many would be surprised to learn that fluoride is a hazardous toxic waste, a by-product of phosphate-based fertilizer and aluminum production. Instead of paying stiff fees for safely disposing of this toxic industrial waste, the industries that generate fluoride make a profit from it by selling it for use in oral care products and to municipal water treatment plants for mass fluoridation.

Some studies have shown that the claims of fluoride's positive effects on dental health are unfounded and that it is actually harmful to health and environment. The same fluoride that's classified as a poison and that can scorch and kill crops and pollute the air on contact, is being regularly added to drinking water and oral care products. Exposure to excessive amounts of fluoride has been linked to brain disorders, birth defects, cancers, reproductive problems, arthritis, and weakened bones and joints. Have you ever noticed the poison warning label on all tubes of fluoridated toothpaste? Avoid the poison on your toothbrush, and seek out nonfluoridated toothpastes instead.

> **In a Nutshell**
>
> In 1975, Tom's of Maine introduced the first natural and cruelty-free toothpaste manufactured in the United States. Tom's of Maine markets several flavors of toothpaste, including nonfluoride formulas, in both adult and child varieties. It also sells several natural mouthwashes and mouth rinses, even alcohol-free varieties. Tom's of Maine does not test on animals.

Try to buy toothpastes and mouthwashes that contain natural cleaners, whiteners, and fresheners, and stay away from the artificially colored and flavored products. Minty freshness is best when it comes from peppermint or spearmint, not a numbered chemical compound.

Also, check your dental floss, as most are coated in beeswax or petroleum-based products. Eco-DenT GentleFloss is a good vegan and cruelty-free dental floss. It uses a blend of essential oils and herbs, plant waxes, and even comes in a plastic-free, biodegradable and recyclable box! Eco-DenT also makes several other vegan and cruelty-free oral hygiene products.

Handling Hair Care

Having healthy skin, nails, and hair is dependent upon a diet rich in B vitamins, especially biotin. Biotin-rich foods such as leafy greens, whole-grains, and beans form the basis of a vegan diet. For a tremendous impact on your outward appearance, get plenty of biotin-rich foods in your diet. Oils high in essential fatty acids—such as omega-rich flax, hemp, avocado, and soybean oils—are also great internal and external lubricants and conditioners.

Eating a well-balanced diet helps give your hair a healthy shine and luster, provides it with moisture, makes it stronger, and reduces hair breakage and loss. Diet helps your hair's inner beauty come shining through, but helping nature along a little doesn't hurt either. Just try to avoid the use of harsh chemical-based products that strip away your hair's natural moisture, leaving dry, brittle, damaged, or fly-away hair.

Read product packaging and labels, and analyze the quality and types of ingredients in your hair care products. Look for natural and organic ingredients first and foremost, and avoid long chemical names you're unfamiliar with, as they may be harsh chemicals or derived from animals. Some common animal-based ingredients that find their way into hair products and other beauty items include the following:

- Hydrolyzed animal protein
- Lanolin
- Nonvegetable glycerin
- Collagen
- Silk protein
- Milk protein
- Honey and bee-based products
- Urea
- Shark and fish oils

For a complete list of animal ingredients in both personal care products and food items, see the excellent and comprehensive book *Animal Ingredients A to Z*, compiled by the E. G. Smith Collective (AK Press, 2004). It's available in libraries and bookstores across the United States.

Hot Potato _____

Sodium laurel sulfate and one of its variations, sodium laureth sulfate, are the most common foaming agents used in shampoos and other foaming personal care products. The good news is that it is chemically derived from coconuts, not from animal ingredients. The bad news is that there's quite a bit of controversy surrounding its safety. Some believe it causes hair loss, skin rashes and irritation, and even cancer. Do some research before selecting products that contain sodium laurel sulfate or sodium laureth sulfate.

After being sure a product does not have any unwanted ingredients, you can move on to looking for some of the ingredients you do want. Herbals and botanicals are wonderful for fragrance, to clean the scalp, and to moisturize. Which ones to choose depends on to whom the product is geared. Flowers such as chamomile, lavender, roses, geranium, passion flower, and citrus scents seem to be more pleasing to the ladies. Mixes of clary sage, rosemary, thyme, and tea tree oil are more often considered "masculine" scents.

More natural conditioners and other styling products have been hitting the market with many of those same natural ingredients and fragrances, along with moisturizing oils and extracts from avocados, sunflower seeds, almonds, flax seed, pumpkin seed, jojoba, soybeans, and sea vegetables. Grain-based proteins from wheat, oats, corn, and rice are also added to give the hair strands strength. Many products are also vitamin fortified.

Soap ... It's Time to Come Clean

We all know that using soap is supposed to make you clean, and some of the new antibacterial varieties are even supposed to kill germs. So why, then, would so many soap companies use slaughterhouse by-products to make a product that's supposed to get you clean? Tallow, the rendered fat from cows and sheep, is used to make many popular brands of soaps, foods, and even candles. Many of the biggest manufacturers rely heavily on the use of tallow as a base for their soaps.

Besides tallow, many of the massively produced brands of soap contain synthetic chemicals, colorants, and fragrances that can be irritating to skin, especially the delicate facial area. Rashes, dry patches, itching, and blistering—these are all common skin reactions to chemical ingredients in soaps. Many of the liquid soaps contain harsh antibacterial and antifungal ingredients that can wash away not only the germs, but your body's natural oils as well. This can leave your skin feeling dry and irritated.

What is a vegan to do to get all clean and sudsy? Look for vegetable glycerin–based soaps or oil-based soaps made with coconut, olive, almond, sunflower, soybean, and hemp oils and sometimes *shea butter*. Note that if a soap doesn't specifically list vegetable glycerin, there's a good chance the glycerin used is derived from animal sources. Most vegan oil-based soaps provide better moisturizing benefits to your skin, result in less clogged pores, and cause fewer skin irritations and breakouts than the conventional tallow-based soaps.

Vegan 101

Shea butter is derived from the shea nut, which grows in many parts of Africa. It is used in the treatment of minor skin problems and irritations such as eczema, dermatitis, psoriasis, sunburn or sun damage, and to soothe dry skin, scalps, and lips. It can be used alone or blended with other ingredients to make hair and skin products, including pomades, salves, lotions, cosmetics, soaps, shampoos, conditioners, and other hair and personal care products.

Saving Your Skin

Having soft, smooth skin depends on having proper moisture and lubrication both inside and out. Start by eating a well-balanced vegan diet containing plenty of nuts, seeds, and healthy oils to provide a little natural protective lubrication from the inside out.

For those who have a beauty regimen, many vegan options exist in the form of tonics, toners, moisturizers, cleansers, and makeup removers. If you like to have a skin care system in place to keep yourself looking young and radiant, you can find several great vegan products by Beauty Without Cruelty, Dessert Essence, and Jason's. Need a lotion to rub on dry elbows or after shaving? When selecting one, be sure to read the labels to ensure an all-vegan product; lanolin, fish oils, and silk and animal proteins are added to many skin products unnecessarily. "Let the buyer beware" and "stay on your toes" are two mottoes for the smart vegan shopper.

Vegan-Friendly Sources

You can find vegan beauty products in many retailers, natural foods stores, through online shopping sources, and from the manufacturers directly. A few quality producers of vegan products follow:

- ABBA
- Aubrey Organics
- Avalon
- Beauty Without Cruelty
- Dessert Essence
- Earth Science
- Ecco Bella
- Jason
- Lamas Beauty
- Nature's Gate
- Paul Penders

You can purchase many vegan cosmetics and personal products online from vegan merchants such as veganstore.com or veganessentials.com. This helps remove any doubt from your mind as to whether or not what you are using is truly cruelty-free and vegan.

As a consumer, you have the option of deciding whether or not to support companies that make mostly animal-based products and only a few vegan products or those that strive to create an all-vegan or veg-friendly product line. How and where you spend your money is a personal decision that often depends on how much of it you have available to spend, so the decision is yours to make.

Brushes and Sponges

Now that you know how to pick out vegan beauty products, you're all set to apply and use them. Uh-oh, wait a minute—take a look at that comb, brush, or sponge you're going to use to style or apply the products. Is it made using animal products?

For centuries, hair combs and brush handles were traditionally made with bone, tortoise shells, mother of pearl, abalone, or even ivory tusks. Animal hair, mostly boar hair, was and is still commonly used to make the bristles of hair and makeup brushes. Many men's brushes used to apply shaving cream are made with badger's hair because it is softer and gentler on their faces.

Fortunately, you don't have to buy an animal-based brush or comb to groom yourself. Many manufacturers make wood- or plastic-handled combs and brushes that are quite sturdy, long-lasting, and suitable for vegans. You can find natural or man-made bristles made from nylon or natural fibers. Many retailers sell vegan-friendly hair combs and brushes. You can find Ecco Bella's vegan makeup brushes at many natural foods stores or online.

Natural sponges may look like they're dried plants because of all their tiny pores, nooks, and crannies, but a sponge is really a multi-celled form of sea animal, a living, eating, water- and oxygen-filtering creature that wants nothing more than to be left alone to live its life. These amazing creatures can anchor themselves to rocks, plants, and other underwater debris or stand free against the ebb and flow of the tide and water currents.

> ### In a Nutshell
>
> Having evolved more than half a billion years ago, sponges, also known as *porifera,* are among the earliest known forms of animal life in existence. They eat plankton and other tiny particles that pass through their body's filtration system. Sponges are hermaphrodites, which means each individual sponge contains both male and female elements.

You can purchase cellulose sponges, made primarily from wood fiber, for use in your household and other cleaning tasks. For applying your makeup, check out synthetic, foam-based sponges available at most retailers.

To clear up any potential confusion, pumice doesn't come from a spongelike animal; rather, it is a piece of volcanic rock. Loofahs, which are also often mistaken for sponges, are actually made from a particular species of dried squash. They help loosen and remove dead skin cells, so use them and scrub to your heart's content. You don't have to give up your loofah once you go vegan!

The Least You Need to Know

◆ Animal testing is a serious issue involving many body care products, and you should take great care to avoid purchasing those that utilize it.

◆ Be sure to read the labels of body care products before buying them, as they can contain many obvious and not-so-obvious animal-based ingredients.

◆ Cosmetics often contain animal ingredients or have been tested on animals, so be sure of what you are buying and from whom you are buying it.

◆ Natural sponges are actually animals, not plants, and cosmetic, shaving, and hair brushes are sometimes made with animal hair bristles. Vegans avoid all these items.

◆ You can purchase vegan, cruelty-free body care and personal items in natural foods stores and online.

Chapter 25

Dressing to Impress

In This Chapter

- ◆ Shopping for animal-free clothing
- ◆ Veganizing shoes and accessories
- ◆ Avoiding non-vegan-friendly materials
- ◆ Putting compassion in fashion
- ◆ Understanding the cruelty of wool and leather

As a new vegan, you've undoubtedly put a lot of time and effort into eliminating animal-based foods and ingredients from your diet and other aspects of your life. But what about the contents of your closet and your dresser drawers? Some non-vegan-friendly items are likely hanging or folded in there. In this chapter, we turn our attention to your wardrobe and the various issues associated with it.

Because many traditional clothing items derive either wholly or in part from animals, a vegan has to be aware of what he or she chooses to wear. Walking into a clothing store and picking out the first thing that appeals to you is not generally an option for people who are making it a point to avoid wearing any and all substances derived from animals.

As is the case with buying vegan food, going shopping for clothing usually involves reading labels and being an informed consumer. Knowing ahead of time what you're looking for and what you want to avoid can save you quite a bit of time in the store. Let's take a look at some of the common clothing items vegans avoid as well as some of the ones they seek out.

"I Wouldn't Be Caught Dead in That!"

In some respects, the issue of what to wear as a vegan is a pretty simple one. Vegans don't wear animal skin, fur, or anything else produced by an animal. The idea is that those items belong to the animals, who had to suffer and eventually die to provide them, and it's both undesirable and wrong to wear them as clothing. Common animal-based clothing materials to avoid include fur, feathers, shells, silk, wool, leather, suede, and other skins taken from animals.

Leather and Suede

The most common animal clothing you encounter will undoubtedly be leather and its roughly buffed variation, suede. Throughout the world, all sorts of animals are used to make leather goods and garments, but in the United States, most leather comes from calves and cattle. Leather seems to be everywhere, but how much do we really know about it?

> **In a Nutshell**
>
> Silkworms produce fine filaments, excreted from openings under their mouths, to spin cocoons in which they will transform into moths. In silk-making, the silkworms are intentionally suffocated inside their cocoons so they won't break the silk threads when they escape. It is estimated that up to 3,000 cocoons are required to produce a single yard of silk fabric.

Leather is used for a variety of clothing and household purposes, and most of it is a by-product of the animal food industry. Animals that are primarily raised as livestock and intended for food or milk production are shared among many different industries at the end of their lives. Their skin or hide is used to make most of the leather goods we encounter so often in our daily lives, from car seats to sporting equipment to living room sofas.

Many animals are killed just for their skin. Calfskin or sheepskin comes from calves and baby sheep that are killed for their soft young skin.

> **CAUTION** **Hot Potato** _____
>
> Leather manufacturers around the world sometimes use skins from other animals such as cats, dogs, horses, pigs, goats, sheep, and deer in the production of their leather products. When purchasing animal skin products, especially discount merchandise produced in other countries, you could get any of these skins as part of a leather or suede purse, shoes, or clothing. "Truth in labeling" laws are virtually nonexistent for leather products.

Factory farming has a negative impact on the environment through waste runoff and the clearing of forests for grazing land, but the environmental impact doesn't stop at the end of an animal's life. The *tanning* industry uses substances such as formaldehyde, mineral salts, coal tars, arsenic, lead, cyanide-based dyes, and chromium. When released into the environment, these substances contaminate water and negatively impact the health of humans and nonhumans alike. When exposed to these substances on the job, tannery workers become susceptible to diseases such as leukemia, lung cancer, and other forms of cancer.

> **Vegan 101** _____
>
> **Tanning** is the process of turning animal hide into pliable, finished leather through exposure to various chemicals, preservatives, and dyes.

Even though vegans don't wear the tanned hides of their fellow creatures, they can still keep warm and dry with natural cloth fabrics, worn alone or in layers. It's easy with some of the new organic hemp, flax, cotton, and blends made into shirts and sweaters. They're soft, light-weight, and snuggly all at the same time. Companies such as Ecolution, Of The Earth, Eco Dragon, Patagonia, Hemptown, and Sweetgrass make it easy to find styles and fashions to suit all tastes. You can also purchase jackets and coats made from these same natural fibers or from man-made nylon, polyester, vinyl, rubber, synthetic ultra suede, micro-fiber, and polar fleece.

Wooly Business

When it comes to obtaining and wearing animal skins, the inherent cruelty is obvious. The cruelty isn't as apparent to most people when it comes to materials such as wool or other animal hair, for which animals aren't always directly killed in the production.

The idea that animals are not harmed in the shearing processes of commercial wool production is a myth. Animal hair used as clothing fibers is generally only acquired after the animals involved have endured tremendous amounts of suffering throughout all aspects of the process. They are treated very roughly when sheared and often have large parts of their skin sliced off with the wool.

For sheep used in the production of wool, large sections of skin around the tail area are often intentionally sliced off without the use of anesthesia. This "mulesing" is done to prevent maggot infestation from flies that are attracted to their specially bred thick folds of skin covered in unnaturally thick amounts of wool. The idea is that the scarred skin that will grow in its place will be more resistant to infestation.

Hot Potato

Male angora rabbits are usually killed at birth due to their hair's lower growth rate. Females are the gender of choice for angora production as they produce up to 80 percent more wool than the males.

Angora rabbits used in the production of angora wool, for use in sweaters and other clothing items, also have it bad. In between shearings, they spend all their time in tiny cages, where the delicate pads of their feet become easily cut on the rough wire mesh of their cages and often become ulcerated and infected.

These examples reflect just the tip of the iceberg of the cruelty associated with the animal fiber industry. Do some research on the web or at your local library to learn more.

Animal Accents

When shopping for clothes or accessories, let your eyes, nose, and fingers be your guide. That's right, ogle the texture or grain, as they say, take a whiff, and finally, give the fabric a good rub between your fingers. Often, you will almost instantly be able to tell if it is made of animal or man-made materials. Then, check the label for the final say in material content. These simple prescreening steps can serve you well when shopping in thrift or secondhand stores, when tags and labels are often missing from the garments.

Be sure to fully inspect items before you buy as sometimes animal-based ingredients are hidden or not mentioned on the label. For instance, a little fur or leather trim could be lurking on a coat or shoes, or down feathers or wool quilting could be inside your parka. You may find a silk lining, instead of cloth, covering the inside of a sports jacket or overcoat, or even a few pearl, bone, or abalone buttons down the front of a shirt. These are just a few of the things that keep a vegan on guard.

Vegan Clothing Options

Fortunately for us, our ancestors learned to weave grasses and fibers into threads and cloth and eventually into clothes, garments, and accessories. The result was that we no longer required the use of animals and animal-based items to clothe us and keep us warm. Today, many nonanimal clothing alternatives are widely available. Materials suitable for vegans include cotton, linen, hemp, polyester, acrylic, nylon, and vinyl, just to name a few.

Vegans seek out clothing made from natural and man-made fabrics over animal skins and other items. Clothing made from natural fibers tends to breathe better and keep you cooler, which makes it ideal for warmer weather conditions.

Man-made fibers tend to trap in warmth and keep out air, so they are better for colder climates and temperatures. For those in need of warm sweaters, coats, scarves, and mittens, there's no need to fret over not wearing wool, angora, or cashmere any more. Popular fleece and micro-fiber fabrics are oh-so-soft, snuggly, and insulating!

> **In a Nutshell**
>
> Pesticides are used in heavy concentrations on many fiber crops, especially cotton. Be a wise shopper and search out organic sources whenever possible for your clothing, footwear, and accessory needs. Hemp is an Earth-friendly alternative to cotton that only requires a fraction of the pesticides and other chemicals and is often grown organically.

Veganizing Your Wardrobe

Buying secondhand items from consignment shops, boutiques, thrift stores, or even garage sales is a great way to get some inexpensive vegan duds to help revamp and veganize your wardrobe quickly and affordably. You'll need to do a bit of searching, so give yourself some time to shop, and you might be amazed at what you find. You may even stumble upon organic cotton, hemp, or linen items for only a few dollars. It's also a great way to recycle unused or unwanted items and keep them out of our overflowing landfills.

For those times when you want something brand new, you'll usually have more luck finding vegan clothing at discount retailers that stock more man-made and cloth-based products than the larger department stores that tend to carry a lot more leather, suede, wool, and fur items. With a little effort, you should be able to find quality vegan apparel ranging from bargain-basement to high-end designer labels.

In a Nutshell

Several designers such as Stella McCartney, Calvin Klein, Anne Klein, Genevieve Gaelyn, and Atom Cianfarani have pledged to not use animal materials in their designs!

It's also a good idea to check your local community for shops and boutiques that sell fair trade clothing items. These are more ethical alternatives to those items mass produced by cheap labor. The Internet can also provide a wealth of sources for fair trade and conventionally produced vegan clothing. Ethicalwares.com is a great site run by vegans. It sells fair trade items, music, accessories, shoes, clothing, and much more.

Pleathering Yourself

Some vegans are so opposed to the thought of wearing animal skins or fur that they even avoid look-alike items that resemble animal products. To do so makes them feel odd, and it can also send the wrong message that wearing animal skins is desirable. If the item looks realistic enough, many people might assume you're actually wearing leather or fur, and you will then be a walking billboard for wearing those items. (If you happen to be wearing fluorescent green pleather, though, that generally won't be an issue.)

Vegans and nonvegans alike have embraced the new fashion creations of pleather, faux (fake) fur, and other synthetically derived animal skin look-alikes. Such items are particularly popular among veg-conscious celebrities, musicians, fashion models and designers, and those who want to dress trendy or flashy without having to buy the farm or add to the suffering that happens on it.

Hot Potato

The drawback to pleather and other petroleum-derived synthetic fabrics is that their production and disposal are not environmentally friendly. Whenever possible, you should choose natural fibers over man-made ones, but when there's no other alternative, many feel it's better than contributing to the suffering of living, feeling creatures.

Pleather is short for "plastic leather," and it's more popular than ever. It's not only used to make clothing, shoes, and accessories but also car and bicycle seats, upholstery, and sports equipment, including basketballs for the National Collegiate Athletic Association (NCAA) and many schools. Pleather is much more affordable and can be just as durable, pliable, easily dyed, and useful as any animal's skin. It's used in the production of boots, shoes, wallets, purses, hats, coats, jackets, vests, pants, shirts, undergarments, and other gear. Vinyl and polyester are also commonly used to make much of the same outerwear and gear.

Designers Genevieve Gaelyn and Atom Cianfarani, creators of the Gaelyn and Cianfarani fashion label, have developed an Earth-friendly clothing material they use in some of their creations. It's handcrafted from recycled bicycle inner tubes and is often mistaken for leather.

Friend or Faux?

The creation of faux furs came about for several reasons but primarily out of the desire to find a more affordable alternative to animal furs. In addition, many animal rights organizations have been busy spreading the word about the cruelty involved in wearing fur. As a result, more and more people are opting to wear faux furs instead of the real thing. The faux versions are more humane, affordable, fashionable, and definitely much more politically correct.

You'll likely be surprised by the variety of faux fur selections. Naturally, you can expect to find imitations of all sorts of furs, with their natural hues and striking patterns or spots, as the basis of garments or as adornments on collars and cuffs. Those who like to draw a little attention to themselves will be excited by faux furs in shades of red, orange, yellow, green, pink, purple, blue, turquoise, and all shades in between. You can actually have a Technicolor faux fur or full-length classic coat if you want one!

You can find faux fur fashions at most retailers, in department stores and boutiques, on the web, and even in the private collections of many top fashion designers.

Shoes and Accessories

Most people have one or more pairs of leather shoes in their closet when they go vegan. It's only natural, as most of us, when growing up, were told about the importance of buying shoes that last, and getting a good value for our money meant buying leather shoes. This applies to dress shoes, work shoes, boots, sandals, and the ever-popular athletic shoes of all kinds, from sneakers, to cleats, gymnast's slippers, and even ice skates. All these were traditionally made from leather, and if we wanted to get our money's worth, this is how we were instructed to shop.

Many new vegans will have a lot to sort out and replace—maybe even most of the shoes, boots, and sandals that they own. But don't despair, you can easily find shoes made from natural and man-made materials in the form of canvas, hemp, linen, cotton, nylon, rubber, polyester, acrylic, vinyl, and even recycled materials. And these man-made varieties can be very durable!

Most retailers and department stores carry non-leather shoes, although you may have to do a bit of searching to find them among the leather stuff. Selection will vary from season to season; more non-leather styles tend to be available in the summer months.

After getting your shoes in order, check out your other accessories, including purses, bags, luggage, and other gear you may have for hauling, carrying, and traveling. Such pieces are often made from leather. Replacing any leather or wool gloves, hats, or scarves with cloth or synthetic alternatives is quite easy. You can purchase cloth, straw, metal, vinyl, pleather, and nylon-based purses, bags, and luggage to replace any animal skin products. As for leather belts, many man-made versions are suitable for vegans, and you can find them all over the place.

Don't forget to check your jewelry box; you may have to do a bit of thinning out there as well. Many earrings, necklaces, rings, bracelets, and other jewelry items can contain obvious animal ingredients. Leather and suede are often used for bands, ties, clasps, and accents on watches, necklaces, and bracelets. Feathers, shells, pearls, abalone, and pieces of bone are often parts of earrings, necklaces, hats, and even hair accessories.

What's wrong with pearls, you may ask? Well, when an irritant like a piece of sand gets inside an oyster's shell, a special liquid called nacre is secreted over it to lessen the pain of having it scratch against its soft tissue. Cultured pearls are those that are created as a result of human intervention. In the process, oysters are forcibly opened, an incision is made, and a bead or other irritant is placed inside. The oysters are kept in cages until the irritant-turned-pearl has reached the desired size.

Compassion in Fashion

By now, you should know that animals don't have to suffer so you can put clothes on your back. You can indeed have compassion in fashion, and we have women to thank for pushing the envelope and helping make widespread change. In particular, the influential Lady Muriel Dowding wasn't content to stand idly by when confronted with the animal cruelty she encountered in her everyday life. During the 1950s in London, she was very active in antivivisection campaigns and as an animal rights advocate in the House of Lords. She did whatever she could to effect positive change on behalf of animals.

Lady Dowding traveled in many influential circles and was appalled at seeing people wearing fur coats and accessories. She encouraged clothing manufacturers that didn't use animal-based products to proudly say so, and in doing so, she developed a "Beauty Without Cruelty" tag for positively describing and promoting such companies' cruelty-free clothing production.

Beauty Without Cruelty began as a simple tag on a garment to signify that no animal had to suffer in its production. Later it became the name of Lady Dowding's cosmetics company, which was one of the first of its kind to employ no animal testing and ensure animal-free ingredients. It still continues to make many fine products suitable for vegans.

Marcia Pearson, former top fashion model, is now the founder of the nonprofit organization Fashion with Compassion. She was greatly influenced by the work of Lady Dowding. After finally meeting face-to-face, the two of them got together and decided to use their celebrity status to help popularize the concepts of compassion in fashion and cruelty-free living. They organized fashion shows and other events to showcase new options in cruelty-free products and clothing items. This started a snowball effect, and now many celebrities eagerly voice their concerns about animal rights, environmental, and vegan/vegetarian issues.

> **In a Nutshell**
>
> In 1991, PETA, with the help of the rock group the Go-Go's, launched their famous ongoing "I'd rather go naked than wear fur" awareness campaign. Many of the ads have featured celebrities in the buff, including Pamela Anderson, Kim Basinger, Dennis Rodman, Melissa Etheridge, Christy Turlington, David Cross, Kristoff St. John, Carnie Wilson, Marcus Schenkenberg, and Dominique Swain.

The Least You Need to Know

- Many people don't realize the suffering and cruelty involved with bringing leather and wool products to our wardrobes.

- Vegans avoid all clothing derived from animal-based sources, including leather, wool, silk, feathers, shells, and bone.

- Replacing leather shoes and accessories is relatively easy, due to the widespread availability of nonleather alternatives.

- Natural and man-made clothing materials suitable for vegans include cotton, linen, hemp, polyester, acrylic, nylon, and vinyl.

26

Other Things to Consider

In This Chapter

◆ Feeding cats and dogs a vegan diet

◆ Exposing the gelatin in film

◆ Veganizing your candles

◆ Finding animal products in the home

◆ Traveling, vegan-style

Throughout this book, we've taken a look at many different issues that surround living as a vegan, from gracefully handling family meals to knowing how to replace the animal ingredients in your recipes. As with everything else in life, being armed with a little bit of knowledge about the issues can make them a lot easier to deal with and can increase your chances of success as a vegan.

This final chapter focuses on a few additional things you need to consider as you continue your voyage into veganism, from taking vegan photos, to lighting animal-free candles, to having vegan dogs and cats!

Vegan Dogs and Cats?

When it comes to animal companions and how to properly care for them, vegans need to be concerned about all the same things nonvegans are concerned about. But some issues are specific to vegans, such as what constitutes an optimal diet for their companions. Because vegans don't like to support animal foods industries, especially factory farming, they are often dismayed at the prospect of having to continue to buy those products for their dogs and cats.

> **Hot Potato**
>
> The meats used in pet foods are often substandard and can even be harmful to your furry friends. There's no mandatory government testing of these meats for safety before they end up in your friend's bowl.

New vegans often want to know if it is safe to feed their faithful companions a vegan diet, foregoing all animal foods. The answer, depending on the species in question, is a qualified "yes." Let's take a look at the two most popular nonherbivorous companion animals, dogs and cats.

Dogs are omnivores that eat both animal and plant foods in their diets. Experts agree that a proper meatless diet, high in protein and other essential nutrients, can easily supply dogs of all breeds and sizes with everything they require to stay healthy and happy. There are a number of commercially available vegetarian dog foods on the market, both moist and dry. Some of the more popular brands are Evolution, Natural Life, Natural Balance, Wysong, and Nature's Recipe. It's also easy to make home-made vegan food for your canine pal, so check the web or your local library for recipe ideas.

Unlike dogs, cats are carnivores and have different nutritional needs. They cannot fulfill all their nutritional requirements on a plant-based diet alone, without supplementation. Most important among the nutrients cats need is the amino acid taurine, found only in animal tissue. Without it, cats can go blind and experience a wide range of other health problems. A synthetic form of taurine is regularly supplemented in conventional nonvegan cat foods as well because most of the taurine originally present in meat is destroyed during the cooking process. It's also vital to supplement vitamins A and D_3, as well as the essential fatty acid arachidonate and a few other nutrients.

Some nutritionally complete, prepared vegan cat foods are available on the market in both canned and kibble form. Most notable are those marketed under the Evolution brand. It's also possible to make your own vegan cat food with the help of the right supplementation. A product called Vegecat makes it easy with their supplement blend. You simply mix the powdered Vegecat supplement in with your homemade vegan cat food, and it adds all the taurine and other nutrients your cat needs.

Feeding your cat a vegan diet involves having faith in the bioavailability of the supplemented forms of the needed nutrients, so it's a decision you shouldn't make lightly. It should also be noted that many people feel the only appropriate diet for carnivores like felines is raw meat, which is what they would naturally eat in the wild. The Internet is rife with success stories of vegan cats, however, and we recommend you do a little research on the topic yourself before coming to any conclusions.

Hot Potato

Onions are toxic to cats (and dogs, to a lesser extent) and should never be included in any form, whether raw, cooked, or powdered, in any of your cat's food. Compounds called sulfoxides and disulfides destroy red blood cells, which leads to anemia. Garlic contains the same harmful compounds, but in lesser amounts.

Capturing the Moment

Are you really into film-based photography? Do you even have your own dark room? Or have you maybe just not gotten around to switching over to digital cameras yet and are still using 35 mm film? Now that you've gone vegan, you do need to be aware of some issues regarding the world of photography.

You may be surprised to learn that gelatin has been used in the production of photographic film since around 1870. Without exception, all modern film contains gelatin. The largest producer of photographic film purchases 80 million pounds of animal bones from the meat industry each year to produce its film. That includes the instant self-developing films, film used for taking medical x-rays, and the kind of film traditionally used to shoot Hollywood movies.

Hot Potato

One note of caution: glossy photographic paper can often contain a gelatin coating as well. This goes for the professional stuff as well as the kind you can purchase for your home printer. Stick with matte (non-glossy) paper unless you know for sure gelatin wasn't used in the glossing process.

Fortunately, more and more movies are being filmed completely digitally, which eliminates the need for gelatin-based film. When theaters make the switch to a completely digital format for showing films, like DVDs or the next generation of digital media, there will no longer be a need to use gelatin-based film in the creation and screening of future movies.

Digital photography is an easy and fun way to avoid the gelatin issue while still being able to exercise the Ansel Adams or Margaret Bourke-White inside you. You can capture your subjects digitally, store them electronically, and if or when you print them out yourself, you will do so without the use of gelatin.

If you're interested in going digital but are intimidated by new technology, have no fear. Many digital cameras are extremely easy to use, and you can find a lot of helpful information and advice via the Internet, your local library, and in numerous magazines devoted to the subject.

Flickering Light

What could possibly not be vegan about something as simple as lighting and enjoying a candle? Well, let's take a look at that match you're planning on using to light it. Most matches use gelatin to bind all the incendiary chemicals together to form the match head. Does that mean you have to go back to rubbing two sticks together to make a flame? Not at all. Just use a lighter.

But wait, before you light your candle, are you sure that wick doesn't contain lead? As recently as 2003, when a small percentage of all candles sold in the United States were found to contain lead-cored wicks, a federal ban was put in place. Zinc is another common component of metal-cored wicks, but unfortunately, this may not be a safe alternative as recent studies have shown zinc-based wicks can cause problems of their own. To be completely sure you are protected, use nonmetallic wicks made from natural fibers like hemp or cotton.

In a Nutshell

The Romans developed the first wick-based candles, which were made from tallow derived from sheep or beef suet. They burned dirty and left a lingering odor. Since the development of paraffin wax in the mid-1800s, the production of pure tallow candles is a rarity. Still, tallow and its derivatives are sometimes used as ingredients in modern candles, either in the wax itself or as a base for additives.

Mind Your Beeswax

For vegans, a major problem with candles is that many of them are made either entirely, or partially, from beeswax. Beeswax is a substance secreted from the abdomen of bees to help form the storage units within the hive, or honeycomb. The honeycomb can contain honey, pollen, or eggs, depending on the particular need. In winter months, the larvae and others in the colony use the honeycomb for food.

When beekeepers collect honey, they smoke the bees out of the hive and slice away the honey-rich honeycomb. After removing the honey, they melt down and purify the honeycomb to form beeswax. Then they mix in scents and other substances and pour the beeswax into molds of all shapes and sizes and form many varieties of candles.

Candles made from paraffin wax, a by-product of the crude oil refinement process, are the most common, cheaper alternative to beeswax candles. Unfortunately, these are not an ideal alternative, as burning paraffin candles has a lot of drawbacks. While in use, they produce a lot of dirty soot, along with many of the same harmful and carcinogenic toxins that are released when burning diesel fuel. And because it is not possible to mix scented, natural essential oils with paraffin wax in the candle-making process, the industry has developed artificial, petroleum-based scents that release even more undesirable chemicals and soot into the air you breathe.

Fortunately, there are healthier vegan alternatives to both beeswax and paraffin-based candles, so let's take a look at some of them.

Soy Candles and Others

Candles based on plant oils such as soy, palm, or hemp, are a safer alternative to petroleum-based candles. These burn just as well as the other kinds—even better in some ways—and don't release harmful toxins and loads of black soot into the air.

Soy candles, made from soy wax, have been growing in popularity during the past decade and are becoming a viable vegan alternative to beeswax and paraffin. Soy wax is produced by adding hydrogen to soy oil molecules in a process similar to that used to create hydrogenated vegetable oils. Although hydrogenated oils, or trans fats, are terribly unhealthy to eat, they make for really good, relatively clean-burning, candles. Just don't eat them, and you'll be fine!

Candles made from palm, hemp, and other plant oils and waxes, alone or in combination, have also become more available in recent years. Like soy candles, these are also

Hot Potato

Like many quality items that are good for you and the environment, alternative wax candles can be pricier than the cheap conventional kind. They are usually also longer-burning, so you usually get your money's worth while treating yourself, the earth, and your fellow creatures more kindly in the process.

nontoxic, cleaner-burning vegan alternatives to conventional candles. You can find them in many stores, natural foods stores and most stores that sell higher-quality candles.

Another vegan alternative to beeswax and paraffin is the humble, old-fashioned oil-based lamp. Some pretty nifty modern versions are available these days, and they can usually even run on olive oil and other vegetable oils. If you get a few small oil lamps with some organic hemp or cotton wicks, they can easily and inexpensively take the place of candles for many years, if not decades.

Other Household Items

If you look closely enough around your home, you will undoubtedly find animal products lurking in the unlikeliest of places. Be on the lookout for sheets and bedspreads made of silk, as well as pillows and comforters that contain down, usually derived from geese or ducks.

Brushes used for oil-based house paints and solvent-thinned finishes are usually made from hog bristles, sometimes called China bristles. Paint brushes used for fine art are usually animal-hair-based and taken from a variety of animals, including sables, squirrels, hogs, camels, oxen, ponies, and goats. A variety of synthetic art brushes are now available, although many purists have been slow in accepting them.

Gelatin is an animal substance you will encounter quite often in your household items, often without even knowing it. Gelatin is used in everything from golf balls to help them roll straight, to the binder used in attaching the abrasive particles to sandpaper, to the glossy coating used on some wallpapers and playing cards. It helps put the crinkle in crepe paper, the shine in glossy papers, and adds to the strength of rag-based papers like the paper money in your wallet or the blueprints for your new home.

In a Nutshell
The most popular brand of glue used at home and school today, Elmer's, actually contains no animal products. In fact, it would be pretty hard for you to find an animal-based glue for everyday use in the home. And according to the U.S. Postal Service, the glue used on stamps is vegan and also kosher. The glue used on envelopes is usually free of animal ingredients as well, so you now have no excuse for not writing to your mother!

These few examples show how animal products are used in everyday household items. It's easy to become overwhelmed when faced with the seeming omnipresence of non-vegan products and ingredients in your everyday life, but relax. Being vegan means doing the best you can to eliminate the use and abuse of animals in your life. It's not an easy task, due to the fact that by-products of the animal foods industry are virtually everywhere. Just do your best, and feel good about making whatever positive changes you can. Every little bit truly does help, and your actions can have a pro-vegan ripple effect on the world around you in unimaginable ways!

Cleaning Products

The biggest issue with products used to clean sinks, toilets, floors, carpet, baths, and windows, is that of animal testing and the presence of toxic ingredients. Just like products used to clean our bodies, many household cleaning products also undergo a great deal of senseless animal testing. The results of animal testing have little connection to how humans would react to the product, which is one of the major flaws in the reasoning behind animal testing.

The best thing you can do to avoid cleaning products that have been tested on animals is to look for a cruelty-free logo and the phrase "no animal testing," on package labels. Also, check out the ingredients to avoid harsh chemicals, detergents, and dyes, and purchase products that contain biodegradable and environmentally friendly ingredients.

You can find products to clean your clothes, dishes, bathrooms, kitchens, floors, and all other surfaces, in most retailers, grocery stores, and natural foods stores, alongside the conventional cleaners. A few notable natural and cruelty-free brands to look for include Bi-O-Kleen, Citra-Sol, Dr. Bronner's, Earth Friendly Products, Ecover, Mountain Green, Planet, and Seventh Generation.

> **In a Nutshell**
>
> Some progressive cleaning products contain natural and organic ingredients such as herbal extracts, essential oils, citrus blends, and vinegar.

You can also make your own household cleaners using simple ingredients such as vinegar, baking soda, and lemon juice. You can get more tips for making homemade cleaners via the Internet or in the excellent book, *How It All Vegan* (Arsenal Pulp Press, 1999), by Sarah Kramer and Tanya Barnard. (See govegan.net or Appendix B for details.)

Travel Tips

As you can see, it can be challenging to be vegan in the comfort of your own familiar surroundings, like your home, your town, and your workplace. But being on the road can take that challenge to a whole new level! Suddenly, you are without your safety nets—your trusty natural foods store, your refrigerator packed full of nutritious and delicious vegan foods, and your local restaurants where you know exactly what is suitable to order and what isn't.

As a vegan, finding yourself in a strange town where you don't know the veg-friendly establishments can be a bit intimidating unless you plan ahead of time and take some precautions.

Planning Ahead

One of the best things you can do as a traveling vegan is to research your destination town or city on the Internet before your trip. You can go online and find a list of vegan, vegetarian, or veg-friendly restaurants, natural foods stores, and even bed and breakfasts in the vicinity.

> **In a Nutshell**
>
> Sites such as vegdining.com and happycow.net are good places to research the vegan options in your destination city. When you find some useful info, be sure to print it out and bring it with you, and don't forget to include directions and a map! Mapquest.com can supply you with those, free of charge.

If you happen to be flying to your destination, call the airline and ask them about vegan meal options that may be available for your flight. Several of the major airlines do offer vegan, vegetarian, kosher, and other special meals on request. Just be sure to request your meal ahead of time because if you wait until you are already on the plane to think of it, it will be too late.

Packing Your Own Food

Bringing your own food with you can be a real lifesaver in the event that you aren't able to find something vegan-suitable on the road, in the air, or at your destination. You could easily find yourself stuck with only a few pieces of iceberg lettuce or a carrot stick at a restaurant or at the mercy of the fast-food restaurants prevalent at most rest areas, terminals, depots, and stations.

You could pack a nut butter and fruit spread sandwich on some whole-grain bread, crackers, or even celery sticks, as these can hold up without refrigeration for a longer period of time. These types of items should provide you with protein, carbohydrates, and sources of vegetables. If you have an insulated lunch bag, you could make some veggie wraps or sandwiches, a big salad, or even a hearty noodle or rice dish with lots of veggies. Just throw in a cold pack or some ice to keep things cool!

Be sure to pack a few pieces of fresh vegetables such as carrots or celery or a piece of fruit like an apple, pear, or banana. These will provide you with live enzymes that help keep you healthy as you travel. It's also a good idea to pack some easy-munching snacks, such as nuts, seeds, raisins, trail mix, crackers, pretzels, or chips. You can make up your own small packages or buy them in small prepackaged sizes through natural foods stores. If you include some items such as protein and nutrition bars, granola bars, fruit leather snacks, and a few juice boxes or bottles of water, you'll be ready for just about anything!

The Least You Need to Know

♦ Dogs can easily thrive on a meatless diet, while vegan cats require supplementation of nutrients such as taurine, vitamins A and D_3, and others.

♦ The best vegan alternative to using conventional gelatin-based photographic film is the digital camera. Beware of glossy photo paper, though, as the gloss often contains gelatin.

♦ Candles based on plant oils—such as soy, palm, and hemp—are healthier vegan alternatives to those made from beeswax or paraffin.

♦ Animal ingredients are found in many products in the home, in many different forms. Don't let it overwhelm you; just do the best you can.

♦ When traveling, it's wise to research vegan options in your destination city ahead of time, and be sure to bring along some convenient and nutritious food just in case.

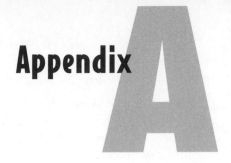

Glossary

arrowroot   A starch obtained from the tubers of the tropical herb *Maranta arundinacea*. It is used primarily as a thickener, but arrowroot tubers are sometimes also eaten whole as a vegetable. *Arrowroot* is derived from the Arawak word *aru-aru*, meaning "meal of meals."

bioavailability   The proportionate amount or level of a certain nutrient contained within a specific food that is actually used or utilized by the body.

compassion   The emotional and sympathetic awareness of another's distress, combined with the motivation and desire to alleviate that distress.

enzyme inhibitors   Present in the seeds or nuts of plants to aid in self-preservation. Enzyme inhibitors protect the seed so it has a better chance to germinate and reach full maturity before being gobbled up. If ingested uncooked or unsprouted, enzyme inhibitors attempt to neutralize the other enzymes in your body, making digestion difficult.

essential amino acids   Our bodies' key protein-building blocks; they must come from dietary sources. Essential amino acids include histidine, isoleucine, leucine, lysine, methionine, phenylalanine, threonine, tryptophan, and valine.

essential fatty acids   Made of alpha-linoleic acid and linoleic acid, which are necessary for the formation and maintenance of our cells. Commonly referred to as omega-3 and omega-6 fatty acids, these classes compete for dominance within your body. Having a greater proportion of one over the other can increase your risks for chronic diseases.

farfalle The Italian word for "butterflies" and also for the pasta of the same shape. The pasta is made from rectangular strips of pasta with zigzag or pinked edges and is crimped in the center. The shape is also often called bow-ties.

gazpacho A cold, tomato-based soup believed to have originated in Andalusia in southern Spain. *Gazpacho* is derived from the Latin word *caspa*, which means "fragments" or "little pieces," a reference to the small pieces of bread found in the classic Andalusian version of gazpacho.

gelatin (also gelatine) A gelling agent made from boiling the connective tissues and skins of animals. It is used in the manufacturing of many products used for consumption and personal use, including foods, beverages, beauty products, pills, and even photographic film.

hummus Hummus originated in the Middle East and Mediterranean. The word comes from the Arabic word for chickpea, known also as the ceci or garbanzo. What most of us know as hummus is really called *hummus bi tahina*, which is made by puréeing or mashing chickpeas with tahini, olive oil, lemon juice, garlic, herbs, and seasonings.

kudzu (also kuzu) A starch-based thickening product made from the tuber of the kudzu plant. In Japan and throughout much of Asia, the leafy foliage is cooked like other greens, and the large tubers are used as a thickening agent. The quick-growing vine was brought from Japan to the southern United States, where it is referred to as "the vine that ate the South" because it now covers nearly 7 million acres of land.

lacto-ovo vegetarian A vegetarian who also includes dairy (*lacto*) and eggs (*ovo*) in his or her diet.

lignans A variety of phytoestrogen, similar to isoflavones, that helps regulate estrogen production in the human body. Lignans have been shown to have cancer-fighting properties that can help inhibit or prevent the growth of breast, colon, and prostate cancers.

living wage A wage sufficient for fulfilling a worker's basic needs, including food, clothing, shelter, education, and health care for the worker and his or her family.

milk In its Standards of Identity, the U.S. Food and Drug Administration (FDA) defines milk as "lacteal secretions from mammals."

miso A pastelike condiment made entirely from soybeans or in combination with other beans or grains such as chickpeas, barley, or rice. Miso ranges from sweet, mild, and mellow with a light beige color, to strong and rich with earthy red tones that sometimes border on appearing black.

oxalates Organic acids that occur naturally in leafy greens, berries, nuts, black tea, and other foods.

phytoestrogens   Naturally occurring plant compounds similar to estradiol, the most potent form of human estrogen. The effects of phytoestrogens are not as strong as most estrogens, and they are very easily broken down and eliminated. They help regulate the estrogen levels in our bodies.

preeclampsia   A condition involving hypertension, retention of fluids, protein loss, and excessive weight gain during pregnancy. Preeclampsia occurs in at least 2 percent of all pregnancies in the United States.

preventive medicine   The field of medicine concerned primarily with helping healthy people stay healthy and providing the tools and information needed to keep disease at bay. It explores the environmental and dietary effects on disease and health and works to determine the root causes instead of reaching for quick fixes.

quinoa   An ancient grain that's made quite a comeback in recent years. Its popularity is due in part to the fact that 1 cup cooked quinoa contains as much calcium as an entire quart of dairy milk.

raita   An Indian salad traditionally comprised of raw veggies, yogurt, and seasonings and served as a cool accompaniment to main dishes.

selenium   A rare mineral, closely related to sulfur, with a distinctive red-gray metallic appearance. In small amounts, it is an essential mineral for mammals and higher plants. In larger amounts, it is toxic. Selenium helps stimulate metabolism and protect against the oxidizing effects of free radicals. These days, most selenium is produced and obtained as a by-product of the copper refining process.

shea butter   Derived from the shea nut, which grows in many parts of Africa. Shea butter is used in the treatment of minor skin problems and irritations and can be used alone or blended with other ingredients to make various hair and skin care products.

sorbet   A usually dairy-free frozen dessert made from puréed fruit, water, and a sweetener. The French have traditionally used sorbet to cleanse the palate between courses of a meal.

tanning   The process of turning animal hide into pliable, finished leather through exposure to various chemicals, preservatives, and dyes.

tahini   A thick paste or butter made from ground sesame seeds. It is often used in Middle Eastern cuisine and features prominently in hummus, baba ghanouj, soups, salad dressings, and many other dishes.

uncooking   The art of preparing or processing raw foods in ways that do not involve the use of heat hotter than 115 degrees Fahrenheit. This leaves vital nutrients and enzymes in the food intact.

veg-friendly   Having an understanding of the basics of vegan and vegetarian dietary guidelines and philosophies and providing vegan or vegetarian options.

vegan   A person who excludes all animal foods and ingredients from his daily dietary intake and who also avoids using any animal-based items and any form of animal exploitation or suffering in all other aspects of his or her life.

vegetarian   A person who chooses to exclude animal flesh from his daily dietary intake.

Resources

Now that you've begun your journey into veganism, where do you turn for information and support on a wide variety of vegan-related issues? Many resources—from books, websites, and organizations—can provide you with the information you need to help maintain your cruelty-free approach to life. This appendix will help you get started in the right direction!

Books

Nowadays, you can find loads of books on a wide range of topics related to vegan living—and that's good news for new vegans! The following sections list some of the books we think will help you the most, in addition to those that were mentioned throughout this book. Happy reading!

Vegan Issues

Adams, Carol J. *Living Among Meat Eaters: The Vegetarian's Survival Handbook.* Continuum International Publishing Group, 2003.

Blair, Linda, and Sunny J. Harris. *Going Vegan!* Sunny Harris and Associates, Inc., 2001.

Lappé, Frances Moore. *Diet for a Small Planet, 20th Anniversary Edition.* Ballantine Books, 1991.

Marcus, Erik. *Vegan: The New Ethics of Eating, Revised Edition.* McBooks Press, 2000.

———. *Meat Market: Animals, Ethics, and Money.* Brio Press, 2005.

Melina, Vesanto, and Brenda Davis. *The New Becoming Vegetarian: The Essential Guide to a Healthy Vegetarian Diet.* Healthy Living Publications, 2003.

Robbins, John. *Diet for a New America: How Your Food Choices Affect Your Health, Happiness and the Future of Life on Earth.* H. J. Kramer, 1998.

———. *The Food Revolution: How Your Diet Can Help Save Your Life and Our World.* Conari Press, 2001.

E. G. Smith Collective. *Animal Ingredients A to Z: Third Edition.* AK Press, 2004.

Stepaniak, Joanne. *Being Vegan.* McGraw-Hill, 2000.

———. *The Vegan Sourcebook.* Lowell House, 1998.

Cooking and Uncooking

Atlas, Nava. *The Vegetarian Family Cookbook.* Broadway, 2004.

Bergeron, Ken. *Professional Vegetarian Cooking.* John Wiley and Sons, 1999.

Brill, Steve. *The Wild Vegetarian Cookbook.* Harvard Common Press, 2002.

Brotman, Juliano, and Erika Lenkert. *Raw: The Uncook Book: New Vegetarian Food for Life.* Regan Books, 1999.

Grogan, Bryanna Clark. *Authentic Chinese Cuisine: For the Contemporary Kitchen.* Book Publishing Company, 2000.

Hagler, Louise. *Tofu Quick and Easy.* Book Publishing Company, 2001.

Klaper, Michael, M.D. *The Cookbook for People Who Love Animals.* Gentle World, 1990.

Kramer, Sarah, and Tanya Barnard. *How It All Vegan!: Irresistible Recipes for an Animal-Free Diet.* Arsenal Pulp Press, 1999.

McCarty, Meredith. *Sweet and Natural: More Than 120 Sugar-Free and Dairy-Free Desserts.* St. Martin's Press, 2001.

McDougall, John A., M.D., and Mary McDougall. *The McDougall Quick and Easy Cookbook: Over 300 Delicious Low-Fat Recipes You Can Prepare in Fifteen Minutes or Less.* Plume Books, 1999.

Newkirk, Ingrid, and PETA. *Compassionate Cook: Please Don't Eat the Animals.* Warner Books, 1993.

Oser, Marie. *The Enlightened Kitchen: Eat Your Way to Better Health*. Wiley, 2002.

Pickarski, Ron. *Eco-Cuisine: An Ecological Approach to Gourmet Vegetarian Cooking*. Ten Speed Press, 1995.

Raymond, Jennifer. *The Peaceful Palate: Fine Vegetarian Cuisine*. Book Publishing Company, 1996.

Robertson, Robin. *Fresh from the Vegetarian Slow Cooker: 200 Recipes for Healthy and Hearty One-Pot Meals That Are Ready When You Are*. Harvard Common Press, 2004.

Stepaniak, Joanne. *The Ultimate Uncheese Cookbook: Delicious Dairy-Free Cheeses and Classic "Uncheese" Dishes*. Book Publishing Company, 2003.

Tucker, Eric, and John Westerdahl. *Millennium Cookbook: Extraordinary Vegetarian Cuisine*. Ten Speed Press, 1998.

Walker, Norman W. *Fresh Vegetable and Fruit Juices: What's Missing in Your Body? Revised Edition*. Norwalk Press, 1981.

Health and Nutrition

Barnard, Neal, M.D. *Food for Life: How the New Four Food Groups Can Save Your Life*. Three Rivers Press, 1994.

Campbell, T. Colin, Ph.D., and Thomas M. Campbell II. *The China Study*. Benbella Books, 2005.

Diamond, Harvey, and Marilyn Diamond. *Fit for Life*. Warner Books, 1987.

Elliot, Rose. *The Vegetarian Mother and Baby Book: Completely Revised and Updated*. Pantheon, 1996.

Klaper, Michael, M.D. *Pregnancy, Children, and the Vegan Diet*. Gentle World, 1988.

———. *Vegan Nutrition: Pure and Simple*. Gentle World, 1987.

Lyman, Howard. *Mad Cowboy: Plain Truth from the Cattle Rancher Who Won't Eat Meat*. Scribner, 2001.

McDougall, John A., M.D., and Mary McDougall. *The McDougall Program for a Healthy Heart: A Life-Saving Approach to Preventing and Treating Heart Disease*. Plume Books, 1998.

Ornish, Dean, M.D. *Dr. Dean Ornish's Program for Reversing Heart Disease*. New York: Random House, 1990.

———. *Eat More, Weigh Less*. New York: HarperCollins, 1995.

Pavlina, Erin. *Raising Vegan Children in a Non-Vegan World: A Complete Guide for Parents*. VegFamily, 2003.

Pinckney, Neal, Ph.D. *Healthy Heart Handbook*. Health Communications, 1996.

Saunders, Kerrie K., Ph.D. *The Vegan Diet as Chronic Disease Prevention: Evidence Supporting the New Four Food Groups*. Lantern Books, 2003.

Stepaniak, Joanne, and Vesanto Melina. *Raising Vegetarian Children: A Guide to Good Health and Family Harmony*. McGraw-Hill, 2002.

Animal Advocacy

Newkirk, Ingrid. *250 Things You Can Do to Make Your Cat Adore You*. Fireside, 1998.

———. *Making Kind Choices: Everyday Ways to Enhance Your Life Through Earth- and Animal-Friendly Living*. St. Martin's Griffin, 2005.

People for the Ethical Treatment of Animals. *PETA 2005 Shopping Guide for Caring Consumers: A Guide to Products That Are Not Tested on Animals*. Book Publishing Company, 2004.

Singer, Peter. *Animal Liberation*. Ecco, 2001.

Kids' Books

Bass, Jules, and Debbie Harter. *Herb, the Vegetarian Dragon*. Barefoot Books, 1999.

Tofts, Hannah. *I Eat Vegetables!* Zero to Ten, 2001.

Vignola, Radha. *Victor, the Vegetarian: Saving Little Lambs*. Aviva! 1994.

———. *Victor's Picnic: With the Vegetarian Animals*. Aviva! 1996.

Zephaniah, Benjamin. *School's Out: Poems Not for School*. AK Press, 1997.

———. *The Little Book of Vegan Poems*. AK Press, 2002.

Websites

Vegan websites abound on the Internet, and the following links will help you successfully navigate your way through vegan cyberspace. They're arranged by category for your surfing pleasure. Don't forget to use a good search engine such as Google to help you discover new vegan sites of your own!

Vegan Issues

EarthSave International
www.earthsave.org

ErikMarcus.com
www.erikmarcus.com

Famous Veggie
www.famousveggie.com

Go Vegan! with Bob Linden
www.goveganradio.com

Grassroots Veganism with Joanne Stepaniak
www.vegsource.com/joanne

John Robbins' the Food Revolution
www.foodrevolution.org

People for the Ethical Treatment of Animals (PETA)
www.peta.org

Veg TV
www.vegtv.com

Vegan.com
www.vegan.com

Vegan Outreach
www.veganoutreach.com

Vegan Village
www.veganvillage.co.uk

Vegetarian Resource Group
www.vrg.org

Vegetarians in Paradise
www.vegparadise.com

VegSource
www.vegsource.com

Vegan Cooking

Beverly Lynn Bennett's "The Vegan Chef"
www.veganchef.com

Kate's (Vegan) Cookery Site
www.earth.li/~kake/cookery

Living and Raw Foods
www.living-foods.com

International Vegetarian Union's Recipes
www.ivu.org/recipes

Marie Oser, the Veggie Chef
www.veggiechef.com

Robin Robertson
www.robinrobertson.com

VeganCooking.com
www.vegancooking.com

VegWeb
www.vegweb.com

Vegetarian Resource Group's Recipes
www.vrg.org/recipes

Vegan Publications

American Vegan
www.americanvegan.org/magazine.htm

The Vegan
www.vegansociety.com/html/
publications

VegNews
www.vegnews.com

Vegan Merchants

A Different Daisy
www.differentdaisy.com

Alternative Outfitters
www.alternativeoutfitters.com

Beauty Without Cruelty
www.beautywithoutcruelty.com

Pangea Vegan Products
www.veganstore.com

Vegan Essentials
www.veganessentials.com

Vegan Store (U.K.)
www.veganstore.co.uk

Vegan Goodies and Treats

Allison's Gourmet
www.allisonsgourmet.com

Alternative Baking Company
www.alternativebaking.com

Chocolate Decadence
www.chocolatedecadence.com

Frey Vineyards
www.freywine.com

Health and Nutrition

Healing Heart Foundation
heart.kumu.org

Institute for Plant Based Nutrition
www.plantbased.org

McDougall Wellness Center
www.drmcdougall.com

Michael A. Klaper, M.D.
www.drklaper.com

Neal D. Barnard, M.D.
www.nealbarnard.org

**Physicians Committee for
Responsible Medicine (PCRM)**
www.pcrm.org

Restaurant Directories

HappyCow's Vegetarian Guide
www.happycow.net

VegDining
www.vegdining.com

Pregnancy and Children

Veg Parenting at VegSource
www.vegsource.com/parent

Vegetarian Baby and Child
www.vegetarianbaby.com

VegFamily
www.vegfamily.com

Animal Companions

Vegancats.com
www.vegancats.com

VegPets.com
www.vegpets.com

Organizations

The American Anti-Vivisection Society
801 Old York Road, #204
Jenkintown, PA 19046
215-887-0816 or 1-800-SAY-AAVS
(1-800-729-2287)
Fax: 215-887-2088
www.aavs.org

American Vegan Society
56 Dinshah Lane
PO Box 369
Malaga, NJ 08328
856-694-2887
Fax: 856-694-2288
www.americanvegan.org

Compassion Over Killing
PO Box 9773
Washington, DC 20016
301-891-2458
www.cok.net

EarthSave International
PO Box 96
New York, NY 10108
718-459-7503 or 1-800-362-3648
Fax: 718-228-2491
www.earthsave.org

Farm Animal Reform Movement
10101 Ashburton
Bethesda, MD 20817
1-888-ASK-FARM (1-888-275-3276)
www.farmusa.org

Farm Sanctuary
PO Box 150
Watkins Glen, NY 14891
607-583-2225
Fax: 607-583-2041
www.farmsanctuary.org

Food Not Bombs
PO Box 744
Tucson, AZ 85702
520-770-0575 or 1-800-884-1136
www.foodnotbombs.net

The Gentle Barn Foundation
26910 Sierra Highway D-8, #318
Santa Clarita, CA 91321
661-252-2440
Fax: 661-251-2440
www.gentlebarn.org

International Vegetarian Union
(See the website for contact information.)
www.ivu.org

North American Vegetarian Society
PO Box 72
Dolgeville, NY 13329
518-568-7970
www.navs-online.org

People for the Ethical Treatment of Animals
501 Front Street
Norfolk, VA 23510
757-622-PETA
www.peta.com

Toronto Vegetarian Association
17 Baldwin Street, 2nd Floor
Toronto, Ontario M5T 1L1
Canada
416-544-9800
Fax: 416-544-9094
www.veg.ca

Vegan Action
PO Box 4288
Richmond, VA 23220
804-502-8736
Fax: 804-254-8346
www.vegan.org

Vegan Outreach
PO Box 38492
Pittsburgh, PA 15238-8492
www.veganoutreach.com

The Vegan Society
Donald Watson House
7 Battle Road
St. Leonards-on-Sea
East Sussex
TN37 7AA
United Kingdom
U.K. phone: 01424 427393
U.K. fax: 01424 717064
U.K. local rate phone: 0845 4588244
International phone: +44 1424 427393
International fax: +44 1424 717064
www.vegansociety.com

Vegetarian Resource Group
PO Box 1463
Baltimore, MD 21203
410-366-8343
www.vrg.org

Vegetarians International Voice for Animals (Viva!)
8 York Court
Wilder Street
Bristol
BS2 8QH
United Kingdom
U.K. phone: 0117 944 1000
U.K. fax: 0117 924 4646
www.viva.org.uk

Index

C

E

M

S

T

W–X–Y–Z